An Introduction to Clinical Immunology and Serology

An Introduction to Clinical Immunology and Serology
Second Edition

Francis K. Widmann, MD
Carol Ann Itatani, PhD

 F. A. DAVIS COMPANY • Philadelphia

F. A. Davis Company
1915 Arch Street
Philadelphia, PA 19103

Printed in the United States of America

Last digit indicates print number: 10 9 8 7 6 5 4 3 2 1

Publisher: Jean-François Vilain
Developmental Editor: Marianne Fithian
Cover Designer: Louis J. Forgione

As new scientific information becomes available through basic and clinical research, recommended treatments and drug therapies undergo changes. The author(s) and publisher have done everything possible to make this book accurate, up to date, and in accord with accepted standards at the time of publication. The authors, editors, and publisher are not responsible for errors or omissions or for consequences from application of the book, and make no warranty, expressed or implied, in regard to the contents of the book. Any practice described in this book should be applied by the reader in accordance with professional standards of care used in regard to the unique circumstances that may apply in each situation. The reader is advised always to check product information (package inserts) for changes and new information regarding dose and contraindications before administering any drug. Caution is especially urged when using new or infrequently ordered drugs.

Library of Congress Cataloging in Publication Data

Widmann, Frances K., 1935–
    An introduction to clinical immunology and serology / Frances K. Widmann, Carol Ann Itatani. — 2nd ed.
        p.   cm.
    Rev. ed. of: An introduction to clinical immunology / Frances K. Widmann. c1989.
    Includes bibliographical references and index.
    ISBN (invalid) 0-8032-0302-9
    1. Immunology. 2. Immunopathology. I. Widmann, Frances K., 1935–   Introduction to clinical immunology. II. Itatani, Carol Ann. III. Title.
    [DNLM: 1. Immune System. 2. Immunity. 3. Serologic Tests—methods.   QW 504 W641i 1998]
QR181.W65 1998
616.07'9—dc21
DNLM/DLC
for Library of Congress   98-11504
                                                                CIP

Preface

This text is an introduction to clinical immunology and serology. Much of the basic information and excellent organization of Dr. Widmann's first edition have been retained.

The second edition has undergone considerable updating and includes many additional serological procedures and applications. A new chapter concerning cancer immunology has been added. Chapter summaries and review questions are now included. Many new figures have been developed and, consistent with the first edition, are simple line drawings meant to convey and enhance understanding of immune concepts. A conscious effort was made to assure that this text remains easy to read and understandable for those with little or no experience in immunology or clinical medicine. Students and practitioners in the health professions as well as any reader seeking to understand recent advances in immunology will find this text useful. Medical technologists and other laboratory personnel, medical and nursing students, students in medical and physicians assisting programs and physicians and instructors in medically related areas will appreciate the close integration of basic immune concepts with clinical applications and laboratory test procedures.

Accordingly, this is the organizational pattern for the text. Part I explains the principles of immune function. Early vaccination procedures and observations by Jenner, Pasteur, Richet, and Hericourt are used to illustrate characteristics of immunity. The structure of proteins, glycoproteins and cell structure and function are included so that immune cell processes can be more easily understood. The essential features of antigens, antigen processing, recognition and adaptive immune responses are then explained. Immunological terms and concepts are introduced and explained before being incorporated into more complex contexts. No matter the sophistication of the reader's background, this section will provide a thorough understanding of how the immune system "works" with important new developments included such as the role of MHC I and II in antigen processing, the genetics of immunoglobulin diversity, and TCR and CD functions.

In part II, "Clinical Applications," immune functions learned in part I are related to normal human defense mechanisms. Then causes and consequences of immune deficiencies, neoplasms of the immune system and diseases due to overreactivity and misdirection of the immune system are explained. Updated sections concerning AIDS, inflammation and immune-mediated diseases are included. Immune activities and ways in which these activities may be manipulated are included in chapters concerning transplantation and cancer immunology. Part II provides a solid clinical foundation for understanding immune-related diseases and future developments in immunology.

Part III, "Laboratory Applications," provides an explanation of the myriad forms of laboratory/serological tests utilizing immune activities. Because of the exquisite specificity of antigen/antibody binding, the detection and quantitation of many different substances is possible. The second edition contains new information concerning immunofixation, Western blots, ELISA techniques, immunohisto-chemical staining, heterogeneous and homogeneous assays and more examples of specific applications of serological test procedures. Dr. Widmann states in the first preface that this section is not merely a manual of laboratory techniques. We both agree that the immunological principles upon which the tests are based are the more important aspects to understand in an introductory text. Not only the personnel who perform these tests, but also those individuals who order and interpret them need to understand how immune principles are applied to laboratory test procedures and the advantages and limitations of the methodology.

This book is written with an emphasis on human clinical applications of immunology. Where appropriate, references to immune-related experiments are included. This is a text for those individuals new to the field of immunology. Careful consideration has been given to a logical, easy-to-remember organization of the text. Unfamiliar terms unique to immunology and some not so unique are presented in bold type and are immediately defined. A Glossary and a list of common abbreviations are provided in the appendices for quick reference. Individual chapters have outlines and introductory paragraphs to guide the reader in understanding the subsequent material. Chapter summaries and student-tested review questions have been added to aid both instructors and students in assessing retention and comprehension.

Many individuals deserve recognition and thanks for their support and assistance in the production of this text. Ms. Pennie Perkins devoted many hours to modifying and perfecting previous figures and sketches for new figures. Valuable comments and suggestions were provided by reviewers who read all or part of the manuscript. My thanks to: Lester E. Hardegree, Jr., MEd, MT(ASCP), Assistant Professor and Program Director of Medical Technology, Armstrong State College, Savannah, GA; Karen S. Long, MS, CLS(NCA), MT(ASCP), Associate Professor, West Virginia University, Morgantown, WV; William E. Meekins, MT(ASCP), SM(AAM), Program Director for Medical Technology, Belleville Area College, Belleville, IL; Susan B. Roman, MMSc, MT(ASCP), SM, Assistant Professor, Georgia State University, Atlanta, GA; Patricia D. Wyatt, MS, MT(ASCP) Assistant Professor, University of Tennessee, Memphis, TN; Julia R. Young, BS, MT(ASCP), MLT Program Director, Pennsylvania State University, New Kensington, PA. Many thanks also to Jean-François Vilain, Marianne Fithian, and the staff of F.A. Davis for their patience and efforts in making this second edition a reality.

RECOMMENDED STUDY TECHNIQUES

This text is an introduction to clinical immunology and serology. I recommend first skimming the chapter, paying close attention to new vocabulary, main topics, and how they are organized. A chapter outline is provided, which is useful for reference and guidance in preparing notes. Check the chapter summaries and review questions to determine how much you have retained and understood after reading the chapter. Immunology is a "high information" subject that cannot be learned and understood as individual bits of information. One piece of information leads to another and soon a "story" can be constructed which then leads to related stories. Understanding the immune system seems a daunting task, but if the "whole" is broken down into related parts, the task becomes surmountable. This is exactly how research in the field of immunology occurs and how research contributes to a growing understanding of how the immune system "works." Have fun! I hope you will find immunology as fascinating as I do.

C.A.I.

Contents

PART I

PRINCIPLES OF IMMUNE FUNCTION

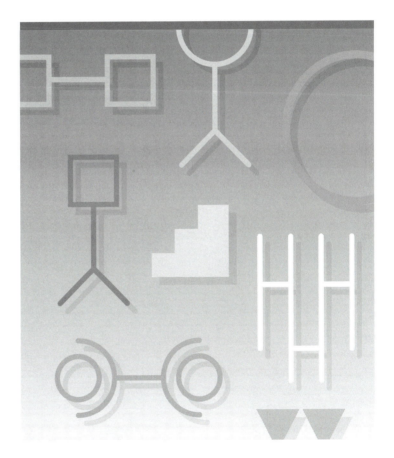

1 Introductory Concepts

The term **immunity** comes from a Latin word that means "exempt" or "free from." Immunity encompasses the body's mechanisms to protect itself from harmful external agents, notably microorganisms and foreign materials; internal abnormalities, such as degenerative changes or tumors; and harmful environmental influences, such as toxins, radiation, and extreme heat or cold. To maintain its equilibrium, the body must have ways (1) to exclude potentially harmful invaders or stimuli, (2) to neutralize or eliminate such stimuli if they succeed in entering, and (3) to repair whatever damage has been inflicted. The first requirement, **exclusion,** depends largely on physical barriers between the body and the environment: intact surfaces, such as skin and mucous membranes, and the secretions that flow over these surfaces, such as saliva, respiratory secretions, urine, intestinal fluid, sweat, and the like. The requirement for **neutralization** or **elimination** of injurious agents depends on activation of the immune system. The remaining requirement of **repair** follows an immune response and embodies an infinite range of cell replication, adaptation, and modification.

Observations that the human body could resist infection or that a person became "immune" after having acquired and survived an infection can be traced back to the ancient Greeks and Peloponnesians. This ability to resist infection on reexposure to the same pathogen is an example of **natural active immunity.** It is also possible to artificially induce immunity, and the development of procedures for immunization has revolutionized modern medicine.

The earliest attempt at immunization was deliberate exposure to the etiologic agent of smallpox, the **variola** virus. Smallpox can range in severity from a relatively mild skin affliction to a rapidly fatal systemic disease. Physicians in China and Asia Minor attempted for centuries to induce protection against the virulent disease by deliberately promoting very mild disease. They injected material from skin lesions of a sick patient into healthy subjects to induce an infection, which did elicit effective immunity. However, the severity of the transmitted disease was unpredictable. Inoculation of material from a mildly ill patient did not guarantee mild illness in the recipient. When this practice, called **variolation,** was introduced into England in the eighteenth century, 2 to 3 percent of those treated developed fatal illness. However, the natural infection caused 20 to 30 percent mortality, so the practice of variolation remained in use.

The future of modern immunobiology was ensured when Edward Jenner (1749–1823) observed that milkmaids who contracted cowpox and developed lesions were thereafter immune to smallpox. In 1796, Jenner injected fluid from a cowpox lesion into a child's arm and 2 months later injected material from a smallpox lesion into the same child. The child developed the mild blistering of cowpox but did not succumb to smallpox! In the twentieth century, the World Health Organization, using essentially the same procedure and a virus similar to cowpox (vaccinia), vaccinated people throughout the world. Smallpox is no longer a threat and has been eliminated throughout the world.

Louis Pasteur extended the concept of vaccination 100 years after Jenner's initial experiments. He had been growing the bacteria that caused chicken cholera and had a culture which, if inoculated into healthy chickens, consistently caused their death. However, one batch of chickens, inoculated with this culture did not die, but remained perfectly healthy. The only factor that differed from previous experiments was that the culture had been left sitting on the laboratory bench for several weeks. Pasteur then grew a fresh culture of chicken cholera bacteria and reinoculated the same batch of chickens. The chickens again did not die! Pasteur realized that the old bacterial culture had performed like a vaccine. Aging the bacteria had reduced the virulence of the culture and had provided protection (immunity) against exposure to a freshly grown virulent culture (Fig. 1–1). Vaccination, as introduced by Jenner and Pasteur, illustrates important characteristics of the immune system: it is possible to induce specific immunity to a disease by injecting a less virulent form (attenuated) of a microorganism. Furthermore, the immune system will "remember" this microorganism and provide protection upon subsequent reexposure. This phenomenon is called **immune memory.**

Pasteur went on to develop a vaccine for **anthrax,** a disease caused by a bacterium that affects sheep, cows, goats, and occasionally humans. Rather than aging the bacteria on the laboratory bench, Pasteur found that growing the bacteria at an elevated temperature could render it safe for use as a vaccine. A few years later, Pasteur developed a rabies vaccine.

Despite the success of his vaccination procedures, Pasteur did not under-

FIGURE 1–1. Chicken "A" dies as a result of exposure to a virulent bacteria causing chicken cholera. Chicken "B" does *not* die, but its immune system is stimulated to recognize antigen associated with the bacteria. Reexposure of chicken "B" to virulent cholera activates its immune system to neutralize toxin and growth capability of the bacteria, whereas unprotected (nonimmunized) control chickens "C" die when innoculated with the same bacteria.

PASTEUR'S CHICKEN CHOLERA EXPERIMENT

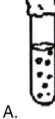 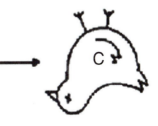

A.
Test tube with
fresh chicken
cholera bacteria

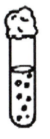 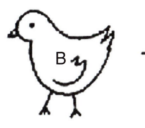 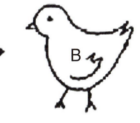

B.
Test tube with
old chicken
cholera bacteria

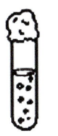 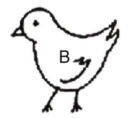 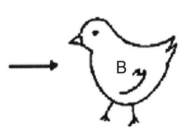

C.
Test tube with
fresh chicken
cholera bacteria

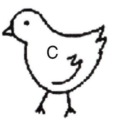

Uninoculated
Control
Chicken

stand *how* an animal or human was protected or became immune to a disease. In 1888, Richet and Herricourt showed that the blood of an immunized animal possessed protective properties. If blood from an animal vaccinated against *Staphylococcus* bacteria was injected into a nonimmunized animal, the nonimmunized animal was protected from immediate infection with this bacteria. Furthermore, if a drop of serum from the immunized animal was mixed with the staphylococci, the bacteria would form clumps or **agglutinate.** If another type of bacteria was mixed with the serum, no agglutination occurred. Likewise, if serum from a nonimmunized animal was mixed with staphylococci, no agglutination occurred. These experiments demonstrated that the protective factors were present in the blood and were highly specific for only the bacteria used to immunize the animal (Fig. 1–2).

In 1890, Emil Von Behring and Shibasaburo Kitasato inoculated animals with diphtheria and tetanus toxin and demonstrated that the serum from inoculated animals would neutralize the toxins. They called the antitoxic factor in the blood **antibodies.** A few years later, Emil Roux showed that patients suffering from diphtheria could be cured by injecting them with serum from a horse immunized against diphtheria. The horse serum contained antidiphtheria antibodies. Transfer of antibodies formed by a person or an animal into a nonimmunized host is called **passive immunity.** Natural passive immunity occurs when antibodies are transferred through the placenta from the mother to an unborn fetus or through breast milk to the infant. This transfer of antibodies provides protection for the child during the first weeks after birth while the child's own immune system becomes progressively functional. The injection of horse serum containing antibodies to diphtheria is an example of artificial passive immunity.

Antibodies are not the only protective agents in serum. Jules Bordet (1870–1961) showed that immune sera could lyse or dissolve certain bacteria, and serum from one person could sometimes lyse red blood cells (RBCs) from other individuals. Bordet called this lysing substance **alexin.** This was later renamed **complement** and together with antibodies provide **humoral immunity** for the body. The term "humoral" refers to the body fluids originally described by the great Greek physician, Hippocrates. Serum is part of the blood, which is a fluid tissue; therefore activities of antibodies and complement are referred to as humoral immunity.

It is customary to divide immune responses into two principal categories: humoral and **cell-mediated** responses. The hallmark of humoral immunity is production of antibodies, proteins uniquely constructed to interact with the stimulating material. Cell-mediated immunity includes a range of activities requiring the presence of activated immune cells (**effector cells**). Material capable of eliciting immune activity is referred to as **immunogenic.** An **antigen,** or immunogen, is defined as material capable of eliciting an immune response when introduced into an immunocompetent host to whom it is foreign. A protective or adaptive immune response requires **recognition** of an antigen. Substances and materials derived from the host's own cells or extracellular substances constitute **self;** anything other than these constituents is **nonself** or **foreign.**

The major features of adaptive immunity are **recognition, memory,** and **specificity.** Immune cells, in various stages of differentiation and activation, perform these functions and are assisted by several other cell types.

AGGLUTINATION

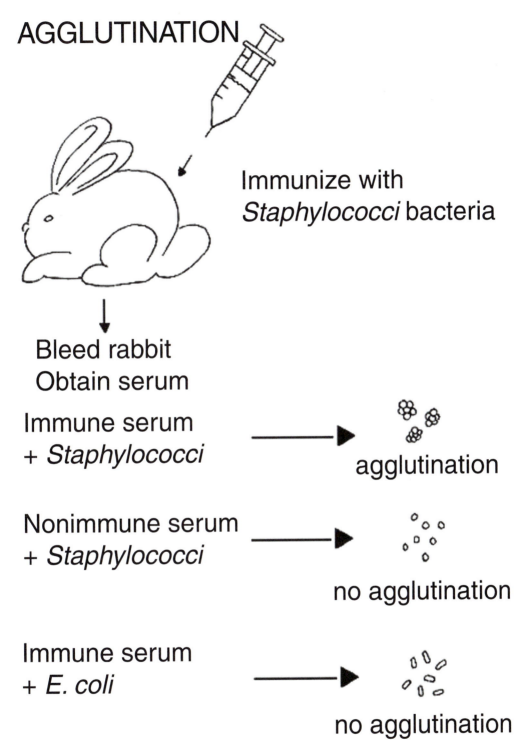

Immunize with *Staphylococci* bacteria

Bleed rabbit
Obtain serum

Immune serum
+ *Staphylococci* ⟶ agglutination

Nonimmune serum
+ *Staphylococci* ⟶ no agglutination

Immune serum
+ *E. coli* ⟶ no agglutination

FIGURE 1–2. A rabbit injected with bacteria will form antibodies to that bacteria. Presence of antibodies in the serum of the rabbit can be demonstrated by mixing a drop of serum with the bacteria. Agglutination occurs only with addition of the original bacteria used for inoculation, thus demonstrating the specificity of the immune response.

INNATE AND ADAPTIVE IMMUNITY

Even the most primitive organisms can defend themselves against injury. Organisms on all rungs of the evolutionary ladder have cells that can surround and engulf molecules or particles, a process called **phagocytosis.** These cells also synthesize products that degrade, denature, or otherwise alter the materials they encounter. Phagocytosis and production of active substances are nonspecific mechanisms; the same weapons are deployed against disturbing agents of all sorts. These ubiquitous nonspecific activities constitute the innate physiologic process called **inflammation.** Discrimination, memory, and modification of physiologic responses according to previous bodily experience constitute **adaptive immunity,** a capacity present only in vertebrates. Table 1–1 summarizes these processes.

Cells Involved

Cells responsible for certain effects are called **effector cells.** Cells that support the activities of effector cells are called **accessory cells.** Effector cells of inflammation, such as the phagocytic cells, often play crucial accessory roles in immune activities.

A cell capable of differentiation into many different cell types is referred to as **pluripotential.** In fetal development, precursor cells from which immune and inflammatory effectors descend originates in the embryonic yolk sac and later migrates to the bone marrow. The pluripotential cell whose descendants include both inflammatory and immune effectors is called the **hematopoietic stem cell.** Progeny of the hematopoietic stem cell differentiate into red blood cells (RBCs); several different kinds of white blood cells (WBCs); megakaryocytes, which generate coagulation-promoting cell fragments called platelets; and phagocytic cells resident in solid tissues (Fig. 1–3). Hematopoietic stem cells are capable of mitotic division and maintain their own cell numbers while also differentiating into precursor cells that are themselves pluripotent: The **lymphoid** precursor cell gives rise to several populations of lymphocytes, the effector cells of specific, adaptive immunity; the **myeloid** precursor cells differentiate into the many cells that perform nonspecific inflammatory activities. Hematopoietic stem cells have enormous capacity for cell division; the differentiated cell lines manifest continuous growth and multiplication throughout life, some within the bone marrow and some at other tissue sites.

TABLE 1–1. **Innate and Adaptive Immunity**

	Innate Immunity (Inflammation)	Adaptive Immunity (Immune System)
Evolutionary distribution	All multicelled organisms	Vertebrates only
Major effector	Neutrophils, macrophages, lymphocytes	Lymphocytes
Major accessory cells	Epithelium, through barrier function	Macrophages
Other accessory influences	Products of immune stimulation	Products of inflammation
Target specificity	Nonspecific	Highly specific recognition
Effect of previous exposure	None	Markedly alters nature of response

DIFFERENTIATION OF CELLS
IN BONE MARROW

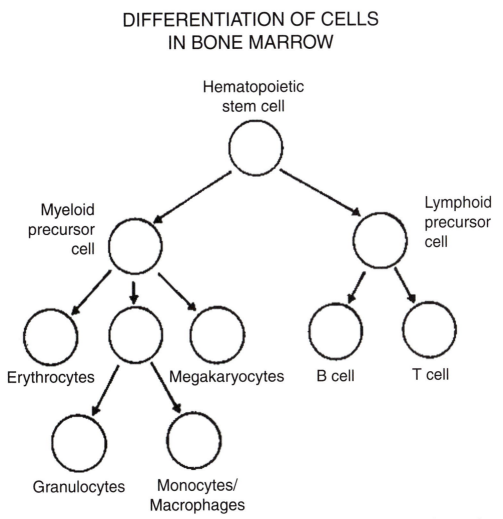

FIGURE 1–3. The pluripotential stem cell divides and maintains its own cell numbers, and its progeny differentiate into lymphoid or myeloid precursor cells that remain and perpetuate themselves in the bone marrow. Normal numbers of circulating blood cells are maintained by continuous division and maturation of these precursor cells. The lymphoid line differentiates into T-cell and B-cell lines. Myeloid precursors differentiate into cells of the monocyte/macrophage population and other cells of the circulating blood. Granulocytes and the monocyte/macrophage line are closely related through descent from a common multipotential precursor.

Characteristics of Cells

Two main types of inflammatory cells evolve from the myeloid precursor: **granulocytes** and mononuclear phagocytic cells called **monocytes.** After leaving the circulation, monocytes enter tissues and differentiate into **macrophages,** or **histiocytes.** Granulocytes have microscopically visible cytoplasmic granules that contain enzymes and other products characteristic of various subtypes, which are described as **neutrophils, eosinophils,** or **basophils,** according to the staining characteristics of the granules. Eosinophils and basophils have highly specialized roles in inflammation that will be described in later sections. Neutrophils have an irregular-shaped multilobed nucleus. Another name for the neutrophilic granulocyte is **polymorphonuclear leukocyte,** often shortened to "PMN," or "poly," or "seg." Monocytes have a large nucleus and abundant cytoplasm that may have a granular appearance but lacks the specific granules that distinguish granulocytes. Both neutrophils and monocytes can move through tissues or across surfaces, a property described as **motility.** These cells engage in phagocytosis when their membranes are suitably stimulated and synthesize a wide variety of proteins, many of which are enzymes capable of cleaving a broad range of proteins.

Descending from the lymphoid precursor are lymphocytes, which characteristically have a round, dense nucleus and relatively scant cytoplasm. Lymphocytes present a relatively uniform appearance on light microscopic examination, but two major subpopulations and several less well-defined categories exist. The major populations are **T lymphocytes** and **B lymphocytes.** Lymphocytes do not exhibit phagocytosis, but they are highly motile. They do synthesize proteins, but few are proteolytic enzymes.

Inflammation

Inflammation is described as nonspecific because the same reactions follow stimulatory events of many varieties. Anything that damages cells or alters normal tissue elements elicits inflammation. Inflammation subsequently involves various proportions of neutrophils and monocytes, as well as vascular changes and many fluid-phase proteins. Table 1–2 summarizes significant features of inflammation. **Acute inflammation** is a short-lived, clearly defined process in which the first visible events are changes in blood vessels induced by damaged cells or products derived from microorganisms or altered tissue. Capillaries and small veins dilate, bringing increased amounts of blood to the area; fluid and proteins leak out of altered vessels into the interstitial fluid. Neutrophils migrate from the blood to accumulate at the site of damage and phagocytize damaged cells and foreign particles. Neutrophilic enzymes degrade phagocytized material and also exert proteolytic effects on material outside the cell, notably cells and proteins at the site of injury. Acute in-

TABLE 1–2. **Acute Versus Chronic Inflammation**

	Acute Inflammation	Chronic Inflammation
Time sequence	Short-term; clearly defined	Prolonged; difficult to determine onset and cessation
Predominant cells	Neutrophils; some macrophages	Lymphocytes; macrophages
Gross appearance of tissue	Reddened, swollen	Pale, retracted
Condition of interstitium	Edema; increased proteins in fluid	Increased collagen; scarring
Condition of tissue elements	Rapid destruction by enzymes from neutrophils	Gradual destruction by enzymes from macrophages

flammation may affect the entire body, resulting in increased bone marrow production of neutrophils, elevated body temperature, and elevated blood levels of several proteins collectively described as **acute-phase reactants.** The goal of acute inflammation is elimination of injurious stimuli and removal of damaged tissue elements.

Chronic inflammation lasts longer and has less sharply defined onset and disappearance than acute inflammation. The predominant effector cells are macrophages, which evolve from monocytes. Vascular dilation and protein-rich interstitial fluid are not conspicuous; normal tissue constituents tend to suffer gradual destruction and replacement by fibrous scar tissue. Macrophages participating in chronic inflammation generate numerous proteins that influence blood coagulation and cell growth, as well as proteolytic enzymes that act less rapidly but more persistently than those of neutrophils.

BIOLOGICALLY SIGNIFICANT MOLECULES

Cells are composed of proteins, carbohydrates, and lipids. Antibodies are composed of proteins. Antigens are usually combinations of the latter. To understand how immune cells function and how antibodies are made and antigens recognized, a brief review of biochemistry is necessary.

Classification and Terminology

Proteins, which are chains of amino acids linked by peptide bonds, are often designated **polypeptides.** The building blocks for mammalian proteins are 20 different amino acids. Like letters of the alphabet combined into words, these 20 units can be combined into an infinite array of large or small proteins. Small polypeptide molecules may contain 10 to 20 amino acids; larger examples include hundreds or thousands of amino acids. Proteins are the working molecules of cells; they confer structure, carry out reactions, control metabolic processes, transport and transform other materials, produce movement, and regulate genetic activity.

Carbohydrates have somewhat less structural and functional diversity. Carbon, hydrogen, and oxygen are the fundamental constituents of carbohydrates. The so-called simple sugars consist of five or six carbons with their associated hydrogen and oxygen atoms joined in characteristic linkages. Simple sugars are frequently polymerized to form chains, and chains that contain a variety of simple sugars are called **polysaccharides.** Carbohydrates provide fuel for metabolism and are incorporated into many structural components of plant and animal cells. Combinations of carbohydrates and amino acids are called **glycoproteins;** carbohydrates with fatty elements are **glycolipids.**

Lipids are hydrophobic, meaning they do not mix with water. The basic building blocks are **hydrocarbons,** carbon and hydrogen residues that combine into chains of various lengths, often with attached side chains of diverse composition. Lipids are incorporated into biologic membranes, which surround and define cells and intracellular structures. Hydrocarbons combined with other chemically defined structures provide a wide range of biologically important materials such as phospholipids, sphingolipids, alcohols, and steroids.

Structure and Shape

The molecules described in the previous text are not just formulas on a page. Complex molecules assume a characteristic three-dimensional configuration that reflects the selection and sequence of constituent parts (Fig. 1–4). The amino acids in a protein are linearly arranged to form a chain, which is called a **primary structure.** Depending on the type and order of the amino acids, they interact with each other and with their environment to fold and coil, forming a unique shape. These proteins

(a) Primary Structure

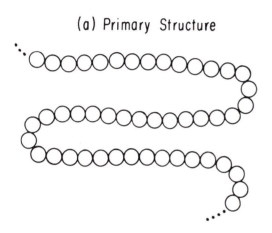

(b) 3-Dimensional Configuration

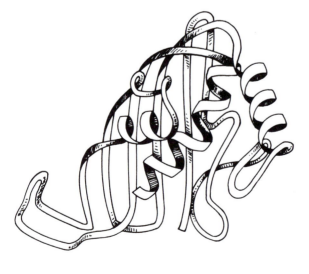

MOLECULAR SHAPE

FIGURE 1–4. The sequence in which constituent parts are assembled is the primary structure of any molecule, schematized in *a*. The attracting and repelling forces inherent in chemical groups impose a three-dimensional shape, shown in *b*. Each molecule of a specific primary composition assumes the same three-dimensional configuration under consistent environmental conditions.

may be integrated into a phospholipid cell membrane. Sugar molecules may be attached to the protein, forming complicated branched structures that extend toward the external environment of the cell. This glycoprotein with its unique structure may have enzymatic activity. Its shape enables it to selectively interact with another molecule and cause a biochemical reaction. The unique shape of this glycoprotein may also be recognized by the immune system as foreign to the body. This same glycoprotein is now an antigen and can cause antibody formation. Such interactions of molecules, as previously described, are predictable and consistent, occurring whenever molecules of complementary configuration encounter each other.

Proteins exhibit enormous diversity of structure and activity. The unique shape of the molecule determines its function and the ways in which it interacts with surrounding materials. Alteration of a single amino acid in a complex protein can radically modify these dependent interactions and cause two molecules—differing only in a single detail—to have completely different functional properties. Sickle cell anemia is an example of a disease in which a single amino acid substitution occurs in the hemoglobin molecule. This substitution causes sickle hemoglobin to be less soluble than normal hemoglobin and under conditions of reduced oxygen tension, sickle hemoglobin precipitates and forms sickle-shaped RBCs. Variations in the number, selection, and sequence of amino acids confer infinitely variable properties on polypeptides.

CELLS AND CELL PROPERTIES

Mammalian cells are enclosed by a membrane that separates the cell from its environment. The nucleus, also enclosed by a membrane, contains the genetic material that controls the cell's structural and functional capacities. Numerous intracellular structures, **organelles,** are responsible for specific cell functions. Fundamental to multicelled existence is the fact that cells can multiply, respond to external stimuli, and synthesize numerous products. All these properties depend on the nature and the actions of the genetic material present in the nucleus.

Genes and Their Actions

A **gene** is the deoxyribonucleic acid (DNA) sequence necessary for production of a single polypeptide (Fig. 1–5). The sequence of amino acids in the protein is determined by the sequence of nucleotides in the DNA helix. Every cell of a single individual contains the same set of DNA sequences arranged into **chromosomes,** which transmit genes from cell to cell during cellular division. Ova and sperm have a single set of 23 chromosomes and are described as **haploid.** All other cell types, **somatic cells,** have 46 chromosomes and are described as **diploid,** meaning that they have two copies of each chromosome. This includes two copies of each of the 22 paired **autosomes** and two **sex** chromosomes. Women have two copies of the X sex chromosome, whereas men have one X and one Y chromosome. One chromosome of each pair is derived from the individual's father and one from the mother. Every cell contains exactly the same genetic material as every other cell; an individual's total genetic endowment is called the **genome.** Although all cells of the body are genetically identical, during development and maturation they assume different appearances and functions through the process known as **differentiation.**

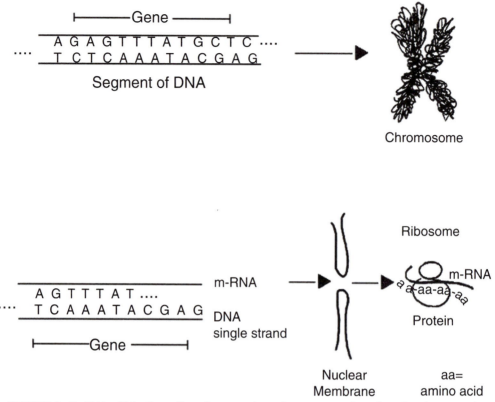

FIGURE 1–5. DNA within the cell nucleus consists of sequences of nucleotides that encode genetic information. "a" gene includes those nucleotides necessary for production of a specific product. Genes are localized as segments along a DNA strand. When a cell is ready to divide, the DNA is duplicated and the long continuous strands are coiled into individual chromosomes. Production of a protein product involves transcription of the genetic code within a gene into messenger RNA (mRNA) and translation of the information within mRNA into a precise sequence of amino acids.

How Cells Differentiate

All cells start with the same potential to produce all the proteins encoded in the genes present, but any one cell synthesizes only those few proteins characteristic of the particular cell type. As cells divide and the embryo develops, DNA undergoes rearrangement and redistribution. Some sequences may be permanently discarded; most sequences persist but exhibit activity only after activation by complex combinations of internal and external stimuli that are not fully understood. Protein synthesis occurs in response to discrete messages that may be present at some times and absent at other times. In most cases, manufacture of structural or functional proteins changes the cell so that it expresses one set of properties but permanently loses the potential for other products or properties. Fully differentiated cells are capable only of a limited number of highly specialized actions. An example of a fully differentiated cell is an RBC that loses even its nucleus. Other cells retain the potential to perform various actions; environmental events determine what course such a cell pursues. Different cell types possess different ranges of potential function; within cell types, differences in maturational stages determine what products each cell manufactures.

Membrane Markers

Structural proteins produced by cells confer shape, motility, contractility, and other properties. Cells also produce metabolically active molecules. Molecules on the cell membrane promote communication between cells and their environment. These molecules may be loosely or tightly associated with the external or internal surfaces of the phospholipid bilayer that makes up the cell membrane (Fig. 1–6). Some molecules traverse the bilayer with parts of the molecule extending from the exterior and into the interior of the cell. The lipid bilayer is highly mobile; it can be likened to a sea of jostling phospholipids with glycoproteins and glycolipids constantly in motion within this thin surface layer. Extensions of membrane marker molecules ensure that exterior signals are received and transmitted to the cytoplasm and eventually to the nucleus for cell reactivity.

Membrane molecules exhibit tremendous diversity. In a single individual, cells of different types display different membrane markers. Membrane markers vary with the stage of cellular maturity, even among cells of a single type. Increasingly sophisticated techniques for identification of membrane markers have expanded our understanding of cell populations and their dynamics.

All cells of all organs of a single individual carry some identical membrane molecules. These help determine the "self" characteristics of that individual. Other molecules characterize cells performing a certain function and serve as markers for that functional capacity. If the activity occurs in a broad range of cells, the marker will be found on many types of cells. Highly differentiated cells have membrane molecules that mediate their specialized functions. Such molecules are present only on cells capable of performing that activity, but the same marker can be present on comparable cells from many different individuals and even from many different species. Cells express a changing selection of membrane molecules; molecules often disappear after performing their function and may or may not reappear with

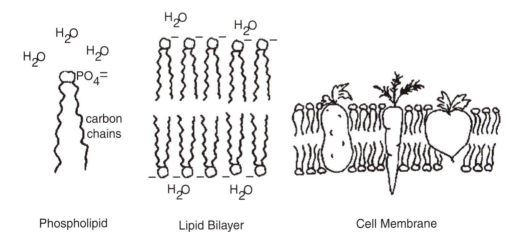

Phospholipid   Lipid Bilayer   Cell Membrane

FIGURE 1–6. The cell membrane consists of a bilayer of phospholipids. The lipid portion of the molecule is hydrophobic while the phosphate group is electrically charged. Therefore, the phospholipids are organized so that the lipid tails face the interior of the membrane. Glycoproteins and glycolipids with various shapes may extend through the membrane and for varying distances from the internal and external surfaces of the cell membrane.

changes in internal and external circumstances. Table 1–3 summarizes categories of markers significant in immune processes.

Receptors and Ligands

A molecule so shaped that it interacts optimally with another molecule is called a **receptor** for that material; the material complementary to the receptor is called a **ligand.** Receptors are often integrated into the cell membrane, and receptor-ligand interactions allow cells to receive instruction or stimulation from their environment. Intercellular communication occurs when one cell manufactures and releases a product that engages the receptor molecule of another cell. The receptor-ligand complex then has physical and physiologic properties different from those of the unbound receptor molecule. The changed state alters the membrane or affects other molecules in the interior of the cell. Sometimes the flexible membrane engulfs the receptor-ligand complex, which ends up inside the cell in a process called **interiorization** or **endocytosis.** Interiorization is an example of the phenomenon called **modulation,** in which cells exhibit altered structural features in response to external events (Fig. 1–7).

Receptor-Ligand Events

In multicelled organisms, a broad range of receptor-ligand events occurs continually. For example, most cells have receptors for insulin. When insulin molecules combine with intact insulin receptors, insulin-mediated metabolic events occur within the cell. For other hormones, only one or a few cell types may possess suitable receptors, and such hormones have rather restricted metabolic effects. In

TABLE 1–3. **Categories of Identifying Features**

Self determinants
    Present on all cells in a single individual
    Determined by genetic constitution
    Different in each individual, except monozygotic ("identical") twins
    May be immunogenic for other members of same species
Species determinants
    Present on cells or proteins of all individuals of a given species
    Determined by genetic information common to the species
    May be immunogenic for individuals of other species
Functional determinants, inherent
    Reflect proteins that perform characteristic functions
    Examples: contractile proteins, enzymes, structural proteins
    Present in all cells, from any species, which perform that function
    Immunogenic only under pathologic or experimental circumstances
Functional determinants, variable
    Reflect phase of differentiation process or activation state
    Membrane receptors may disappear after interacting with ligand
    Stimulation of one receptor may initiate appearance or disappearance of others
    Immunogenicity may be part of a physiologic network of immune regulation

RECEPTOR-LIGAND INTERACTION

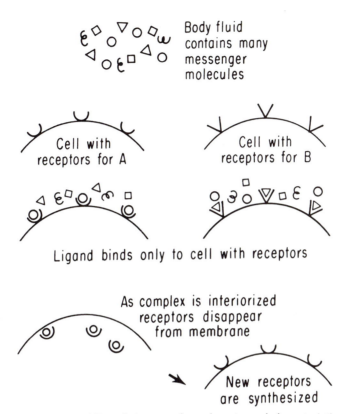

Body fluid contains many messenger molecules

Cell with receptors for A

Cell with receptors for B

Ligand binds only to cell with receptors

As complex is interiorized receptors disappear from membrane

New receptors are synthesized

FIGURE 1-7. Receptors and ligands interact through reciprocal characteristics of their configurations. Mediator molecules convey messages only to cells possessing the complementary receptor molecule. If the receptor-ligand complex is incorporated into the interior, the membrane remains bare of receptors and unable to receive new messages until additional receptor molecules are expressed.

neural transmission, stimulation passes from cell to cell when neurotransmitter substances generated by the sending cell interact with complementary receptors on the receiving cell. Many types of cells produce various growth-promoting factors that stimulate multiplication of cells that have suitably configured receptors. Phagocytosis occurs when membrane receptors of inflammatory cells interact with molecular complexes of other cells or particles. Each cell has many different receptor molecules, enabling it to respond to various stimuli as they occur. A cell unable to manufacture a particular receptor does not respond to the presence of the complementary mediating substance, no matter how high its concentration.

Interiorization of the receptor-ligand complex leaves the cell without receptors and unable to respond to additional ligand, a condition described as being **refractory** to further stimulation. Reappearance of newly synthesized receptors reestablishes a responsive state. Many receptor-ligand interactions, however, provoke internal changes that cause the cell to synthesize different products or to express different capabilities. This may cause a different set of receptors to appear, initiating avenues for stimulation and function different from those originally present. The genetic composition of the cell is unchanged, but structure and function can change dramatically with changing external events.

Cell Replication

For cell replication to occur, genetic material present in the diploid nucleus must undergo duplication. **Mitosis** is the asexual process whereby duplicated chromosomes are then segregated so that the resulting two new cells each receive an identical set. Occasional mishaps occur as chromosomes replicate and divide, but daughter cells are, for all practical purposes, identical with the cell of origin. With appropriate stimulation, the daughter cells can divide and their offspring can divide in geometric expansion to produce a cell population genetically identical with the original cell. A **clone** is a cell population that evolves without sexual recombination; if all cells in a population derive from successive divisions of a single cell, the population is described as **monoclonal.** When many different cells divide, the accumulating cells embody the differing genetic properties of diverse progenitor cells. A cell population that reflects division of many different cells is called **polyclonal** (Fig. 1–8). Polyclonal cell multiplication occurs when an extensive growth stimulus affects several or many individual cells. Monoclonal expansion occurs when some stimulus activates the receptors only of a single cell or when defective internal regulation enables an individual cell to divide in the absence of any external growth stimulus.

   Meiosis is the form of cell division whereby an original diploid cell evolves into four haploid cells, each containing a single copy of the 22 autosomes and a single sex chromosome, either X or Y. The **germ cells,** ova and sperm, are the only haploid cells in normal individuals. During meiosis, genetic material often exchanges between duplicated copies of individual chromosomes in a process called **crossing over** or between segments of different chromosomes in a process called **translocation.** As the complex nucleic acid molecules undergo replication, the sequence of

Cellular Aggregates

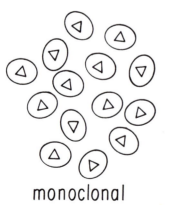

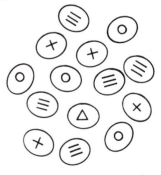

monoclonal   polyclonal

FIGURE 1–8. A group of cells is described as monoclonal if every member derives from a single progenitor; all cells have identical genetic constitution. In a polyclonal aggregate, many different cells of origin are represented, and the genetic constitution of the accumulated cells manifest many differences, some of them subtle and some pronounced.

nucleotides may be changed, causing new genetic information to develop, a process called **mutation.** Mutation may result in loss or acquisition of cell activities that may or may not be detrimental to cell function.

SUMMARY

1. Immunity includes the ability to exclude harmful invaders of the body; if protective surfaces or other defense mechanisms are breached, then the immune system is able to neutralize or eliminate the injurious agent. Innate immunity refers to nonspecific responses such as phagocytosis or inflammation. Adaptive immunity refers to specific activation of immune cells and secretion of antibodies to counter a specific antigen.

2. Induction of an adaptive immune response to smallpox was first practiced by physicians in China and Asia Minor and was called variolization. In 1796, Edward Jenner observed that milk maids who contracted cowpox were immune to smallpox. He then conducted the first vaccination procedure against smallpox using cowpox. Pasteur serendipitously observed that a microorganism could be attenuated and used to induce immunity.

3. Subsequently, the blood of an immunized animal was found to contain protective properties that could be transferred to an unimmunized animal (passive immunity). It was also discovered that the protective property was highly specific. The protective property was identified in the serum and called an antibody.

4. Activation of cells capable of providing protection is called cell-mediated immunity. Production of protective antibodies is referred to as humoral immunity. The cells responsible for immune activity are derived from a pluripotential cell called a hematopoietic stem cell. This cell undergoes mitosis and differentiation to produce RBCs, all the various WBCs, and platelets. The WBCs, neutrophils, and monocytes provide protection by phagocytosis. T lymphocytes and B lymphocytes are the WBCs responsible for cell-mediated and humoral immunity, respectively.

5. Important molecules for understanding immune cell responses include proteins, which are made of amino acids linked by peptide bonds to form polypeptides. Polysaccharides are sugars linked to one another to form chains and complex branched structures. Glycoproteins and glycolipids are combinations of polysaccharides linked to proteins or fats. These molecules are produced according to information contained within genes and have distinctive three-dimensional structures. Distinctive structure is crucial to the functions of these molecules. Important functions include enzyme activity, serving as membrane receptors and cell recognition markers. A receptor binding to its ligand enables a cell to respond and interact with its external environment.

6. Immune cells respond to their environment through receptor-ligand binding. When a receptor-ligand complex is formed, increased cell activity, secretion of growth-promoting factors, and mitosis may occur. A responsive immune cell with a specific receptor will undergo mitosis to form a clone and thereby expand the number of reactive cells.

REVIEW QUESTIONS

1. An example of natural, active immunity is _____.
    a. tetanus vaccination
    b. immune serum injection into an unimmunized animal
    c. recovery from a measles infection
    d. administration of anti–snake venom
    e. acute inflammation

2. Earliest attempts to develop immunization procedures were by _____.
    a. Chinese physicians
    b. Edward Jenner
    c. Louis Pasteur
    d. Emil Roux
    e. Jules Bordet

3. Serum from an animal immunized with staphylococci and mixed with *Escherichia coli* will cause _____; if mixed with streptococci will cause _____.
    a. no agglutination . . . agglutination
    b. no agglutination . . . no agglutination
    c. agglutination . . . agglutination
    d. agglutination . . . no agglutination

4. Humoral immunity refers to the activities of _____.
    a. antibodies
    b. complement
    c. phagocytosis
    d. a and b
    e. a, b, and c

5. A macrophage is derived from a circulating white blood cell called a _____.
    a. megakaryocyte
    b. monocyte
    c. lymphocyte
    d. eosinophil
    e. basophil

6. Predominant effector cells of chronic inflammation are _____.
    a. neutrophils
    b. basophils
    c. eosinophils
    d. megakaryocytes
    e. macrophages

7. A glycoprotein is composed of _____.
    a. carbohydrates
    b. amino acids
    c. lipids
    d. a and b
    e. a, b, and c

8. Consequences of receptor-ligand binding may include _____.
    a. endocytosis
    b. phagocytosis
    c. mitosis

d. a and b

e. a, b, and c

ESSAY QUESTIONS

1. Louis Pasteur introduced the term vaccination in honor of Edward Jenner. What was significant about Jenner's observations and how did Pasteur extend these observations concerning vaccines and the use of attenuated microorganisms?

2. What is a hematopoietic stem cell? Explain its function and why it is important to the immune system.

3. Describe the structure of the cell membrane and how a membrane protein is produced by a cell.

SUGGESTIONS FOR FURTHER READING

Lodish H, Baltimore D, Berk A, Zipursky SL, et al: Molecular Cell Biology, 3rd ed, New York: Scientific American Books. 1995:52–100 (Protein structure and function); 101–140 (Nucleic acids, the genetic code and the synthesis of macro molecules); 141–188 (Cell organization, subcellular structure, and cell division)

Quesenberry PJ: Hemopoietic stem cells, progenitor cells and cytokines. In: Beutler E, Lichtman MA, Coller BS, Kipps TJ, eds: Williams Hematology, 5th ed. New York, McGraw Hill, 1995:211–228

Silverstein AM: History of Immunology. London: Academic Press, 1989

Voet D, Voet JG: Biochemistry, 2nd ed. New York: John Wiley & Sons, 1995:105–140 (Covalent structures of proteins); 141–190 (Three dimensional structures of proteins); 251–276 (Sugars and polysaccharides); 277–329 (Lipids and membranes)

REVIEW ANSWERS

1.	c	5.	b
2.	a	6.	e
3.	b	7.	d
4.	d	8.	e

2 The Immune System

A brief overview of immunity is necessary to provide a context for description of the cells, tissues, and organs that constitute the immune system. Later chapters will discuss in greater depth the concepts introduced here.

NATURE OF IMMUNE REACTIONS

The essential features of immunity are **recognition** of specific antigen and **adaptive responses** to later encounters with the same material. Under normal conditions, immune responses occur only to "foreign" materials, with configurations that differ from those of the host's cells and cell products.

Antigen Recognition

Lymphocytes are the cells that recognize foreign material as potentially antigenic and respond to its presence with cellular and humoral changes characteristic of an immune response. Responsive lymphocytes that have receptor molecules configured to interact optimally with a single antigen are said to exhibit **specificity** for that material.

Interaction between antigen and receptor is a complex process. Antigenic materials enter the body usually through breaks in the skin layer or the thinner epithelial layers of the digestive or respiratory tracts. To ensure efficient stimulation of a receptive lymphocyte, the antigen must undergo modification, called **antigen processing.** Cells that process antigen are **accessory** or **antigen-presenting** cells and are frequently macrophages or related cells (Fig. 2−1). Macrophages also secrete many products that stimulate and modify lymphocytes and other cells involved in

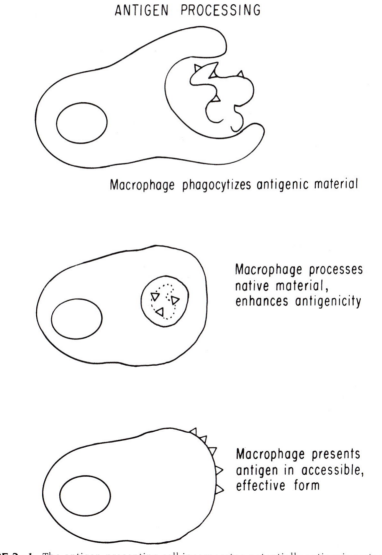

ANTIGEN PROCESSING

Macrophage phagocytizes antigenic material

Macrophage processes
native material,
enhances antigenicity

Macrophage presents
antigen in accessible,
effective form

FIGURE 2−1. The antigen-presenting cell incorporates potentially antigenic material, modifies its chemical or physical characteristics, and presents the altered material in a manner that facilitates interaction with the antigen-specific receptor of a lymphocyte. Macrophages and specialized epithelial cells perform most antigen processing and presentation.

immunity and inflammation. Cell products that influence the actions of other cells are called **cytokines.** Cytokines derived from macrophages and from lymphocytes have crucial regulatory roles in the immune process.

Response to Antigenic Stimulation

Contact between antigen and cell membrane receptor activates intracellular message systems that prepare the cell for replication. A lymphocyte that has never encountered its antigen is described as a **resting cell;** antigenic stimulation causes transformation into an **immunoblast,** a lymphocyte beginning to undergo multiplication. Multiplication involves replication of nuclear material and division into successive generations of cells. A variety of cytokines, many of which come from accessory lymphocytes activated by the same antigen, influence these processes. A complex sequence of cytokine production, receptor interactions, and modulation of membrane receptors orchestrates the generation of identical cells cloned from the original stimulated cell. Cells responding to recent antigen contact and expressing receptors for various cytokines exist in a state of **activation.**

As activated antigen-specific cells proliferate, individual members of the clone experience contact with any of several cytokines at various concentration levels. The result of these varied influences is that immune cells may exhibit a range of different membrane and internal products. Many of these cells evolve into effector forms that produce antibodies or initiate the cell-to-cell activities described as cell-mediated immunity. Most of these highly differentiated effector cells survive only for hours or days, performing their functions and then disappearing. Some activated cells do not become effector cells; they cease active division and become quiescent, although maintaining intracellular changes that reflect prior activation. These become **memory cells,** retaining a state of heightened reactivity such that subsequent encounter with antigen provokes rapid proliferation. Figure 2–2 illustrates the changes that follow contact with antigen.

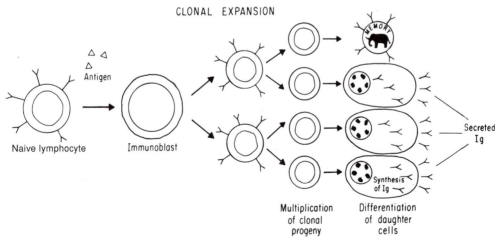

FIGURE 2–2. The naive lymphocyte transforms into an immunoblast after stimulation of the idiotypically unique receptor molecule. Clonal expansion generates progeny that are genetically identical but evolve into different effector cells after contact with mediators of different sorts.

Immune Cell Populations

Macrophages do not recognize specific antigenic configurations. They are very efficient phagocytic and antigen-presenting cells. Another antigen-presenting cell type is the **dendritic cell.** These cells are large and irregular-shaped with long filamentous cytoplasmic extensions called **dendrites.** Dendritic cells are located throughout the body, but particularly in lymphoid organs. Several types of dendritic cells are found in the body: Langerhans' cells located in the skin and interdigitating and follicular dendritic cells in lymphoid tissue.

Lymphocytes, unlike macrophages or dendritic cells, have exquisitely specific receptors for binding to and therefore "recognizing" specific antigen. Two major types of lymphocytes are capable of specific antigen recognition: T lymphocytes (T cells) and B lymphocytes (B cells).

Human and other mammalian B lymphocytes are exposed very early to the maturational effects of yolk sac, liver, and bone marrow. B cells undergo gene rearrangements that confer the ability to manufacture immunoglobulins, the proteins with antibody activity. Activation and subsequent differentiation cause antigen-stimulated B lymphocytes to evolve into **plasma cells,** which secrete the antibody into body fluids. After activation, B lymphocytes evolve either to short-lived antibody-producing plasma cells or to long-lived memory cells that are capable of rapid multiplication but are not actively synthesizing antibody.

Several different populations of T cells with different functions normally exist in the body. Precursor forms of T cells undergo differentiation in the thymus by a process completely different from that of B cells. T lymphocytes recognize antigen and participate in regulation of the immune response. Different T-cell populations can be identified by antibodies against characteristic membrane markers.

ORGANS OF THE IMMUNE SYSTEM

Lymphocytes, macrophages, and other antigen-presenting cells are capable of migration and are dispersed throughout the body. Large numbers of these cells are concentrated in immune organs including the bone marrow, lymph nodes, spleen, liver, thymus, and elements of the mucosal lining of the alimentary, respiratory, and, to a lesser extent, genitourinary tracts. Many of these tissues perform additional functions besides immune reactivity.

Circulatory Patterns

Lymphocytes and macrophages lead a nomadic existence, traveling continuously through tissues, blood, and lymphatic fluid. The body has several fluid compartments, all in dynamic equilibrium with one another. Sixty percent of body weight is water. Of this volume, approximately 60 percent is inside cells; the fluid part of blood constitutes 5 to 7 percent of the total water in the body. Water that is neither inside cells nor inside blood vessels is called **interstitial fluid;** this surrounds and bathes cells in all organs and tissues and is the medium across which gases and metabolites pass as they enter and leave cells, blood, and the external environment. In performing their inflammatory and immune functions, lymphocytes, macrophages, and granulocytes move between blood and interstitial fluid.

Lymphatic System

The heart and blood vessels can be considered a closed circulatory system, in which the plasma and cells of blood remain confined unless trauma or abnormal permeability occurs. This is not *strictly* true. Water and metabolites enter and leave the blood across capillary walls. Lymphocytes enter and leave the blood at different sites, and certain proteins of blood origin can accumulate to substantial concentrations in the interstitial fluid. The lymphatic system is necessary to clear tissues of accumulated fluid, protein, and cells.

The **lymphatic system** is open-ended. It consists of lymphatic vessels, lymph nodes, and lymph fluid. Lymph fluid or **lymph** originates from the interstitial fluid. The smallest lymphatic vessels are funnel-like traps in the interstitium, into which fluid, particles of all sorts, and wandering macrophages and lymphocytes are pushed when tissue pressures rise. The flow of lymph fluid is **centripetal,** meaning from the periphery toward the center of the body. In its centripetal course, lymph passes through **lymph nodes,** aggregates of tissue located in large numbers in the neck, axilla, and groin. As lymph fluid exits a lymph node, it enters larger vessels. The largest lymphatic vessel, the thoracic duct, receives lymph from the entire body and empties it into the bloodstream in one of the two veins that returns blood to the heart for repeated circulation. The fluid and cells present in lymph mingle with the blood and reenter the circulatory cycle.

Sinusoidal Flow

An important aspect of lymphatic flow is sinusoidal drainage through lymph nodes. **Sinusoids** are channels of relatively wide caliber, with irregular contours and thin walls. Fluid passing through these broad, meandering paths moves relatively slowly, so that material carried in the fluid has prolonged and intimate contact with cells and membranes that line the sinusoids. Lymph fluid enters lymph nodes through **afferent** lymphatics at the periphery; it percolates through sinusoids toward the center of the node, where a slightly larger **efferent** vessel continues the centripetal route that leads eventually to the bloodstream. Macrophages and dendritic cells line sinusoids or lie immediately beneath the walls, where they may experience prolonged contact with material present in the lymph fluid. Particulate matter such as microorganisms, bits of foreign material, or debris from the body's own cells is cleared from the tissues by entering the lymphatics; it is cleared from lymph by sinusoidal macrophages. Macrophages either degrade the material permanently or process it for presentation to immune effector cells.

In several portions of the cardiovascular system, the bloodstream passes through sinusoids, allowing comparable contact of macrophages with the contents of flowing blood. In the spleen, liver, and bone marrow, flowing blood has intimate contact with macrophages associated with the walls of sinusoids. If the blood contains cellular, particulate, or molecular material with antigenic properties, macrophages can extract these elements and process them as needed. Sinusoidal macrophages also have repeated contact with circulating cells and act to remove aging or damaged blood cells from the circulation.

Lymph Nodes

Lymph nodes are round to bean-shaped structures present in clusters along the routes that lymphatic vessels follow before joining the bloodstream. They are ideally located to filter out any foreign material carried in the lymph. Lymph nodes consist of a fibrous network of reticular and collagen fibers packed with lymphocytes, macrophages, and dendritic cells. Afferent lymph fluid flows into a subcapsular sinusoid just beneath a connective tissue capsule and flows toward the interior of the node. The outer portion of the node is called the **cortex.** The cells in the cortex are predominantly B cells and are arranged into nodules called **primary follicles.** After antigenic stimulation, B cells in a follicle undergo clonal expansion. The follicle enlarges to become a **germinal center** or **secondary follicle.** Germinal centers are sites where B cells undergo a process called **somatic mutation,** whereby the binding capabilities of B cells for antigen change at random. Those cells that become more efficient at binding antigen are stimulated to undergo further clonal expansion and will subsequently produce a more specific antibody. These cells may also migrate via blood or lymph to other lymphoid organs to form secondary follicles.

T lymphocytes cluster around the follicles and are a major population in the deeper portions of the lymph node, the paracortical area. Deeper still, in the **medulla,** B cells and their differentiated plasma cell progeny are the predominant cells, along with the macrophages that hug the walls of sinusoids. Figure 2–3 shows a schematized lymph node.

Bone Marrow

Bone marrow occupies the central portion of nearly all the 206 bones in the body, but in adults, most marrow spaces contain a large percentage of fat, with little productive activity. Active bone marrow is the site of **hematopoiesis,** the production of

ARCHITECTURE OF LYMPH NODE

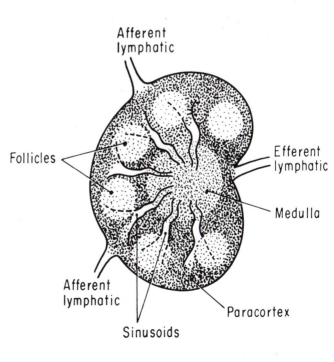

FIGURE 2–3. Lymph fluid enters the periphery of the lymph node through the afferent lymphatics and percolates through the sinusoids to emerge from the node through the centrally located efferent lymphatic vessel. Follicles, which consist largely of B cells, are conspicuous in the outer cortex. Around the follicles and in the slightly deeper paracortical portions of the node, T cells predominate. In the central portion, the medulla, there is a mixed population of lymphocytes, in which B cells and plasma cells are the most numerous.

blood cells, including lymphocytes. Hematopoietic and lymphoid tissue occupies more marrow space in the fetus than in postuterine life and more in young children than in adults. In normal adults, active bone marrow is almost entirely confined to the vertebral column, the breast bone, and the bones of the pelvis. However, both physiologic and pathologic stimuli can reexpand adult bone marrow activity to the ribs, the long bones of the extremities, and the bones of the skull.

Bone marrow consists of sinusoids surrounded by macrophages. Between the sinusoids are masses of proliferating erythrocytes, granulocytes, monocytes, and platelets. Mature cells enter the blood by migrating across the sinusoidal walls into the circulating blood. Macrophages resident in the bone marrow phagocytize particulate material and damaged cells and secrete cytokines that affect both hematopoietic and immune cells. Normal-functioning bone marrow is critical to a normal immune system as a source of lymphocyte precursor cells and as a site of lymphocyte maturation and antibody production.

Spleen and Liver

The **spleen** is a fist-sized organ in the upper left quadrant of the abdominal cavity and relative to its size, receives a substantial amount of blood. Blood circulating through the spleen pursues a tortuous course. The arterial tree branches into arterioles that run adjacent to follicles of lymphocytes. B cells occupy the centers of follicles; T cells occupy the periphery of these follicles. Blood traversing the spleen leaves the arterial side and percolates slowly through venous sinusoids, allowing intimate contact with splenic macrophages. During this interaction, aging or damaged cells are removed from the circulation, and antigenic material is extracted for processing and presentation. The spleen contains many **dendritic cells,** in close association with follicular B cells. The normal spleen is the major site for blood filtration, serving a function comparable to the cleansing effect that lymph nodes exert on lymphatic fluid. If the spleen is absent or splenic circulation is impaired, liver and bone marrow can take over these activities.

Like the bone marrow, the **liver** has substantial lymphoreticular elements in an organ that serves other functions. Between the macrophage-lined sinusoids of the liver lie **hepatocytes,** cuboidal cells of epithelial origin that constitute most of the approximately 1500 g (about 3 lb) that the liver weighs. Hepatocytes synthesize many blood proteins and perform metabolic conversions that manufacture and degrade most body constituents. Blood that traverses the hepatic sinusoids comes largely from the gastrointestinal tract and other abdominal organs, bringing with it antigenic material as well as the nutrients essential for continuing metabolism. The combined actions of hepatocytes and Kuppfer's cells, hepatic macrophages, regulate antigenic exposure from the many substances entering the body as food and drink. The normal liver contains very few lymphocytes and appears to generate very little immune effector activity.

Thymus

The thymus and bone marrow are considered **primary lymphoid organs.** They are sites absolutely necessary for the formation of competent T and B cells. **Secondary**

lymphoid organs include the lymph nodes, spleen, and other sites in the body in which mature lymphocytes encounter antigen and become effector cells. The thymus, a fleshy, lobulated organ in the anterior chest, is at its largest and most active during intrauterine life and early childhood. It almost disappears in older children and adults, but its early presence and activity are crucial for immune system development. The thymus is demarcated into a highly cellular outer portion called the **cortex** and a smaller central area, the **medulla.** Early in fetal life, lymphoid precursor cells from the marrow enter the outermost portion of the cortex and acquire the markers characteristic of T cells. Progressive maturation and proliferation occur as the cells migrate through cortex and medulla to emerge as circulating T lymphocytes. These events are discussed more fully in Chapter 5 and illustrated in Figure 5–3. Lymphocytes within the thymus are called **thymocytes;** they become **peripheral T cells** after leaving the thymus. Differentiation and subsequent maturation are mediated by hormones, including **thymosin** and **thymopoietin,** produced by thymic epithelial cells. A lifetime supply of dedicated T-cell precursors develops during the migration and proliferation that occur in the large, active thymus of early existence.

Mucosa-Associated Lymphoid Tissue

Approximately one-third of the body's lymphocytes are found in superficial mucosal locations. Large numbers of lymphocytes and plasma cells lie beneath surface epithelial cells in the respiratory and alimentary tracts, close to the cells that metabolize incoming material and secrete the fluids that bathe these surfaces. The superficial portions of the genitourinary system have a smaller lymphoid component. Lymphocytes in these locations are collectively described as the **mucosa-associated lymphoid tissue (MALT).** Lymphocytes—mostly B cells—form follicles in the upper portions of the respiratory and alimentary tracts. These are most easily seen as the tonsils, adenoids, and Peyer's patches of the small intestine. A thick layer of lymphocytes is diffusely arranged among the epithelial elements in most segments of these mucosal surfaces. These lymphocytes express a very strong functional sense of place. Cells initially present in specific mucosal locations consistently return to these sites after their migrations. Figure 2–4 depicts the major sites of lymphoid tissue.

Lymphocyte Circulation

Lymphocytes travel continuously through the tissues, the lymphatic system, and the bloodstream. "Naive" T cells, antigen-specific lymphocytes that have not yet encountered antigen, leave the bloodstream and enter lymph nodes through venules in the paracortex. These venules have tall endothelium and are therefore called **high endothelial venules (HEV).** The amount of HEV in a lymph node is controlled by local immune activity and the presence of antigen. Circulating T cells have **homing receptors** which bind to surface proteins on high endothelial cells called **addressins.** Once these are loosely bound, they migrate between the endothelial cells and enter the lymph node. More circulating naive lymphocytes are therefore at-

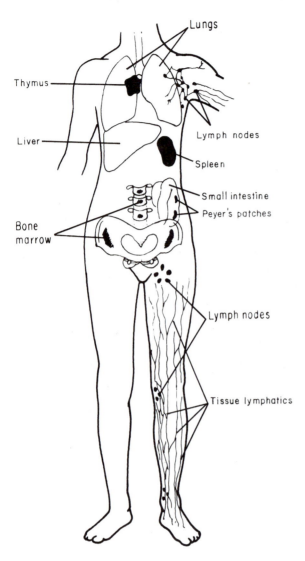

FIGURE 2–4. Elements of the immune system are present throughout the body with lymphatic vessels draining every organ and tissue. On its way to join the bloodstream, lymph fluid passes through lymph nodes at many sites. The spleen, liver, and bone marrow are important immune organs at all stages of life, whereas the thymus is prominent only in fetal life, infancy, and early childhood. The respiratory and gastrointestinal tracts contain most of the mucosa-associated lymphoid tissue.

tracted to an active immune site. Different types of addressins are present on endothelial cells of different lymphoid tissues; therefore, lymphocytes "home" to specific sites in the immune system. Once in the lymph node, lymphocytes may undergo immune activation, remain in the lymph node for a period of time, die, or leave again via the efferent lymph. Lymphocytes thereby reenter the bloodstream and can recirculate in some cases for years. Lymphocytes also leave the bloodstream by migrating through conventional endothelium and are then carried to lymph nodes by afferent lymph (Fig. 2–5).

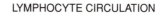

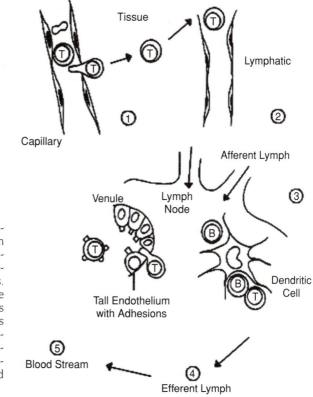

FIGURE 2–5. Many more T lymphocytes than B lymphocytes circulate in the blood. Lymphocytes may enter tissues by migrating between endothelial cells of capillaries and venules. Lymphocytes as well as other white blood cells demonstrate chemotaxis and are selectively attracted to sites in the body by cytokines and the presence of addressins and homing receptors. Unlike granulocytes, lymphocytes are capable of migrating and recirculating multiple times.

THE MONONUCLEAR-PHAGOCYTE SYSTEM

Macrophages, which are intimately involved in the processes of antigen recognition, immune stimulation, and the tissue consequences that follow immune stimulation, have different lineage and functional properties from those of lymphocytes.

Bone Marrow Origin

Development and replenishment of mononuclear phagocytic cells occur continuously throughout life. Macrophages and granulocytes descend from a common bone marrow precursor. The two populations then diverge into immature precursor forms: **monoblast** and **myeloblast.** Under the influence of local growth factors and cytokines, monocytes and granulocytes mature and develop from these precursors and enter the circulating blood. In inflammatory conditions, certain factors promote increased monocyte development, and others reduce this activity when the stimulus ceases.

Monocytes enter the circulation within 24 hours of their generation. They constitute approximately 3 to 8 percent of peripheral white blood cells. Circulating monocytes are cells that have not reached full differentiation. Further development into macrophages occurs at the various tissue sites to which the blood carries them.

Locations and Functions in Tissue

The mononuclear-phagocyte population occupies many tissue sites and exhibits a wide range of differentiated appearance. Features common to cells of this overall category include the presence of several cytoplasmic enzymes, notably **nonspecific esterase** and **lysozyme.** Several membrane receptor molecules consistently occur on macrophages but are not lineage-specific, being present on other cell types as well. Particularly important in immune activity are the receptors for immunoglobulin molecules, the **Fc receptor** and the **C3 receptor** (which binds one of the proteins in the complement system) (see Chapter 8). Therefore, mononuclear phagocytes have the capability of phagocytizing particles, especially those coated with antibody or complement proteins (Fig. 2–6).

PHAGOCYTOSIS

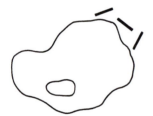 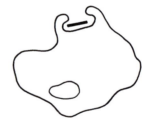 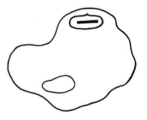

Macrophage surrounds and engulfs particle

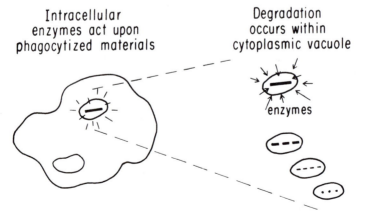

Intracellular
enzymes act upon
phagocytized materials

Degradation
occurs within
cytoplasmic vacuole

enzymes

FIGURE 2–6. Phagocytosis begins with surface contact between the particle and the cell membrane, which invaginates to enfold the material and incorporate it into the cytoplasm. A complex system of enzymes and energy-requiring reactions causes degradation of the phagocytized material.

Differentiation into Macrophages

On leaving the bloodstream, monocytes migrate to tissue locations and remain as **resident macrophages.** We have already mentioned macrophages in lymph nodes, spleen, and liver. Additional populations of resident macrophages include (1) **alveolar macrophages,** which live in the lungs; (2) macrophages that monitor and protect the **peritoneal** lining around abdominal organs and the **pleural** surfaces that surround the lungs; (3) **osteoclasts,** which perform degradative activities in bone; (4) macrophages in the central nervous system, sometimes called **microglia;** (5) **histiocytes,** macrophages that are free in connective tissue; (6) **Langerhans'** or **dendritic cells,** often found in the skin; and (7) macrophages in joint linings and in renal glomeruli. Compared with circulating monocytes, macrophages have a wider repertory of internal enzymes, a greater phagocytic capacity, and the ability to synthesize a wide range of cytokines and other proteins. Macrophages in tissue retain some capacity to multiply, but this potential is exercised only after pronounced stimulation. Under normal conditions, macrophage populations are replenished from the bone marrow.

Resident macrophages occupy predictable locations within each tissue. After a stimulus to inflammation, macrophages become activated and may accumulate as **exudate macrophages.** Activated macrophages secrete cytokines that activate other cells of the immune system and influence other aspects of inflammation. In turn, the lymphokines from antigen-specific lymphocytes cause macrophages to manifest heightened reactivity. Stimulated by immune cytokines, activated macrophages become larger, exhibit more numerous and more active organelles, engage in more effective phagocytosis with the production of bactericidal metabolites of oxygen and nitrogen (O_2-NO) and even hypochlorite or bleach (HOCl). Other products of activated macrophages include proteolytic enzymes and numerous proteins that affect coagulation, complement activity, and multiplication of cells that generate new tissue and repair damaged tissue.

SUMMARY

1. The essential features of an immune response are recognition of a specific antigen and adaptive responses to that antigen. Antigen recognition requires lymphocytes with specific receptors and may also require prior antigen processing by macrophages or other antigen presenting cells. Cytokines, which activate immune cells, are also necessary for an immune response to occur.

2. Two major types of lymphocytes are capable of antigen recognition: T lymphocytes (T cells) and B lymphocytes (B cells). Each of these cell types has specific receptors for binding to antigens. Binding of antigen to a specific lymphocyte induces conversion from a resting cell to an immunoblast that undergoes proliferation and differentiation to effectors cells capable of making antibody or participating in cell-mediated immunity. Some activated lymphocytes become memory cells capable of responding with heightened reactivity upon reexposure to the same antigen.

Continued on following page

3. Lymphocytes, macrophages, and other antigen-presenting cells migrate and are dispersed throughout the body. They can also be found concentrated in immune organs such as the bone marrow, thymus, lymph nodes, spleen, liver, and the mucosal lining of the gut and respiratory system. Lymphocytes circulate in the blood and lymphatic system and can enter and leave lymph nodes located along the lymphatic vessels. Afferent lymph flow may carry lymphocytes as well as antigen into a lymph node. Macrophages in the lymph node process and present antigen to T cells and B cells clustered in primary follicles in the cortex of the lymph node. Upon antigenic stimulation, lymphocytes undergo clonal expansion and form germinal centers or secondary follicles.

4. The thymus and the bone marrow are considered primary lymphoid organs because these are sites absolutely necessary for the formation of competent T and B cells. After competent lymphocytes are formed, they disperse into secondary lymphoid organs, where they encounter antigen and become effector cells. Although secondary lymphoid organs such as the spleen and liver have other functions to perform, they are also important to the immune system because antigens in the blood can be trapped by resident macrophages and presented to local lymphocytes.

5. Lymphocytes circulate and are localized to mucosa-associated lymphoid tissue (MALT). Aggregates of lymphocytes are present in the walls of the respiratory and alimentary tracts, where they provide immune protection for these thin vulnerable surfaces.

6. Macrophages are derived from monocytes, which are produced in the bone marrow. Once released from the bone marrow, monocytes travel through the bloodstream and migrate to tissue locations, where they become resident macrophages. As resident macrophages, they are referred to by various names, but all have the ability to phagocytose antigens and produce degradative cytoplasmic enzymes to aid in antigen processing and will have common membrane receptor molecules—some of which aid in binding antigen (Fc receptors, C3 receptors). Involvement in inflammation causes activation of macrophages. Macrophages secrete cytokines, which activate other immune cells. Activated macrophages become larger, display increased metabolic activity, and engage in more effective phagocytosis with increased production of bactericidal metabolites.

REVIEW QUESTIONS

1. Which cells are capable of presenting antigen to lymphocytes?
   a. Macrophages
   b. Dendritic cells
   c. Plasma cells
   d. Neutrophils
   e. a and b

2. Organ(s) in the adult in which blood is normally produced is/are _____.
   a. liver
   b. bone marrow
   c. spleen
   d. lymph nodes
   e. a and b

3. If lymphatic vessels become plugged, what will happen?
   a. Accumulation of interstitial fluid (edema)
   b. Dehydration of tissues
   c. Blood clot formation
   d. Blood vessel contraction
   e. Blood vessel dilation

4. Which of the following is NOT a function of a lymph node?
   a. Filter blood
   b. Filter lymph
   c. Trap bacteria
   d. Trap cancer cells
   e. Promote macrophage–T-cell interaction

5. Which of the following is a macrophage localized to the liver?
   a. Plasma cell
   b. Monocyte
   c. Kupffer's cell
   d. Microglial cell
   e. Dendritic cell

6. Which of the following is NOT a function of macrophages?
   a. Secretion of cytokines
   b. Phagocytosis
   c. Antigen presentation
   d. Antigen recognition
   e. Enzyme production

7. Which lymphoid organ(s) is(are) considered primary lymphoid organ(s)?
   a. Bone marrow
   b. Thymus
   c. Spleen
   d. Liver
   e. a and b

8. Lymphocytes enter lymph nodes from the bloodstream primarily through _____.
   a. arterioles
   b. venules
   c. high-endothelial venules
   d. capillaries
   e. lymphatic vessels

ESSAY QUESTIONS

1. What is a sinusoid and where are sinusoids found? Why are sinusoids found in these organs?

2. How do lymphocytes *circulate continuously* through the tissues, the lymphatic system, and the bloodstream. Why do they do this? Describe the pathway of a lymphocyte, beginning in the bloodstream.

SUGGESTIONS FOR FURTHER READING

Butcher EC: Cellular and molecular mechanisms that direct leukocyte traffic. Am J Pathol 1990;136:3–12

Gallin, JI, Goldstein IM, Snyderman R: Inflammation: Basic Principles and Clinical Correlates, 2nd ed. New York: Raven Press, 1992

Gorlin JB, Stossel TP: The phagocyte system: Structure and function. In: Nathan DG, Oski FA, eds: Hematology of Infancy and Childhood, 6th ed. Philadelphia: WB Saunders, 1993:882–903

Groom AC, Schmidt EE: Microcirculatory blood flow through the spleen. In: Bowdler, AJ, ed: The Spleen: Structure, Function and Clinical Significance. London: Chapman & Hall, 1990:45–102

Mackaness GB: Reflections on the history of the macrophage. In: Lopez-Berestein G, Klostergaard J, eds: Mononuclear Phagocytes in Cell Biology. Boca Raton, FL: CRC Press, 1993:1–6

REVIEW ANSWERS

1. e   5. c
2. b   6. d
3. a   7. e
4. a   8. c

3 Major Histocompatibility Complex: The HLA System

Crucially important in immune regulation are several classes of membrane glycoproteins, collectively designated **major histocompatibility molecules.** All mammalian species possess a cluster of genes called the **major histocompatibility complex (MHC complex),** which determine the composition and specificity of these membrane molecules. In humans, the MHC complex is called the **HLA system** (human leukocyte antigens) because these molecules were first detected on white blood cells. The MHC plays a central role in the development of humoral and cell-mediated immunity. T cells recognize only antigen that is presented in association with MHC molecules. In fact, the function of MHC molecules is antigen presentation. Differences in individual expression of MHC molecules influence the ability of T cells to recognize antigen and therefore the body's susceptibility to disease and the development of autoimmunity. The MHC is also important for compatibility of organ or tissue transplantation. If

MHC molecules in a donor are different from those of the recipient, the donor MHC molecules will be recognized as foreign antigen and immunologically rejected.

ORGANIZATION AND INHERITANCE OF HLA

Alleles and Polymorphism

The amino acid sequence of a polypeptide is a direct reflection of the nucleotide sequence in chromosomal deoxyribonucleic acid (DNA). DNA sequences may undergo substitutions, transpositions, additions, or deletions. These changes (called **mutations**) cause predictable changes in amino acid sequence of the corresponding protein. For some proteins, any alteration in amino acid sequence destroys functional capacity. If the function of that protein is essential for survival, the affected cell or organism does not survive to transmit the altered DNA to offspring. Many mutations, however, induce protein alterations that do not affect reproductive capacity, and offspring of the original individual exhibit the same genetic trait. Different forms of a gene, occupying the same chromosomal location and determining variant forms of the same product, are called **alleles.** The structural differences that result are called **allotypic variants.** Figure 3–1 depicts the effects of allelic variation.

Some proteins have exactly the same structure in every individual; the gene for these products is presumably the same in everyone. For many proteins, slight structural variations exist, and individuals expressing different forms of the polypeptide possess different alleles. The existence of many different alleles for a given characteristic in a population is described as **polymorphism,** from Greek words meaning "many forms." The HLA system is highly polymorphic, with numerous alleles that determine subtle differences among cells from different humans.

ALLELIC DIFFERENCES

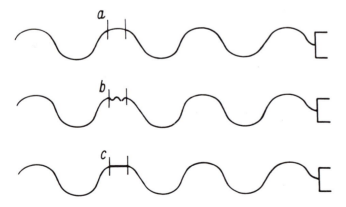

Same protein
Different allelic characteristics

FIGURE 3–1. Alleles are alternative genes for the production of a single protein. Differences in DNA sequence cause the resulting proteins to differ in amino acid sequence at localized sites. For the protein shown at left, the products of three different alleles (designated *a, b,* and *c*) differ in structure at a single segment. The overall nature of the protein is the same, but the allelic characteristics may affect functional or antigenic properties of the molecule.

Significance of Polymorphism

Allelic variants may determine products that vary in functional efficiency. For example, certain variants of the hemoglobin molecule cause significant health problems; genetically aberrant enzymes cause diseases of many sorts. Other allelic differences have few or no apparent physiologic effects. HLA molecules modify how immune effector cells interact with both accessory and target cells. Inheritance of specific alleles may confer advantages or disadvantages, and continuing research has revealed some associations of immune-related disease with the presence of certain alleles.

HLA molecules differ sufficiently in structure, so that exposure of a host to cells with foreign HLA molecules can provoke an immune response. Thus, HLA molecules can function as antigens and are involved in graft rejection. HLA and transplantation immunology are discussed later in this chapter and in Chapter 13. Characterization of the highly polymorphic HLA system resulted from observations made in women exposed to the foreign HLA antigens of the fetus they carried, in patients exposed to transfused cells, and in experimental tissue-grafting systems.

Chromosomal Organization and Haplotypes

Genes performing a given function occupy the same position on the same chromosome in all individuals of a species; that position is called the **locus** (plural: **loci**) for that gene. Loci for many human genes have been identified. For example, genes for manufacture of immunoglobulin chains reside on chromosomes 14, 2, and 22; those for ABO red blood cell (RBC) antigens are on chromosome 9. Genes controlling the HLA molecules are on chromosome 6 (Fig. 3–2).

Diploid cells possess two copies of every chromosome except the sex chromosomes; hence, they have two copies of every gene. If the locus on both chromosomes is occupied by the same allele, the cell is said to be **homozygous** for that gene. If each chromosome has a different allele, the cell is **heterozygous** for the

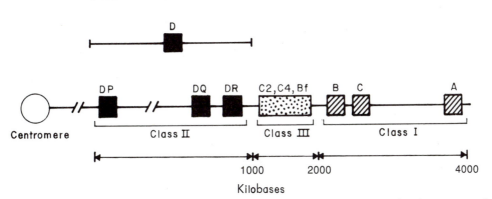

FIGURE 3–2. The major histocompatibility complex (MHC) on chromosome 6 has been mapped in detail. Discrete portions encode the class I products (HLA series A, B, and C), the class II products (HLA-D and DP, DQ, and DR series), and the class III products, largely proteins that participate in the complement system.

gene. Heterozygotes express two different sets of HLA-bearing molecules. Homozygotes, who have the same allele on both chromosomes, do not produce twice as much of that material; their cells simply display molecules of a single antigenic structure.

Manner of Transmission

When chromosomal material is apportioned to germ cells during meiosis, genes located very close to one another tend to remain together. Genes some distance apart on a chromosome may become entangled with strands of condensed chromosomal material and **crossover** from one chromosome to the opposite member of the pair. The alignment of genes on the resulting chromosomes is therefore different from that in the original cell. Genes so close together that crossing-over rarely occurs are inherited as a consistent unit of genetic material, called a **haplotype.** MHC genes pass from one generation to the next in predictable haplotypes, although crossing-over occurs occasionally.

HLA molecules on cell surfaces display at least six different categories of activity, designated **series,** which are identified by letters. Each series is determined by alleles at a specific site within the MHC. The combined sequence of genes within that segment of chromosome 6 makes up the MHC haplotype on that chromosome. Each individual possesses two haplotypes—one from each parent. When the parents reproduce, each offspring will receive one (and only one) of those haplotypes. No matter how many different alleles exist in a population and how many ways these alleles can align into haplotypes, the offspring of a single mating can express only those haplotypes present in the original couple. Starting with two maternal haplotypes and two paternal haplotypes, each child will express one of only four possible combinations (Fig. 3–3).

Classes of MHC Products

The HLA system or MHC complex is a collection of 40 to 50 genes in a continuous stretch of DNA located on the short arm of chromosome 6. The genes and their protein products are organized into three classes: **class I, class II,** and **class III.** Class I genes encode the information for MHC molecules present on nearly all nucleated cells. MHC class I molecules present antigen necessary for activation of a subclass of lymphocytes called **cytotoxic T cells.** Cytotoxic T cells are instrumental in cell-mediated immune responses. Class II molecules are expressed by phagocytic cells and other cells capable of phagocytosis and antigen presentation. Class II molecules are necessary for activation of another subclass of T cells called **helper T cells.** Class III genes encode for a mixture of non-HLA products, which include some of the complement proteins, enzymes, and the cytokines TNF-α and β.

STRUCTURE AND FUNCTION OF MHC MOLECULES

Antigen Processing

An immune response first involves the processing of foreign antigen. An antigen is fragmented and is presented in combination with "self antigen" or MHC molecules.

TRANSMISSION OF HLA HAPLOTYPES

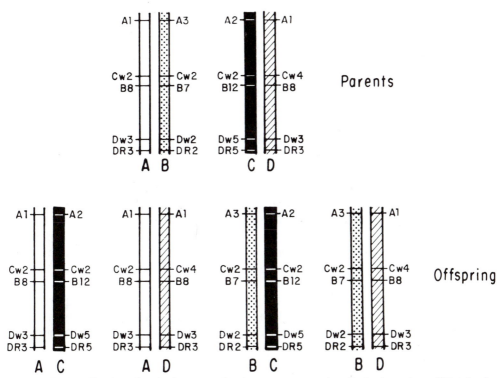

FIGURE 3-3. Offspring of a single parental pair can express only a limited number of HLA haplotypes. In the mating shown above, one parent will transmit *either* the A or the B haplotype; the other will transmit *either* C or D. Combination occurs at random, but only four different combinations are possible.

The foreign antigen and MHC must then be recognized by T cells, and, on binding of antigen to receptors on responsive T cells, immune cells are activated, effector cells formed, and humoral or cell-mediated immunity results.

Humans are exposed to many different kinds of antigens. Antigens can be grouped according to their origin. **Exogenous antigen** is antigen that enters the body, is free in the circulation or tissues for a short period of time, and is then phagocytosed. An example of exogenous antigen is bacteria. **Endogenous antigen** is made within the body. For example, a virus may invade a cell and take over. New viral proteins are made within the cell, and because they are foreign proteins, they constitute endogenous antigen. Or, cancer cells may develop within the body. These mutated cells make new altered proteins, which may or may not be treated as endogenous antigen.

MHC Class II

MHC class II glycoproteins are important for presentation of exogenous antigens. These proteins are products of a region of the MHC complex called HLA-D. Within the HLA-D region are five loci called DN, DO, DP, DQ, and DR. Class II glycoproteins are expressed primarily on professional antigen-presenting cells. Monocytes/

macrophages and mature B lymphocytes express large amounts of class II molecules. Cytokines that enhance reactivity cause MHC II expression to increase. Resting T lymphocytes express weak or nondetectable activity, but activated T cells may have strong class II expression.

MHC class II molecules are surface membrane-bound glycoproteins consisting of two chains: alpha and beta. The alpha chain is slightly larger than the beta chain, with molecular weights of 34 kD and 29 kD, respectively. Both alpha and beta chains have looped segments called **domains.** The looped segments extend into the external environment of the cell. Another portion of the chains passes through the membrane and is referred to as the **transmembrane domain.** A cytoplasmic portion (cytoplasmic domain) anchors the glycoprotein in the cell membrane (Fig. 3–4). Each chain has two external domains designated alpha-1, alpha-2 and beta-1, beta-2. The alpha-2 and beta-2 domains are nearest the cell membrane and have amino acid sequences similar to those of antibodies. Proteins that share similar amino acid sequences are said to be **homologous** and are related. Class II glycoproteins and antibodies belong to the **immunoglobulin superfamily** of molecules.

The alpha-1 and beta-1 domains extending farthest from the cell membrane form a peptide-binding groove or cleft for processed antigen. In the alpha-1 and beta-1 domains, the greatest amount of polymorphism occurs. This results in slight changes in amino acid composition in the peptide-binding groove and therefore slight changes in the shape and ability of the cleft to bind and present processed antigen fragments. MHC genes have a high mutation rate with many different alleles existing for each gene locus. This high mutation rate aids and enhances the ability of the MHC molecules to interact with processed antigen.

Antigen Presentation With MHC Class II

Professional phagocytic cells that express MHC II are capable of phagocytosing or pinocytosing antigenic materials into phagosomes or endosomes. These cells produce **lysosomes** (membrane-enclosed vesicles containing degradative enzymes), which aid in the breakdown of phagocytosed material. The MHC II glycoproteins are likewise produced and packaged into vesicles. The MHC molecules are incorporated into the membrane of the vesicles. When phagocytosis occurs, lysosomes fuse with a phagosome and digestion of antigen results. MHC vesicles then fuse with the

STRUCTURE OF MHC PRODUCTS

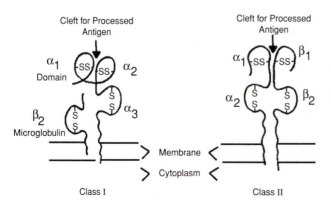

FIGURE 3–4. MHC class I molecules are composed of one alpha chain and β_2 microglobulin. Structure of the large alpha chain is determined by genes of the MHC. The β_2-microglobulin chain is the same in all class I molecules; its production is directed by a gene on chromosome 15. In class II molecules, both chains are products of genes in the MHC. The chains are similar in size and configuration.

phagosomes containing partially digested antigenic fragments. The antigenic fragments bind to the groove formed by the alpha-1 and beta-1 domains. Vesicles containing MHC molecules and antigenic fragments move toward the cell surface, where they then fuse with the cell membrane revealing MHC II molecules with bound antigenic peptides (Fig. 3–5).

MHC Class I

T cells recognize foreign antigen only in association with MHC molecules. Exogenous antigen is presented in association with MHC class II molecules. Endogenous antigen is presented in association with MHC I. Endogenous antigens originate within the body. They may include such materials as normal cellular breakdown products, excess regulatory proteins, or viral proteins. MHC class I molecules are

PROCESSING AND PRESENTATION OF ANTIGEN

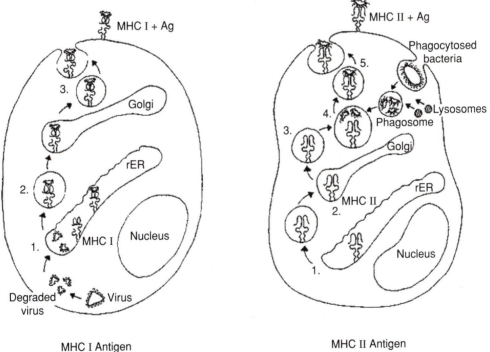

MHC I Antigen
Presentation

MHC II Antigen
Presentation

FIGURE 3–5. Pathways for processing of endogenous- and exogenous-derived antigens. MHC class I molecules are necessary for presentation of endogenous peptides and MHC class II is needed for exogenous antigen (Ag) presentation. Polymorphism and the existence of multiple alleles of MHC I and II ensure diverse antigen-binding capabilities. Pathway for endogenous antigens: (1) degraded viral peptides (Ag) transported into rough endoplasmic reticulum (rER), (2) vesicles containing MHC I and Ag transported to Golgi, (3) vesicle with MHC I and Ag transported to surface membrane. Pathway for exogenous antigens: (1) production of MHC II molecule in rER, (2) vesicle transport of MHC II for Golgi processing, (3) vesicle release of MHC II, (4) fusion of phagosome with MHC vesicle, and (5) transport of MHC II and exogenous Ag to surface membrane.

found on the cell surface of almost all nucleated cells. Macrophages and lymphocytes can also express MHC class I molecules.

Class I molecules can be divided into two groups: **MHC class Ia** molecules, which are highly polymorphic, and **MHC class Ib,** which are much less polymorphic. MHC Ia genes occupy loci called **HLA-A, HLA-B,** and **HLA-C.** MHC Ib loci are called **HLA-E, HLA-F, HLA-G, HLA-H, HLA-J,** and **HLA-X.** MHC Ia consists of a single alpha chain encoded by genes within the A, B, or C locus and another smaller chain called β_2 **microglobulin,** which is encoded by a gene on chromosome 15. The alpha chain contains the polymorphic sites for antigen presentation. The β-microglobulin component is unvarying with a looped configuration and molecular weight of 12 kD. The β-microglobulin polypeptide also exists as an independent fluid-phase molecule in serum and urine, but its function is unknown. The larger alpha chain has 338 amino acid residues and a molecular weight of 44 kD. Its configuration includes three external domains, a transmembrane domain, and a cytoplasmic tail.

Endogenous cellular materials marked for antigen presentation are degraded within the cytoplasm. The resulting peptides are transported across the membrane of the rough endoplasmic reticulum (rER), where they bind to newly synthesized MHC class I alpha chains. Peptide-bearing alpha chains then associate with β_2-microglobulin. MHC I molecules bearing antigenic peptides, similar to MHC II, are incorporated into membrane-bound vesicles that make their way from the rER to the Golgi cells and then move through the cytoplasm to fuse with the surface cell membrane. Fusion with the cell membrane results in presentation of MHC I with bound antigen to the exterior of the cell. Figure 3–5 depicts antigen processing and presentation.

Cytotoxic T cells recognize MHC class I molecules and destroy a virally infected cell only when the infected cell has MHC I and associated viral antigen on its surface. Thus, cytotoxic T cells are referred to as being **MHC-restricted.** Association of MHC I with viral antigen ensures effective stimulation of cytotoxic T cells and controls the amount of antigen that is presented. Excessive amounts of viral antigen can result in saturation of T-cell receptors and paralysis of cell function.

Each type of class I molecule (A, B, or C), because of its polymorphic configuration, binds a unique set of peptides. A single nucleated cell can express thousands of class I molecules, which can bind many different endogenous peptides. A similar diversity of MHC molecules and binding capabilities occurs with MHC II. Thus, immune responses to a huge diversity of antigens are possible.

HLA Nomenclature

Early workers assigned idiosyncratic names and numbers to the antigens they discovered. Subsequently, HLA antigens were named according to the concept that they derived from separate genetic loci. Antigens of the series designated "A" reflected alleles at one locus; those of the B series, another. Numbers were assigned to those antigens with clearly defined serologic characteristics. Antigens about which uncertainty existed received a number prefixed by "w," standing for "workshop." Succeeding workshops have incorporated newly discovered antigens into this scheme, removing the "w" as ambiguous findings were clarified.

After the establishment of the A and B series in 1970, additional genetic loci have been discovered and new antigenic series established. The first workshop worked with many antigens already established in the vocabulary, and it seemed undesirable to assign numbers arbitrarily to each series as parallel sequences. Instead, the numbers 1, 2, and 3 went to A antigens; 4, 5, 6, 7, and 8 to B antigens; 9 and 10 to A antigens, and so on. The A and B series continue to share a single numeric sequence as new observations are incorporated; for example, numbers 41 and 42 are B-series antigens, whereas 43 is an A antigen. As new antigenic series emerged, however, later workshops assigned new letters and a sequence starting with 1, continuing the w designation until full characterization of each antigen was achieved. Current practice requires that HLA specificities be correlated with specific DNA sequences; therefore, the w designation will no longer be used. All new serologic specificities will be named for their ability to identify a protein encoded by an identified DNA sequence. For example, the new serologically defined specificity of HLA-A2, corresponding to the allele sequence HLA A*0210 is designated as HLA-A210. The "w" is retained for C-locus specificities to distinguish them from complement components. Other exceptions include the Dw and DPw specificities and Bw4 and Bw6. Table 3–1 lists letters and numbers that constitute the HLA system as of 1995.

TABLE 3–1. **Complete Listing of HLA Antigens**

HLA-A	HLA-B	HLA-B	HLA-C	HLA-D	HLA-DR	HLA-DQ	HLA-DP
A1	Bw4*	B48	Cw1	Dw1	DR1	DQ1	DPw1
A2	B5	B49 (21)	Cw2	Dw2	DR103	DQ2	DPw2
A203	Bw6*	B50 (21)	Cw3	Dw3	DR2	DQ3	DPw3
A210	B7	B51 (5)	Cw4	Dw4	DR3	DQ4	DPw4
A3	B703	B5102	Cw5	Dw5	DR4	DQ5 (1)	DPw5
A9	B8	B5103	Cw6	Dw6	DR5	DQ6 (1)	DPw6
A10	B12	B53	Cw7	Dw7	DR6	DQ7 (3)	
A11	B13	B54 (22)	Cw8	Dw8	DR7	DQ8 (3)	
Aw19	B14	B55 (22)	Cw9 (w3)	Dw9	DR8	DQ9 (3)	
A23 (9)	B15	B56 (22)	Cw10 (w3)	Dw10	DR9		
A24 (9)	B16	B57 (17)		Dw11 (w7)	DR10		
A25 (10)	B17	B58 (17)		Dw12	DR11 (5)		
A26 (10)	B18	B59		Dw13	DR12 (5)		
A28	B22	B60 (40)		Dw14	DR13 (6)		
A29 (19)	B27	B61 (40)		Dw15	DR14 (6)		
A30 (19)	B35	B62 (15)		Dw16	DR1403		
A31 (19)	B37	B63 (15)		Dw17 (w7)	DR1404		
A32 (19)	B38 (16)	B64 (14)		Dw18 (w6)	DR15 (2)		
A33 (19)	B39 (16)	B65 (14)		Dw19 (w6)	DR16 (2)		
A34 (10)	B3901	Bw67		Dw20	DR17 (3)		
A36	B3702	B70		Dw21	DR18 (3)		
A43	B40	B71 (70)		Dw22	DR51		
A66 (10)	B41	Bw72 (70)		Dw23	DR52†		
A68 (28)	B42	B73		Dw24	DR53†		
A69 (28)	B44 (12)	B75 (15)		Dw25			
A74 (19)	B45 (12)	B76 (15)		Dw26			
	B46	B77 (15)					
	B47						

Numbers in parentheses indicate the original specificity from which the listed antigen was split.
*Bw4 and Bw6 are broadly specific antigens whose expression is associated with many other specificities.
†DR52 and DR53 are broadly specific antigens whose expression is associated with many other specificities.

Significance of Test Methods

White blood (WBC) cell antigens were first discovered through agglutination reactions induced by serum antibodies. In **agglutination,** interaction between antibody and surface antigen causes cells that express the antigen to clump together. Agglutination was used to test WBCs because it was so satisfactory for studying RBC antigens; however, agglutination proved less well suited for leukocytes. Other techniques were developed that used different end points for the specific interaction between antibody and antigen, but all used serum antibody as the indicator. The term **serologically defined** was applied to leukocyte antigens identified by reactions in a serum system.

With increasing understanding of cellular immune events, new test methods were adopted that exploited cell-mediated immunity. In test systems that used tissue culture–grown lymphocytes, new patterns of membrane reactivity emerged. Antigens could be observed that provoked predictable cellular changes, but for which no identifying antibodies existed. This series of antigens, assigned the letter D, was described as **lymphocyte defined.** The HLA-D antigens have been characterized from the behavior of carefully standardized reagent lymphocytes.

GENETIC AND CELLULAR SIGNIFICANCE

The presence of a combination of three class I and three Class II alleles on a chromosome constitutes the HLA haplotype, two of which are in all somatic cells. Inasmuch as HLA genes produce detectable products when present in either homozygous or heterozygous expression, an individual's cells can express up to 12 different HLA molecules. The combination of detectable traits that an individual expresses is called the **phenotype;** the composite of genetic material in the nucleus is the **genotype.** "HLA typing" means testing with available reagents to generate information necessary for clinical investigations, research purposes, or matching of tissue in paternity or criminal cases. Complete phenotyping is seldom performed. The antigens for which reagents are most widely available and from which the most useful clinical and investigational information is derived are those of the A, B, and DR series. From the antigens detected, it is usually possible to infer which alleles are present, but phenotyping cannot illuminate how the alleles are distributed in haplotypes. That information can come only from family studies, which show groups of alleles transmitted as consistent units. Figure 3–3 depicts the arrangement of alleles into haplotypes and the way in which these traits are transmitted to progeny.

Cellular Expression of Antigens

All cells possess all HLA genes, but expression varies among cells. Class I antigens have far wider distribution than class II antigens. Almost all nucleated cells express HLA-A, HLA-B, and HLA-C antigens, with the probable exception of ova and sperm. Mature RBCs have no nucleus and do not have consistent HLA reactivity. Free molecules of HLA-active material exist in blood plasma, and unpredictable amounts of fluid-phase material may adsorb to RBCs and platelets. HLA expression on circulating RBCs and platelets is clinically significant because transfusion of these components may immunize the recipient to the donor's HLA antigens. When organs are transplanted, the HLA antigens on solid tissue and bone marrow cells cause continuing antigenic stimulation.

MHC class II antigens are expressed primarily on immunologically reactive cells. Mature B lymphocytes and monocyte/macrophages manifest MHC class II molecules at all stages of maturity; cytokines that enhance overall reactivity cause MHC II expression to increase. Resting T lymphocytes express weak or nondetectable activity, but activated T cells have fairly strong class II expression. Functional cells of most other tissues and organs have little class II antigenic activity, but, because solid tissues include variable numbers of monocyte/macrophages, most organs express appreciable class II activity.

Selection of Target Cells

HLA molecules are identification markers for cellular specificity, serving as a target to focus T-cell reactivity. To recognize antigen, T cells with helper functions require that the antigen-presenting cell express class II antigens on its surface. T cells with suppressor or cytotoxic actions recognize antigens only if presented simultaneously with class I antigens. Helper cells interact primarily with antigen-presenting macrophages and antigen-stimulated B lymphocytes, cells that strongly and consistently express class II activity. Class II expression may also occur during states of altered immune reactivity on tissue cells normally devoid of these molecules. Class I molecules, which engage cytotoxic T cells, are a consistent membrane component of cells of all types (Table 3–2).

Expression in Populations

Genes for the HLA antigens exhibit striking differences in geographic distribution and provide markers useful for determining parentage and, on a larger scale, for evaluating migrations of population groups. There are marked differences among populations in frequency of different alleles; such differences increase the power of these markers in evaluating parentage. If an allele rare in a given population proves to be present in a child and in the man alleged to be the father, the probability of paternity becomes high. If the allele that child and man share is widespread in the population, the common finding could be a chance occurrence.

TABLE 3–2. **Comparison of MHC Class I and Class II**

	Class I	Class II
Loci	HLA-A, -B, and -C	HLA-DN, -DO, -DP, -DQ, and -DR
Distribution	Most nucleated cells	B cells, macrophages, other antigen-presenting cells, activated T cells
Function	To present endogenous antigen to cytotoxic T cells	To present exogenous antigen to helper T cells
Detection	Serologically	Serologically and cultured lymphocyte reactions

HLA genes often manifest **linkage disequilibrium,** a phenomenon in which alleles at different loci occur in the same haplotype—either more often or less often than the absolute frequency of each allele would predict. The most notable example is the combination of A1 with B8. The independent occurrence of each allele in the white population would predict a frequency of association of 0.0124 (i.e., 124 persons out of 10,000). Instead, the observed frequency is nearly five times the predicted value—0.0609. Less striking but still significant associations have been observed between A3 and B7, A30 and B13, and A26 and B38.

CLINICAL SIGNIFICANCE

Transplantation

A major impetus for studying the HLA system has been tissue transplantation. Animal experiments and, later, human transplantation made obvious the fact that genetic constitutions of donor and host affect the survival of transplanted tissue. Early work with leukocytes made it clear that antigens on WBCs reflect genetic properties significant for successful transplantation. Two decades of experience with human kidney grafts demonstrated that congruence for HLA types improves graft survival. This is especially striking when donor and recipient are closely related. Among siblings or parent-child pairs, shared HLA antigens indicate that the same MHC haplotype is present. Unrelated individuals whose two A and two B antigens are the same could not be expected to share all the remaining material of the MHC. "Matching" A and B antigens of unrelated individuals leaves much genetic disparity at other loci that affect histocompatibility. As techniques for HLA testing change and post-transplantation immunosuppressive regimens improve, the significance of HLA matching for tissue transplantation seems to exert a less striking effect. However, HLA-compatible matches are still most desirable.

Transfusion

RBCs express HLA antigens weakly and inconsistently. Although repeated RBC transfusions can elicit HLA immunization, the resulting antibodies do not affect survival of RBC transfused later. Platelets consistently display HLA material and are far more immunogenic for these antigens than RBCs. Recipients of multiple and repeated platelet transfusions often develop antibodies to several or many HLA antigens, and transfused platelets expressing these antigens survive poorly. It is more difficult to type donors and patients for HLA groups than for RBC antigens, and pre-transfusion procedures to establish compatibility have been less successful for platelet transfusions than for RBCs. Methods to select optimum platelet donors and to achieve the best possible post-transfusion survival continue as subjects of intense investigation.

Association with Disease

The MHC genes inherited by an individual regulate immune responsiveness by means of their ability to influence antigen binding and recognition by lymphocytes. Each individual has a unique set of MHC molecules, and therefore individuals may respond differently to disease. It has also been observed that many diseases of immune origin correlate with the presence of certain HLA antigens. This need not mean that the HLA molecules themselves are responsible for the occurrence, magnitude, or direction of immune responses. Many other factors (many still unknown) are also involved. These disease associations are far from absolute. Persons possessing the antigen will not inexorably manifest the disease, nor does every person with the disease express the antigen. Degrees of association vary, some being striking and others merely suggestive or modestly greater than chance would predict.

B27 and Skeletal Inflammation

The firmest association of specific antigen and specific disease is B27 and the inflammatory condition of the vertebral column called **ankylosing spondylitis.** In patients of all races with this disease, 70 to 95 percent possess the B27 antigen. The prevalence of B27 in the white population is only 8 to 9 percent; for blacks and Asians, it is even lower. The relative risk, which is the degree to which possessing the trait predicts present or future disease, is extremely high in Asians, among whom the B27 antigen is very uncommon; it is somewhat lower in blacks. In whites, the relative risk for ankylosing spondylitis is considered moderate, inasmuch as the antigen is present in many healthy individuals who never acquire the disease. There is no plausible explanation for this association; the B27 antigen is associated, but less impressively, with several other immune-mediated diseases that involve the skeletal system.

Other Associations

The form of diabetes termed **insulin-dependent diabetes mellitus (IDDM),** or type I diabetes, is strongly associated with DR3 and DR4. Both genetic and environmental factors affect development of IDDM, and the association with the HLA system is far from straightforward. One interpretation is that the gene-promoting development of IDDM is either the same as or closely linked to the genes that produce DR3 and DR4. Oddly enough, the likelihood of developing IDDM is greater in heterozygotes carrying both DR3 and DR4 than in homozygotes who have two expressions of either DR3 or DR4 alleles. Several other DR antigens have apparent association with immune-related diseases, among them DR2 with a particularly aggressive form of leprosy; DR4 with rheumatoid arthritis; DR3 with the intestinal condition called celiac disease; and DR2 with an antibody-mediated disease of lung and kidney called Goodpasture's syndrome. The combination of A3 and B14 carries a high relative risk for idiopathic hemochromatosis, a disorder of iron metabolism. See Table 3–3.

TABLE 3–3. **Association of HLA Inheritance With Selected Diseases**

Disease	HLA Allele	Relative Risk*
Joint diseases		
Ankylosing spondylitis	B27	87
Reiter's syndrome	B27	37
Rheumatoid arthritis	DR4	5
Endocrine disorders		
Insulin-dependent	DR3/DR4	20
diabetes mellitus	DR3/DQw8	100
Graves' disease	B8/DR3	4
Subacute thyroiditis	B35	14
Neurologic diseases		
Multiple sclerosis	DR2	4
Dermatologic diseases		
Psoriasis vulgaris	Cw6	13
Dermatitis herpetiformis	DR3	15
Pemphigus vulgaris	DR4	14
Systemic diseases		
Idiopathic hemochromatosis	A3, B14	8,5
Myasthenia gravis	DR3, B8	3,3
Sjögren's syndrome	DR3	10
Goodpasture's syndrome	DR2	16
Systemic lupus erythematosus	DR3	6

*Relative risk refers to how frequently a disease occurs in a group of individuals carrying an allele compared with a group lacking it.

SUMMARY

1. Mammalian species possess a cluster of genes called the major histocompatibility complex (MHC). The MHC contains the information necessary for membrane glycoproteins whose functions are crucial to immune recognition and regulation. In the human, the MHC complex is called the HLA system (human leukocyte antigens). T cells recognize antigen only when presented in association with MHC molecules, and therefore differences in MHC molecules can influence the body's susceptibility to disease and development of autoimmunity.

2. MHC genes are highly polymorphic and are passed from one generation to the next in predictable haplotypes. MHC genes are located on chromosome 6 and can be grouped into three classes: class I, II, and III. Class I genes encode the information for MHC molecules present on almost all cells of the body and are necessary for activation of cytotoxic T cells. Class II molecules are found primarily on phagocytic cells and other professional cells capable of antigen presentation. Class II molecules are necessary to activate helper T cells.

3. MHC class II molecules aid in the presentation of exogenous antigen. Antigen taken in by a phagocytic cell is enclosed in a phagosome and will be partially digested. MHC II molecules produced in the rough endoplasmic reticulum (rER) are enclosed in a vesicle, which will fuse with the phagosome. Antigenic fragments bind to the groove formed by the alpha-1 and beta-1 domains of the MHC II protein subunits. Vesicles containing the MHC molecules with bound antigen move toward the cell surface. Fusion of vesicles with the cell membrane results in display of MHC with antigen. Helper T cells with appropriate receptors are now able to recognize and bind the processed antigen.

4. MHC class I molecules are necessary for presentation of endogenous antigen. Endogenous cell materials marked for antigen presentation are degraded in the cytoplasm of the cell, and resulting fragments are transported across the rER where they are bound to newly synthesized MHC I alpha chains. Alpha chains then associate with β-microglobulin. Complete MHC I molecules with bound antigen are then incorporated into vesicles that are transported to the cell membrane. Fusion of vesicles with the cell membrane results in display of MHC I and antigen at the cell surface. Cytotoxic T cells recognize MHC I and can destroy virally infected cells if the infected cell displays MHC I and associated viral antigens on the cell membrane.

5. MHC/HLA antigens can be detected and identified by serologic and cell-mediated immune techniques. Expression of HLA antigen has clinical significance because every person has a unique combination of HLA antigens. If a recipient of donor cells is exposed to HLA antigens different from their own, the recipient's immune system will be activated. Transfusion of platelets may immunize the recipient to the donor's HLA antigens. Organs for transplantation purposes will express HLA antigens that can affect acceptance or tolerance of the graft.

6. Genes for HLA antigens exhibit striking differences in geographic distribution and can be useful markers for determining parentage. The presence of specific alleles is also associated with autoimmune disease. MHC genes inherited by an individual regulate immune responsiveness by their ability to influence antigen binding and recognition by lymphocytes. Therefore, it may be possible that induction of immune responses to self antigens (autoimmune disease) is influenced by inheritance of certain MHC genes.

REVIEW QUESTIONS

1. Processing of exogenous antigen occurs mainly in _____.
   a. T cells
   b. B cells
   c. macrophages
   d. virally infected cells
   e. endothelial cells

2. _____ is important for presentation of endogenous antigen.

3. _____ is important for production of some complement proteins.
   a. MHC I
   b. MHC II
   c. MHC III

4. MHC class II molecules are composed of _____.
   a. one gamma and one delta chain
   b. one alpha and one beta chain
   c. one kappa and one lambda chain
   d. two alpha chains
   e. one alpha and one β_2-microglobulin

5. Which of the following is *not* true concerning HLA?
   a. HLA consists of over 50 genes.
   b. HLA genes are located on chromosome 17.
   c. HLA genes are organized into three classes.
   d. HLA genes have a major role in transplantation of organs.
   e. HLA genes determine individual differences in disease susceptibility.

6. MHC class I molecules are found on _____.
   a. B cells and macrophages
   b. human erythrocytes
   c. neutrophils, T cells, and B cells
   d. embryonic cells
   e. all nucleated cells

7. Mother's HLA type is A1 A3 B7 B8 Cw2 Cw2
   Baby's HLA type is A1 A4 B7 B12 Cw2 Cw4
   Putative father's HLA type is A1 A4 B8 B9 Cw2 Cw4
   Could this man be the father?
   a. Yes
   b. No

8. _____ are MHC-restricted and recognize only MHC I.
   a. Helper T cells
   b. Cytotoxic T cells
   c. B cells
   d. Macrophages
   e. Neutrophils

9. Which MHC gene products are highly polymorphic?
   a. MHC Ia
   b. MHC Ib
   c. MHC II
   d. a and b
   e. a and c

10. The highest correlation of specific HLA antigen association with autoimmune disease occurs with _____.
    a. diabetes
    b. ankylosing spondylitis
    c. rheumatoid arthritis
    d. Goodpasture's syndrome
    e. myasthenia gravis

ESSAY QUESTIONS

1. Describe the structure of the MHC II molecule. How does its structure contribute to its function? Where does antigen bind?

2. How do antigen processing and antigen presentation with MHC I differ from those with MHC II?

SUGGESTIONS FOR FURTHER READING

Bodmer JB, Marsh SGE, Albert ED, et al: Nomenclature for factors of the HLA system. Tissue Antigens 1992;39:161–175

Charron D: Molecular basis of human leukocyte antigen Class II disease associations. Adv Immunol 1990;48:107–159

Dabey D: Quantitative aspects of HLA. In: Rose NR, DeMacario EC, Fahey JL, et al, eds: Manual of Clinical Laboratory Immunology, 4th ed. Washington, DC: American Society for Microbiology, 1992:867–876

Goldberg AL, Rock KL: Proteolysis, proteosomes and antigen presentation. Nature 1992;357:375–379

Neetjes JJ, Pleogh HL: Intracellular transport of MHC Class II molecules. Immunol Today 1992; 13:179–183

Reisher G: Human leukocyte and platelet antigens. In: Beutler E, Lichtman MA, Coiler BS, et al, eds: Williams Hematology, 5th ed. New York: McGraw Hill, 1995:1611–1617

Steinman L: Autoimmune disease. Sci Am 1993;269:107–114

REVIEW ANSWERS

1. c	5. b	9. e.
2. a	6. e	10. b
3. c	7. b	
4. b	8. b	

4 Principles of Immune Activation

An antigen is any material that elicits an immune response in an immunocompetent individual. Between exposure to antigen and detectable presence of the immune response lie many variables. This chapter primarily considers the events that influence antibody production. This arm of the immune response has been more fully characterized than the cellular and molecular events of cell-mediated reactions. The principles underlying the two arms of the immune response are similar, but cell populations and mediator substances differ.

DETERMINANTS OF IMMUNITY

Nature of Antigen

The general term for material that elicits immunity is **immunogen.** The smallest biochemical unit capable of eliciting an immune response is called an **epitope.** Some epitopes are very small, such as polypeptides, with just a few amino acids or certain simple sugars. The molecular weight of discrete epitopes may be less than 1 kD, but, under most circumstances, very small molecules do not elicit immunity without assistance. Epitopes are characteristically part of a larger molecule with substantial total mass (Fig. 4–1). A small epitope that cannot stimulate immune reactivity as a freestanding molecule may become immunogenic if joined to a larger molecule, called a **carrier.** The carrier molecule may or may not have immunogenic properties, but the complex of epitope plus carrier has the mass and configuration sufficient to initiate immune recognition.

Material that stimulates immunity only when complexed with a carrier is called a **hapten.** Once antibody has been generated, independent molecules of hapten can combine with immunoglobulin (Ig) without the need for a carrier. Hapten-carrier models are useful in experimental immunology and also occur in nature. Many small molecules in the environment elicit a primary immune response only if complexed to certain proteins in the host's body. The small foreign molecule can later provoke immune reactions by itself. Poison ivy reactions are a familiar example of this phenomenon, which is depicted schematically in Figure 12–10. Penicillin is another example of a clinically important hapten-carrier immune response. Penicillin is a very small molecule that is not immunogenic by itself. However, it is degraded in the body to form a "penicilloyl" group, which binds to carrier proteins such as albumin. The penicilloyl-albumin conjugate may now be recognized as foreign in individuals with a genetic predisposition to form antibodies to penicillin. Subsequent reexposure to penicillin can provoke a life-threatening allergic reaction.

Shape and Immunogenicity

Immune events reflect contact between three-dimensional receptors on effector cells and the ligand with an optimally complementary configuration. The three-dimensional shape of a molecule reflects its primary chemical structure and also the intramolecular attractions and repulsions that occur among individual constituents. Altering ionic composition or pH of the medium can alter these intramol-

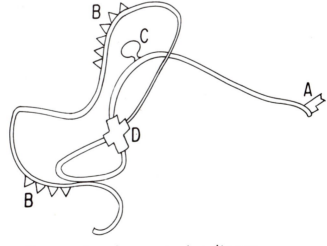

FIGURE 4–1. In a complex molecule, different portions of the three-dimensional structure may have different antigenic attributes. In the molecule shown, configurations at each of the several lettered locations may interact with individual cells with receptors of the corresponding idiotypes. An epitope frequently exists at several locations in the same molecule, as shown at right for B.

One molecule, several epitopes

ecular events and change the shape of a molecule without disrupting its primary structure. Such configurational changes may enhance the ability of the molecule to stimulate an immune response or, conversely, may abolish effective interaction with immune receptors. Molecules of consistent configuration are more immunogenic than those with shapes easily modified by changing ambient conditions. For example, gelatin, which is structurally unstable, is a poor immunogen. Proteins and complex polysaccharides are consistently effective immunogens. Most lipids have little or no independent immune activity, but, if combined with protein or polysaccharide (lipoprotein or lipopolysaccharide), the molecule can be immunogenic. Molecules that cannot be degraded or broken into fragments for presentation to lymphocytes may not be immunogenic. For example, artificial joints composed of stainless steel or plastic do not trigger immune responses.

Route of Administration

Material from the antigen-laden environment can enter the host in many ways. Most foreign elements enter the body across intact mucosal surfaces of lungs or alimentary tract or across epithelium damaged by trauma, infection, or chemical abnormalities. Antigens can be introduced into blood or interstitial fluid by intravenous, intramuscular, or subcutaneous injection.

Within limits, the larger the dose of antigen, the greater the likelihood of initiating an immune response. Because antigen must be presented by accessory cells and because most cells interact more effectively with particles than with soluble molecules, particulate or cellular antigens are more immunogenic than soluble antigens. Aggregating individual molecules into a complex or attaching them to a surface makes them more antigenic (Fig. 4–2). Contact with antigen-presenting cells occurs in lymph nodes or in tissues with large populations of resident macrophages or accessory immune cells. Immunization tends to occur more rapidly when antigens enter tissues directly than when they enter the bloodstream.

Immunization can often be enhanced by introducing, along with the antigen, substances that heighten immune responsiveness, called **adjuvants.** Adjuvants act primarily by prolonging exposure to an antigen and by promoting an inflammatory response, attracting macrophages and lymphocytes to the area, and accelerating the interaction between effector and accessory cells. Examples of adjuvants are insoluble aluminum salts, such as aluminum hydroxide, aluminum phosphate, and aluminum potassium sulfate (alum). **Freund's complete** and **incomplete adjuvant** is another example. Freund's adjuvant is composed of an antigen emulsified in oil and water droplets to which killed *Mycobacterium tuberculosis* can be added (complete), forming a particularly potent vaccine. M. *tuberculosis* contains a compound called muramyl dipeptide (N-acetyl-muramyl-L-alanyl-D-isoglutamine), which promotes macrophage production of interleuken-1 (IL-1). IL-1 is an intercellular messenger molecule (cytokine) that stimulates cells of the immune system and thereby enhances immunity.

Recognition as Foreign

The whole point of immunity is protection against the outside world. However, many physical and chemical configurations in the mammalian body are also present

ENHANCING ANTIGENICITY

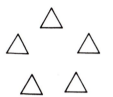

Unmodified antigen

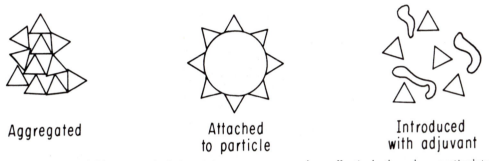

Aggregated   Attached   Introduced
                          to particle   with adjuvant

FIGURE 4–2. Soluble material elicits an immune response less effectively than does particulate material. Immunogenicity of an antigen can be increased by aggregating it into a macromolecular complex, by attaching it to the surface of an inert carrier, or by introducing it with an adjuvant substance that alters local tissue conditions.

in the outside world in many different combinations and permutations. An example is the identical combinations of simple sugars in certain bacterial cell walls and in the A and B antigens of human red blood cells (RBCs). The presence of identical or similar epitopes such as these on unrelated cells is called **cross-reactivity** and may result in the formation of a **heterophile antibody.** Thus, a person of blood type A makes antibodies to blood type B because of exposure to intestinal bacteria with B epitopes. No exposure to type B RBCs is necessary.

Some configurations of plants, animals, or microorganisms are similar or identical with host configurations, but others are very different. In general, the more completely an agent differs from materials in the host, the more likely it is to elicit an immune reaction. To provoke an immune response, materials that differ only modestly from host elements may require a larger dose, more frequent exposure, or a more effective route of administration than the immunizing conditions for massively dissimilar material.

Origin of Antigens

It is useful to classify the relationships between antigenic material and host constituents. Immune responses may develop against antigens arising within the host's own body. This is an abnormal process called **autoimmunity** or an **autologous re-**

TABLE 4–1. **Types of Immunogens**

Source	Descriptive Term for Antigen	Descriptive Term for Immune Response	Example
Material from host	Autoantigen	Autoimmune Autologous	Antibodies to hormones Cellular attack on liver cells
Material from some other human	Alloantigen	Alloimmune Homologous Allogeneic	Antibodies to transfused blood cells Cellular attack on transplanted organ
Material from plants microorganisms, chemicals, other animals	Heteroantigen	Heterologous Xenogeneic	Antibodies to bovine or porcine insulin Cellular response to poison ivy

sponse, and the responsible antigen is described as an **autoantigen.** Immunity against material from other members of the host's species is called **alloimmunity** or a **homologous response;** the immunity is directed against features that derive from allelic differences, and the antigens are considered **alloantigens.** Antigenic material coming from outside the host species can be considered completely foreign; descriptive terms are **heterologous** or **xenogeneic** response, from Greek words meaning "different" and "foreign," respectively. These terms are summarized in Table 4–1.

Mammalian hosts ordinarily mount less intense immune responses against allogeneic material than against the comparable substance from other species. Most antibodies used as laboratory reagents are produced by injecting antigen from one species into another species. This can occur spontaneously as well as under laboratory conditions. An example is development of anti-insulin antibodies in humans repeatedly exposed to insulin from pigs or cows, whereas insulin derived from humans is far less immunogenic.

THE NATURE OF RECOGNITION

A unique characteristic of an immune response is its specificity toward an antigen. MHC molecules, because of their polymorphism, can bind many different antigenic molecules. The specificity of the immune response is a result of recognition of antigen by receptors on lymphocytes. A highly specific ligand-receptor interaction must occur to obtain a specific immune response. Other cell types have receptors that stimulate cell responses; however, their receptors do not bind to antigen. Only lymphocytes have the ability to respond to foreign antigen.

The Cell-Surface Receptor

Both T lymphocytes and B lymphocytes express receptor molecules of unique configuration specific for antigen recognition. The receptors on T and B cells have different structures, but their functions are similar. The differences in configuration of receptors restrict optimal binding of any one receptor to one specific molecular ligand. Differences in amino acid sequence at defined portions of the receptor polypeptide chains produce these differences in configuration. The unique amino acid sequence of the receptor is called the **idiotype** of the molecule and is the structure that confers specificity for recognizing a unique antigen.

Differences Between T and B Receptors

B lymphocytes, which are cells destined for antibody secretion, have molecules of antibody on the exterior of their membranes, where they recognize and react with antigen. Antibodies are proteins with a common structure described as **immunoglobulin (Ig).** This structure has four chains arranged as two pairs of identical chains in a longitudinally symmetric pattern. The larger chains are called **heavy chains;** the smaller ones, **light chains** (Fig. 4–3). The decisive event whereby B-cell precursors differentiate from the pluripotent lymphoid stem cell is rearrangement of chromosomal deoxyribonucleic acid (DNA) in a way that commits each cell to man-

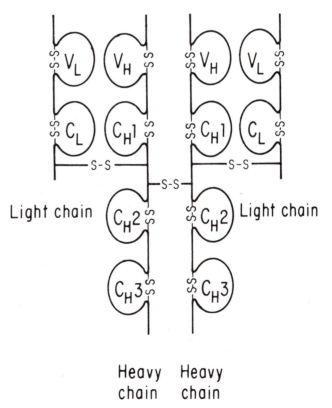

Immunoglobulin Monomer

Light chain

Light chain

Heavy chain

Heavy chain

FIGURE 4–3. All immunoglobulins consist of two identical heavy chains and two identical light chains. Each heavy chain is linked through a disulfide bond to one light chain; the two heavy chains are linked by one or several disulfide bonds through the hinge region, which gives the molecule longitudinal symmetry.

ufacturing Ig of a single idiotype. As the cell matures, it synthesizes the two kinds of polypeptide chains, links them into the four-chain Ig molecule, and then positions the Ig molecules on the exterior of the cell membrane. **Membrane immunoglobulin (mIg)** serves as receptors for antigenic activation; it is a sample of the product that will later be secreted.

The T-cell receptor consists of two idiotypically unique polypeptide chains synthesized after rearrangement of chromosomal DNA. Interaction between receptor and antigen is more complicated for T cells than for B cells because T cells must also recognize the major histocompatibility complex (MHC) class I or II molecules that are presenting antigen. The T cells from an individual recognize only the MHC products of that individual's HLA phenotype, so that T cells respond to antigen only when the antigen-presenting cell is of the host's HLA type. Antigen recognition by T cells is said to be **MHC-restricted.** Antigens presented without MHC products or in combination with the wrong MHC products will not initiate immune activity. (See Chapter 3 for more detailed discussion of MHC products and HLA phenotype.)

Exposure to Self Determinants

Every individual has unique MHC or HLA molecules that are antigenic to nearly everyone else. Why are these HLA molecules not immunogenic to the host, or why are they not autoantigens? T cells and B cells acquire their idiotypes early in fetal life and are exposed to prolonged, intense contact with all antigenic configurations present in the individual. Immunocompetent cells with idiotypes specific for autologous antigens are formed. However, during differentiation and maturation those cells that are capable of responding to autoantigens are eliminated or suppressed to prevent self-destruction or autoimmune disease. Failure to display a response for which innate capability exists is called **tolerance.** Early exposure to self constituents produces tolerance to self.

The mechanisms of self tolerance are not fully understood. One possibility is that early exposure to its target material causes cell death or inactivation of the cell expressing that idiotype. This theory does not explain how pathologic autoimmune reactivity can later develop, nor does it explain persistence of tolerance in cells produced late in life by the mature individual. Another theory is that contact with self determinants stimulates suppressor cells with idiotypes that recognize autoantigens. In this view of tolerance, self-specific suppressor cells respond to continuing antigenic contact by exerting continuous suppressive action against self-specific effector cells that could produce antibodies or autoaggressive cellular activities. These two concepts are not mutually exclusive. Deletion or inactivation of self-responding cells could occur before, or in addition to, ongoing immunosuppression. The consequence of self tolerance is that the normally functioning immune system does not exhibit actions against autologous cells or cell products. Everything else is a potential target for immune activity.

PRIMARY EXPOSURE TO ANTIGEN

Antigens enter the body after eating, drinking, breathing, or touching. Digestive enzymes and enzymes from inflammatory cells degrade complex entities into smaller fragments suitable for metabolic conversions, but further changes are necessary before immune reactions occur. The potential antigen becomes immunogenic only after **processing** and **presentation.**

The Antigen-Presenting Cell

Antigen-presenting cells possess the enzymes necessary for proteolytic cleavage of antigen. Although macrophages are not the only cells with suitable enzymes, their propensity to encounter and engulf foreign material makes cells of this lineage the most numerous of the antigen-presenting cells. **Dendritic** and **Langerhans' cells** in skin and lymph nodes also present antigens encountered in these tissues. Some macromolecules are immunogenic without processing; presumably their epitopes are sufficiently accessible and concentrated that molecular reorganization or fragmentation is unnecessary.

Interactions With Receptors

Whether processed or effective in an unprocessed state, antigen must bind with a matching receptor before an immune response occurs. B lymphocytes have specific antibodies on their membrane surfaces that serve as receptors for antigen. T cells have slightly more complicated receptors with two functions. The idiotypic portion of the T-cell receptor (TCR) recognizes and binds to epitopes of the antigen. The other portion of the TCR must recognize the antigen-associated MHC molecules. Helper T cells respond to antigen presented by MHC class II molecules. Cytotoxic T cells respond to antigen presented by MHC class I molecules (Fig. 4–4). Macrophages, along with dendritic and Langerhans' cells, are the major antigen-presenting cells and consistently express MHC class II molecules. B cells also express class II products and can assist in presenting antigen to some populations of helper cells.

Individual T and B lymphocytes have many copies of one antigen-specific receptor molecule on their exteriors. Effective antigen exposure requires numerous copies of epitope to engage simultaneously with numerous copies of receptor. When a binding substance reacts simultaneously with contiguous molecules, the receptor is said to be **crosslinked.** Crosslinking of receptor molecules stimulates cell responses (Fig. 4–5).

Events in Activation

Cells that have not yet encountered their antigen are called **naive** or **resting lymphocytes.** Both T cells and B cells recirculate continuously. Constant circulation brings idiotypically specific cells into contact with antigen-presenting cells at many different sites. Idiotypic specificity develops as a random, independent genetic event in the normal development of mature T cells and B cells. Both T cells and B cells develop idiotypes of the same specificities. Activation of most B cells requires simultaneous activation of helper T cells specific for the same epitope. T-cell responses do not require activation of B cells.

Binding of antigen to the TCR or Ig on B cells activates migration and interaction with other membrane-bound molecules, which stabilize the ligand-receptor bond. These molecules help stabilize the ligand receptor between antigen-present-

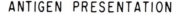

ANTIGEN PRESENTATION

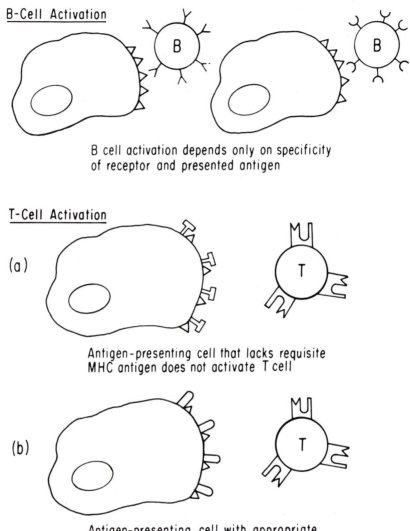

B-Cell Activation

B cell activation depends only on specificity
of receptor and presented antigen

T-Cell Activation

(a)

Antigen-presenting cell that lacks requisite
MHC antigen does not activate T cell

(b)

Antigen-presenting cell with appropriate
MHC antigen does activate T cell

FIGURE 4–4. Activation of a B lymphocyte requires only that the antigen-presenting cell express antigen of the correct epitopic configuration, as shown in the top panel. The cell on the left will recognize and respond to the antigen, but the one on the right will not. Activation of T cells requires that the antigen be presented in the context of the appropriate MHC product. In *panel a*, activation will not occur despite complementary epitope and receptor, because the presenting cell expresses the wrong MHC antigen. In *panel b*, the same antigen is presented by a cell with the MHC antigen corresponding to the receptor on the T cell.

ing cell and effector cell and ensure that the antigen-binding signal is relayed to the interior of the responding lymphocyte. The process of relaying the antigen-binding signal to the interior of the cell and activating the nucleus is called **signal transduction.** A host of membrane-bound molecules, cytokines, and a series of cytoplasmic molecules are needed for effective signal transduction to occur.

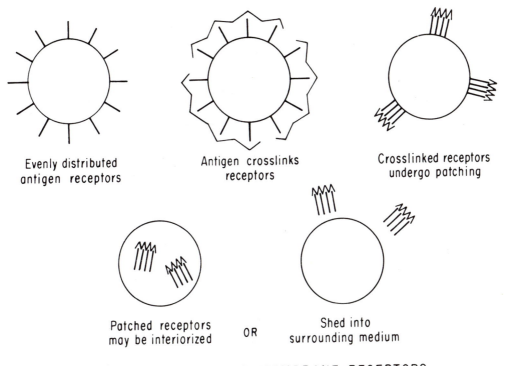

Evenly distributed antigen receptors

Antigen crosslinks receptors

Crosslinked receptors undergo patching

Patched receptors may be interiorized   OR   Shed into surrounding medium

ANTIGEN CROSSLINKS MEMBRANE RECEPTORS

FIGURE 4–5. On a resting cell, receptors are distributed throughout the membrane. Crosslinking brings them together into aggregates, a process called *patching*. The patched antigen-receptor complexes are often incorporated into the cell cytoplasm, but may sometimes be shed into the surrounding medium as nonreactive macromolecular complexes.

The most conspicuous evidence of lymphocyte activation is a change in appearance called **lymphoblast transformation.** Lymphoblasts are larger than resting lymphocytes primarily because of enlargement of the nucleus, where new DNA is synthesized preparatory to division into daughter cells. Lymphoblasts are recognized morphologically by their size and nuclear appearance and functionally by the metabolic activity that incorporates the nucleotides necessary to construct new DNA. Contact with antigen is the physiologic stimulus to lymphoblast transformation, but other events can induce the same functional change.

Other Receptors

In addition to antigen-specific receptors, both T cells and B cells have membrane receptors for molecules that induce **mitosis,** the process of cell division. Nonantigens that combine with receptors to induce mitosis are called **mitogens.** Mitogens induce lymphoblast transformation and cellular division but do not promote a functional immune response. The lymphocytes are nonspecifically stimulated. T cells and B cells also can be activated by antibody directed against the antigen-specific receptor molecules. Antibodies that recognize the unique aspects of receptor molecules are called **anti-idiotype antibodies.** Other antibodies may react with structural elements common to receptor molecules of various specificities. Crosslinking by anti-idiotype or antistructural antibodies is a useful laboratory tool to induce transformation and other cellular responses (Fig. 4–6). It is thought that anti-idiotype antibodies develop under physiologic conditions and play an important role in regulating immune activity.

After stimulation, the activated cell may express a set of receptor molecules on the membrane different from those molecules present in the resting state. These receptors do not affect idiotype specificity; their function is to recognize various mediator molecules. Expression of new receptors enables the cell to respond to changing environmental conditions (Fig. 4–7). The presence of antigen provokes changes in the environment through effects on antigen-presenting cells and inflammatory cells as well as on immune cells. As environmental conditions change, the nature and number of mediator substances change, and the responsive capacities of the stimulated cell change.

Differentiation of Daughter Cells

Lymphoblast transformation is the first in a series of steps leading to **clonal selection and expansion.** Mature B cells and T cells with their respective antigen receptors are committed to recognize only a specific epitope. Binding of antigen to a specific receptor on B cells and T cells triggers mitotic division of the responsive lymphocyte. Successive mitotic divisions produce a population of genetically identical activated cells specific for the same initiating antigen—a **clone.** A variety of growth and differentiation factors modulate these steps. The presence of antigen induces macrophages and other lymphocytes to release these mediators. Macrophages produce the broadly reactive mediator, IL-1 (see p. 128). T cells of the CD4 phenotype elaborate products that enhance growth, multiplication, and differentiation of B cells and other T cells (see p. 129). IL-1 production occurs without regard to antigenic specificity.

The antigen-stimulated B cell matures further into antibody-producing plasma cells under the influence of growth-promoting factors (lymphokines) generated by

WAYS TO CROSSLINK RECEPTORS

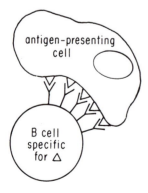

Receptors are crosslinked by presented antigen

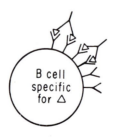

Receptors are crosslinked by antibody to receptor idiotype

FIGURE 4–6. Crosslinking of the idiotypically specific receptors on a cell membrane can occur through combination with suitably presented antigen or through interaction with antibody reactive against the receptor molecules. The antibody may be directed against the idiotypic part of the molecule (anti-idiotype antibody) or against structural features of the receptor.

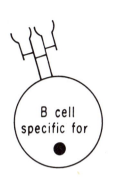

ANTIGEN-STIMULATED B CELLS
EXPRESS RECEPTORS FOR VARIOUS MEDIATORS

FIGURE 4–7. Activation causes the clonal progeny to synthesize molecules not produced by the resting cell. Membrane receptors appear, which enable the activated cells to interact with mediators that would have no effect on unstimulated cells.

helper T cells that have recognized the same antigen that activates the B cell. Except for the antigens described as **T-independent** (see later section in this chapter), antibody production occurs only when activated B cells receive help from comparably stimulated T cells. Lymphokines from the T cell bind to receptors newly expressed on the activated B cell. These provoke further changes that induce cell division, followed by differentiation into cells capable of synthesizing and secreting huge numbers of antibody molecules. Because antigen "selects" the particular responsive lymphocytes, this process of antigen driven proliferation and differentiation is called **clonal selection.**

Types of Response

All members of a clone are genetically identical, but they may encounter different concentrations of mediators that influence separate aspects of multiplication and differentiation. This is shown schematically in Figure 4–8. Cells that become plasma cells lose the capacity to multiply. They survive for only a few days, generating many thousands of specific antibody molecules and secreting them into the body fluids. Multiplying cells that do not evolve into plasma cells may cease dividing and resume the appearance of the unstimulated cell, but they do not return to the naive state. They retain the activated state induced by antigen contact and are called **memory cells.** Memory cells survive and circulate for months or years in a state of suspended animation. Second exposure to only small amounts of the same antigen stimulates them to resume activity.

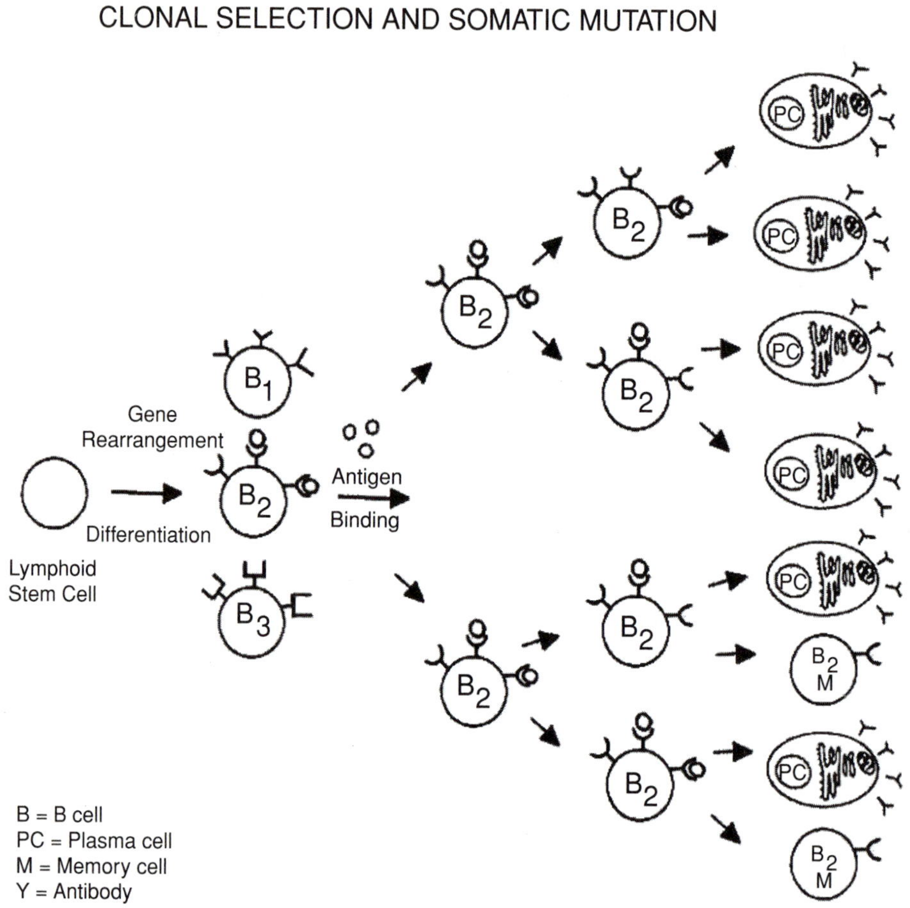

CLONAL SELECTION AND SOMATIC MUTATION

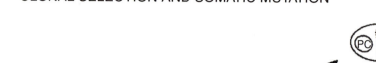

B = B cell
PC = Plasma cell
M = Memory cell
Y = Antibody

FIGURE 4–8. After antigen selection, mitotic division occurs to form a clone of lymphocytes capable of responding to the inciting antigen. Each of the clonal progeny also develops other receptors to different types of growth factors and mediators, resulting in differentiation to plasma cells and production of different classes of immunoglobulin. Small changes in DNA sequences governing the precise fit of receptor to antigen also occur. Lymphocytes with improved receptors are stimulated by antigen to form new clones, which produce better antibody. This process is called *somatic mutation*.

Helper T cells secrete mediator products (lymphokines) that influence not only B cells but also the T lymphocytes active in several cell-mediated immune events, notably cytotoxicity and delayed hypersensitivity (see pp. 134–136). T-cell activities are thus essential for production of most antibodies and for most manifestations of cell-mediated immunity. Some of the growth- and differentiation-promoting mediators that antigenically specific T cells produce will act only on effector cells specific for the same antigen. Others are not antigen-restricted and react with any cell possessing receptors for that mediator molecule (Fig. 4–9). By inducing formation of these nonrestricted mediators, stimulation by one antigen or organism can affect the reactivity of cells specific for other antigens. In addi-

T-CELL SECRETION OF LYMPHOKINES

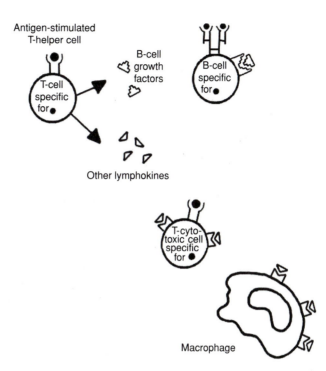

FIGURE 4–9. Antigen-stimulated T cells secrete many different lymphokines. Some of these are capable of interacting only with cells that recognize the same antigen; others are broadly effective for any cell that has a receptor for the lymphokine molecule.

tion, many T-cell products enhance the functions of macrophages, which never express antigenic selectivity.

T-Independent Antigens

Certain antigens elicit antibody formation without conspicuous participation of T cells. Antigens characterized by a well-defined epitope in multiple, closely repeated copies can stimulate target B cells through crosslinking alone, inducing transformation, multiplication, and plasma-cell differentiation without the usually identified T-cell mediators. Such antigens are called **T-independent.** Polysaccharide antigens of bacterial cell walls are the most notable examples and are thought to affect B lymphocytes through specialized antigen-presenting cells that are particularly numerous in the spleen. T-independent antigens never provoke cell-mediated immunity, and they elicit antibodies only of restricted Ig characteristics. T-cell factors appear to be necessary for production of other antibody classes and for evolution of memory cells.

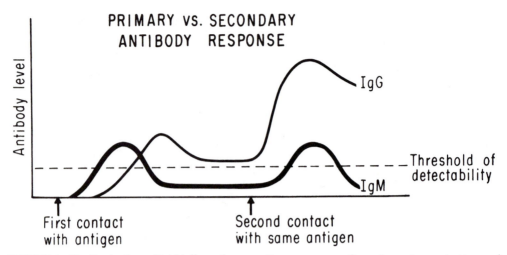

FIGURE 4–10. Production of IgM follows the same time sequence after primary immunization and after all subsequent contacts with the antigen. Establishment of IgG-producing cells engenders memory. In the primary response, substantial time elapses between antigenic contact and appearance of IgG, but subsequent contact with the same antigen elicits rapid increase in antibodies of this class.

Time Sequence

Between the first encounter with antigen and the appearance of detectable antibody or cell-mediated activity, days or weeks may elapse. The nature and dose of the antigen, the route of administration, and the host's overall metabolic state influence the rate of immunization, but a minimum of several days is necessary.

The earliest antibody class to appear is immunoglobulin M (IgM, see Chapter 6), followed in days or weeks by IgG antibody, which has the same idiotype but different structural features. IgM production tapers off promptly if the antigen disappears, but IgG production persists somewhat longer. The antibody sequence in primary immunization is early appearance of IgM, later appearance of IgG, subsequent disappearance of IgM, and fairly prolonged manufacture of IgG (Fig. 4–10). All protein molecules are subject to enzymatic degradation. Individual antibody molecules survive only for several weeks. Unless plasma cells continue to produce new molecules, antibody of a particular specificity disappear from body fluids after all the molecules with that idiotype have been degraded.

SUBSEQUENT EXPOSURE TO ANTIGEN

Immune events that follow the host's first exposure to an antigen are the **primary immune response,** which usually generates memory cells in addition to the measurable immune products. Later contact between memory cells and additional examples of antigen produces a **secondary** or **anamnestic** immune response. "Anamnestic" reflects the same linguistic origin as "amnesia"; it means that there has not been forgetting.

Timing in Secondary Responses

The anamnestic response occurs more rapidly than the primary response. Whereas days, weeks, or even months may pass before measurable antibody develops in a primary response, second and subsequent exposures boost antibody levels in a matter of hours. Several factors contribute to this acceleration. Because memory cells have already undergone some of the intracellular events necessary for immune activity, fewer differentiating events are needed after repeated antigen contact. In addition, previous clonal expansion has generated a larger number of cells capable of recognizing the antigen; following activation of memory cells, geometric expansion of each available cell rapidly generates effective numbers of plasma cells. Figure 4–10 contrasts antibody levels in the primary and anamnestic immune responses.

Obvious benefits accrue from the rapidity of anamnestic reactions. Once the host has immune memory for a pathogenic organism, later exposures can provoke anamnestic protection that attacks the organism before it can cause full-blown disease. Often, the initial encounter with an organism causes clinical disease, from which the host recovers after mobilizing inflammatory defense and an effective primary immune response. With elimination of the organism, immune activity becomes quiescent, but if the organism is prevalent in the environment, the host will encounter it again and again. These later exposures do not cause disease; they promote anamnestic responses that prevent the organism from establishing itself. Promotion of an anamnestic response is the reason a vaccination is often followed by a booster shot.

Nature of the Response

Antibody molecules can belong to any of five classes of Ig (to be discussed in detail in Chapter 6), and the distinction between IgG and IgM is mentioned briefly here. IgM is the first antibody class that a newly stimulated B cell produces. In most T-dependent reactions, lymphokines induce some daughter cells to switch to IgG production, and some of these become memory cells. IgM-producing memory cells do not develop. Secondary contact with antigen can stimulate memory cells to prompt IgG production, but there is no memory mechanism for IgM. In second and subsequent exposures, the time between antigen contact and the detectable presence of IgM is as long as it was for the primary event. Whereas IgM precedes IgG by days or weeks in the primary immune response, anamnestic responses can be identified through the appearance, in 12 to 24 hours, of rising IgG levels. T-independent antigens cannot evoke anamnestic responses because they elicit the production only of IgM.

Accelerated immune events also occur for some cell-mediated reactions (see discussion of the tuberculin reaction, p. 136). Effector cells responsible for the "delayed-type hypersensitivity" of cell-mediated immunity exhibit accelerated activity after previous antigenic exposure. A clonally expanded population of specific responsive helper T lymphocytes will activate cytotoxic T cells as well as nonspecific effector cells, such as macrophages and neutrophils.

SUMMARY

1. Materials that elicit an immune response are called immunogens, and the smallest biochemical unit still capable of such a response is referred to as an epitope. An epitope may be so small that it must be attached to a carrier molecule to be immunogenic and is then called a hapten. Factors such as ionic composition or pH of the surrounding media may affect the three-dimensional configuration and the ability of an immunogen to stimulate an immune response. Other factors affecting immunogenicity are route of administration, dose of antigen, aggregation or attachment of an antigen to a surface, and presence of adjuvants.

2. Similar epitopes may occur on unrelated cells resulting in cross-reactivity of heterophile antibodies. Antigenic material from outside the host species (heterologous) is generally more immunogenic than autologous or homologous.

3. Individual T cells and B cells possess unique receptors capable of binding antigens. Antigen receptors on B cells are antibodies. Antibodies are proteins with a common four-chain structure referred to as immunoglobulin (Ig). As B-cell precursors undergo differentiation and maturation, rearrangement of DNA occurs, which commits each cell to manufacturing Ig of a single idiotype. That Ig is then inserted into the cell membrane of a mature competent B cell. T cells have receptors capable of recognizing antigen in association with MHC. Helper T cells recognize antigen and MHC II. Cytotoxic T cells recognize antigen and MHC I.

4. Antigen "selects" those lymphocytes with receptors capable of binding to the antigen and induces clonal expansion. Clonal expansion results in T cells capable of secreting lymphokines, which activate other cells. Upon binding antigen, B cells become plasma cells capable of secreting large amounts of Ig. T cells and B-memory cells are formed capable of enhanced reactivity on reexposure to the same antigen in the future.

5. Most antigens require T-cell interaction before cell-mediated or humoral responses occur. A smaller number of antigens are called T-independent antigens; these antigens are capable of crosslinking membrane Ig on B cells and thereby stimulate humoral immunity directly. T-independent antigens stimulate production of only IgM type immunoglobulin and do not promote memory cell formation. T-dependent antigens promote humoral and cell-mediated responses. In a primary immune response, IgM is produced first followed by IgG production. Subsequent exposure to the same antigen stimulates a secondary or anamnestic response characterized by activation of memory cells and accelerated and heightened IgG production.

REVIEW QUESTIONS

1. Which one of the following is *not* a factor influencing antigenicity of a molecule?
   a. Conformation
   b. Ionic composition
   c. Stability
   d. Color
   e. pH of surrounding media

2. With penicillin allergy, the penicillin acts as a(n) _____.
   a. antibody
   b. antigen
   c. carrier
   d. hapten
   e. adjuvant

3. A hapten is a(n) _____.
   a. carbohydrate side chain
   b. amino acid side chain
   c. small molecule attached to a protein
   d. large molecule attached to a protein
   e. antibiotic

4. _____ require MHC II for antigen recognition.
   a. B cells
   b. Helper T cells
   c. Cytotoxic T cells
   d. Macrophages
   e. Dendritic cells

5. T-independent antigens _____.
   a. require antigen processing
   b. bind directly to B cells
   c. stimulate B-memory cells
   d. stimulate T-memory cells

6. Substances that heighten immune responsiveness to an antigen are called
   _____.
   a. enhancers
   b. adjuvants
   c. aggregators
   d. heterophile antigens
   e. haptens

7. Which of the following is an example of a heterologous or xenogeneic antigen?
   a. Baboon heart transplanted into a human infant
   b. Porcine insulin used by a human
   c. Human red blood cells transfused to a human
   d. a and b
   e. a, b, and c

8. Infectious mononucleosis (IM) is caused by the Epstein-Barr virus. The principle of the monospot test for diagnosis of IM is detection of antibodies able to bind and agglutinate particles coated with bovine red blood cell antigens. The antibodies detected with this test are _____.
   a. cross-reactive antibodies
   b. heterophile antibodies
   c. heterologous antibodies
   d. a and b
   e. a, b, and c

9. Binding of antigen to a specific T cell leads to activation and mitosis of this cell. This process is called _____.
   a. the mitotic response
   b. antigen activation
   c. clonal selection and expansion
   d. clonal reproduction
   e. clonal initiation

10. B-cell antigen receptors are _____.
    a. genetically determined
    b. composed of immunoglobulin
    c. composed of alpha and beta chains
    d. composed of gamma and delta chains
    e. a and b

ESSAY QUESTIONS

1. Explain why these materials differ in their immunogenicity: Knox gelatin, tetanus toxoid, contact lenses.

2. If you were in charge of developing a vaccine to a new bacterial toxin that is a very small molecule, what would you do to make this toxin more immunogenic?

3. What is the difference between a primary and a secondary antibody response?

SUGGESTIONS FOR FURTHER READING

Ada GL, Nossal G: The clonal-selection theory. Sci Am 1987;257(2):62–69
Arnon R, Van Regenmortel MHV: Structural basis of antigenic specificity and design of new vaccines. FASEB J 1992;6:3265–3274
Barber LD, Parham P: Peptide binding to major histocompatibility complex molecules. Annu Rev Cell Biol 1993;9:163–206
Cohen IR: The self, the world and autoimmunity. Sci Am 1988;258(4):52–60
Tizard I: Immunology: An Introduction. Philadelphia: Saunders College Publishing, 1995:39–48 (Antigens and Antigenicity)

REVIEW ANSWERS

1. d   6. b
2. d   7. d
3. c   8. d
4. b   9. c
5. b   10. e

5 Lymphocyte Populations

The rich diversity of lymphocyte populations is a relatively new concept in cell biology. Neutrophils and macrophages have been studied since the introduction of the microscope, but lymphocytes remained an enigma long after inflammatory cells were clearly characterized. Until the 1950s, little more was known about these small, round cells than their association with immune events and with chronic inflammation. The past 30 to 40 years have disclosed a diversity of lymphocyte functions and populations far greater than those of inflammatory cells.

HOW TO IDENTIFY CELLS

To understand how cells function, it is essential to identify them. Increasingly discriminating methods of examination can uncover distinguishing features in seemingly similar tissues, cells, or molecules. Some of these techniques are illustrated in Figure 5–1.

Structure and Function

The morphology, or appearance, of a cell or tissue is the simplest means of identification. With light microscopic examination, the location and number of lymphocytes can be determined in blood and tissue. Lymphocytes differ sufficiently

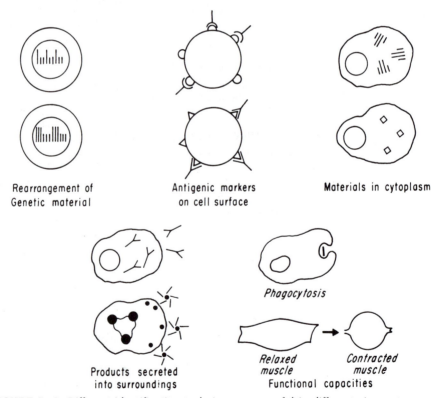

WAYS TO IDENTIFY CELLS

Rearrangement of
Genetic material

Antigenic markers
on cell surface

Materials in cytoplasm

Phagocytosis

Products secreted
into surroundings

Relaxed
muscle

Contracted
muscle

Functional capacities

FIGURE 5–1. Different identification techniques are useful in different circumstances. Genetic probes illuminate differences in DNA sequence, the most fundamental difference between cells. Consequences of genetic constitution include antigenically distinctive molecules on the cell surface, nature and location of cytoplasmic constituents, composition and volume of secreted products, and functional activities that can be observed and measured.

from plasma cells in size, shape, and staining characteristics that these populations are easily identified. Resting lymphocytes can be differentiated from lymphoblasts by their light microscopic appearance. Other microscopic techniques include transmission electron microscopy, which reveals details of intracellular structures, and scanning electron microscopy, which casts surface characteristics into sharp relief.

Important for studying function is the ability to isolate individual cells or purify cell populations and to propagate them in cell culture. Activity can be determined by examining which materials the cells remove from the culture medium and what substances they secrete. Mitotic activity in transformed immunoblasts, for example, is identified by uptake of radiolabeled deoxyribonucleic acid (DNA) precursors; production of lymphokine or antibody is documented by harvesting these proteins from the supernatant fluid. Introducing agents that selectively inhibit or enhance metabolic steps allows identification of cells with differing intracellular processes. Study of viable cells permits delineation of dynamic events like growth, changes in morphology, motility, and responses to environmental agents.

Immunologic Markers

Antibodies binding to antigens can be used to locate and study cell constituents. The critical factor for such methods is development of antibodies that react specifically and exclusively with the desired target. Information derived from immune reactions is only as good as the identification and specificity of the antibody involved. Early experimenters introduced whole serum or other complex materials into a rabbit, guinea pig, or other immunologically responsive hosts and then attempted to purify the polyspecific serum by manipulation to remove unwanted reactivities. Current immunization protocols use highly purified antigens and sophisticated techniques to separate and to concentrate the resulting antibodies.

Monoclonal antibodies have greatly expanded the scope of immunologic study. They are derived from individual immunoglobulin-producing cells stimulated to multiply indefinitely in cell culture. The cell producing the monoclonal antibody is a hybrid of two very different cells. Normal plasma cells resulting from clonal selection are fused with myeloma cells (cancerous plasma cells). The resulting hybrid cells are called **hybridomas.** The myeloma cell, as a cancerous cell type, contributes its properties of uncontrolled growth, and, because the hybridoma is also derived from a single plasma cell, the clone produces an immunoglobulin of a single idiotype. These cells are capable of multiplying indefinitely in cell culture and producing large quantities of antibody of a single specificity.

The hybridoma cells are isolated, and grown into a clone, and the monoclonal antibody produced by each clone is tested. Any harvested antibody from a single clone will be exquisitely specific. Once the specificity has been shown to recognize a desired antigen, it is relatively easy to prepare large quantities of antibody with consistent behavioral properties (Fig. 5–2). Much of our current knowledge about surface antigens has come from studies with monoclonal antibodies. These antibodies can also be used to identify and to localize materials within the cell.

MONOCLONAL ANTIBODY PRODUCTION

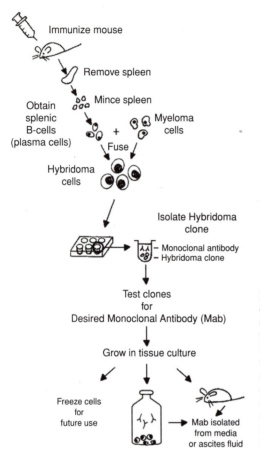

FIGURE 5-2. Monoclonal antibodies are produced by clones of hybridoma cells. Hybridoma cells are selectively grown in a culture medium that inhibits growth of nonfused cells. The hybridoma cells are diluted and placed into individual tissue culture wells. After a few weeks, the supernatant fluid can be tested for the presence of antibody. Those clones producing the desired antibody are grown further in culture. Hybridoma cells can be frozen for future use or grown in mice and antibody obtained from the ascites fluid.

Clusters of Differentiation

The use of monoclonal antibodies has allowed detailed characterization of cell surfaces. Membrane molecules expressed by immune cells of different lineages and maturational stages can be identified by specific binding with monoclonal antibodies. Initially, individual researchers used their own designations for these membrane markers, which led to much confusion, especially if the same membrane molecule had numerous names. Through international collaboration, a uniform nomenclature of membrane molecules was developed.

All the monoclonal antibodies reacting with a membrane molecule were grouped together to form a **cluster of differentiation** or **cluster determinant, (CD).** Well-characterized CDs receive numbers; as with the HLA nomenclature, the letter "w," which stands for workshop, precedes a number until the specificity is fully characterized. Rather than assigning dedicated alphanumerics to different cell lines or receptor functions, the workshops have assigned sequential numbers to characteristics as they are identified. Antigens receive a noncommittal designation like CD1 or CD10 or CDw26; correlation of antigens with different cell lines or different developmental phases cannot be inferred from the number. Many membrane markers that received CD numbers were already known by one or more other names. These names are still in use, although CD terminology is assuming increasing prominence. Table 5–1 presents some selected CD antigens and their correlation with other cellular features.

Molecular Genetic Techniques

Most molecules subjected to immunologic investigation are proteins or related complex structures, such as nucleoproteins. Proteins consist of amino acids joined through peptide bonds. It is possible to exploit the known behavioral characteristics of certain polypeptide sequences or associated chemical groups or side-chain linkages to characterize the molecules in which they appear. Chemical reactions and physical events such as precipitation, migration through electrical fields, or crystallization have been useful for generations. An increasingly useful analytic tool is selective action of enzymes, which cleave only specific peptide bonds between specific amino acids. Certain enzymes act only on peptide bonds that include some single amino acid. If that amino acid appears many times in a polypeptide, the enzyme will divide the molecule into that number of fragments. If the amino acid is present only once or twice, treating the protein with enzyme generates only a few, fairly large fragments or if the amino acid is not present, enzyme treatment will not affect the protein.

With well-characterized enzymes and suitable techniques to analyze the resulting fragments, the precise structure of individual proteins can be determined. Each constituent amino acid need not be identified; generating fragments of predictable behavior often provides adequate analytic information.

Significance of Paired Nucleotides

Enzymes with predictable activity against DNA are also available. With techniques to isolate and to manipualte DNA, it has become possible to examine the DNA sequences that constitute individual genes. The enzymes, called **restriction endonucleases** or just **restriction enzymes,** target specific sequences within nuclear DNA. The resulting fragments, **restriction fragments,** can be analyzed in several ways. The most ingenious analyses exploit the fact that nucleic acids are double-stranded molecules that reproduce themselves by pairing restricted, predictable combinations of purines and pyrimidines in rigidly prescribed complementary relationships. Reagent sequences of known nucleotide composition can be exposed to restriction fragments. Because the constituent elements pair only with complementary structures (adenine to thymine; guanine to cytosine), the structure of the restriction fragments can be inferred from the structure of the known sequences with which they combine. The known sequences are called **gene probes.**

Differences of one or a few nucleotides in a gene can produce differences in protein structure that may exert profound physiologic effects. Even if the full nucleotide sequence in a gene is not identified, the existence of variant sequences can be demonstrated by observing which gene probes match which restriction fragments. Sequence differences in genetic material at a single locus are called **restriction fragment length polymorphisms (RFLPs).** Gene probe examination has demonstrated substantial rearrangements in sequence when chromosomal segments that direct manufacturing processes switch from potential to activated func-

TABLE 5–1. **Selected Cluster Differentiation Antigens**

CD No.	Other Name	Distribution	Function, if known
1	T6	Thymocytes, Langerhans' cells, brain astrocytes, dermal cells	Ligand for CD58, CD59, accessory molecule, role in signal transduction
2	Sheep red blood cell receptor leukocyte function antigen-2 (LFA-2)	Thymocytes, T cells, some natural killer (NK) cells	Signal transduction
3	T3	T cells	Assist MHC II recognition; signal transduction
4	T4, Leu-3	Helper T cells	Ligand for CD72, involved in cell activation or adhesion or both
5	Tp67, Leu-1	T cells, thymocytes, some B cells	Signal transduction
6	T12	T cells, thymocytes	Possible receptor for Fc-μ
7		Thymocytes	Assists MHC I recognition
8	T8, Leu-2	Cytotoxic/suppressor T cells	Signal transduction
9	p24	Monocytes, pre–B cells eosinophils, basophils, activated T cells	
10	Common acute lymphocytic leukemia (CALLA)	1% of normal marrow cells, early T-cell and B-cell precursors	Zinc metalloprotease
11a	LFA-1	All leukocytes	Cell adhesion
11b	Mac-1, CR3	Monocytes, granulocytes NK cells, expression increases with inflammation	Receptor for C3bi, cell adhesion to endothelium; facilitates chemotaxis, phagocytosis
13	Aminopeptidase gp150	Myeloid cells	Zinc-binding metallo-protease
14	gp55, GPI-linked glycoprotein	Monocytes, macrophages, neutrophils	Receptor for lipopolysaccharide; signal transduction leads to oxidative burst or synthesis of TNF-α
16		NK cells, macrophages	Low-affinity receptor for Fc-γ
18		All leukocytes	Signal transduction
20		B cells	Calcium channel
21	EBV (Epstein-Barr virus) receptor	B cells dendritic cells, some thymocytes, some T cells	Signal transduction, possible receptor for IFN-α

CD	Common Name	Cellular Distribution	Function
25	Tac-antigen	Activated T and B cells, some thymocytes, myeloid precursors	Low-affinity receptor for IL-2
28	Tp44 antigen	95% CD4 T cells, 50% CD8 T cells, most plasma cells	Ligand for CD80, enhances transcription of IL-2
31	Platelet endothelial cell adhesion molecule (PECAM-1)	Myeloid cells, platelets, endothelial cells, NK cells, monocytes	Induces respiratory burst, leukocyte migration through intercellular junctions of endothelial cells; possible role in signal transduction, monoclonal antibodies
34	My10	Pluripotential stem cells immature hematopoietic cells	Available for isolation of stem cells and use in bone marrow transplantations
35	CR1	B cells, granulocytes, monocytes, dendritic cells	Receptor for C3b, facilitates phagocytosis of immune complexes
40	gp50	B cells, monocytes,dendriti cells, epithelial cells	Signal transduction, activation, proliferation, differentiation
45	T200 Leukocyte common antigen (LCA)	All leukocytes	Signal transduction
54	Intercellular adhesion molecule (ICAM-1)	Leukocytes, endothelial cells inducible and up-regulated on lymphocytes, dendritic cells, keratinocytes, chondrocytes, fibroblasts, epithelial cells	Member Ig super family, ligand for LFA-1, MAC-1; receptor for rhinovirus
55	Decay-accelerating factor (DAF)	All hematopoietic cells and spermatozoa	Neutralizes complement activation, absent or defective in paroxysmal nocturnal hemoglobinuria
95	APO-1; FAS	T-cell and myeloid cell lines	Crosslinking may induce cells to undergo apoptosis
102	ICAM-2	Endothelial cells, platelets	Ligand for LFA-1; may facilitate recirculation of T-memory cells
w116		Monocytes, granulocytes, endothelial cells, dendritic cells, fibroblasts	Receptor for granulocyte-macrophage colony-stimulating factor (GM-CSF)
120a		T cells, thymocytes, chondrocytes, synovial cells, endothelial cells, fibroblasts, keratinocytes, and hepatocytes	Receptor for IL-1

Information presented in this table was obtained from the 5th International Workshop and Conference on Human Leukocyte Differentiation Antigens and adapted from Kipps TI: The cluster of differentiation (CD) antigens. In: Beutler E, Lichtman MA, Collen S, Kipps TI, eds: William's Hematology. 5th ed. New York: McGraw-Hill, 1995:113–140. Data compiled from the above conference resulted in the classification of over 125 CD antigens.

tion. Cells destined to synthesize different protein products display differences in DNA sequence at the relevant loci.

An isolated gene may be copied innumerable times by a molecular technique called the **polymerase chain reaction (PCR).** Because of the complementary pairing of nucleotides, a single DNA strand may serve as a template for synthesis of a matching strand. This double strand of DNA may then be denatured so that separation into individual strands occurs and a new round of amplification or production of two new double-stranded DNA molecules ensues. PCR can be used in the diagnosis of many genetic disorders. It can be used to detect microorganisms that are present in numbers too few to be isolated or cultured or whose growth characteristics prevent timely identification. Gene amplification with PCR has provided and will continue to provide valuable information about genes and molecules essential for immune function.

After a gene has been identified, it is also possible to inject this gene into a fertilized egg of a mouse. If successful, the resulting embryo will undergo normal development and the adult mouse will express the gene product or demonstrate some type of detectable change. This mouse is referred to as a **transgenic mouse.** Likewise, it is possible to specifically inactivate a single gene and produce a "knock-out" mouse. Observation of loss or gain of a specific CD marker, HLA allele, cytokine production, or other cellular function, contributes to the understanding of essential components of the immune system.

DEVELOPMENT OF LYMPHOCYTES

The Hematopoietic Stem Cell

All cells of marrow origin are thought to derive from a single progenitor. Irreversible developmental changes in progeny of this multipotential cell direct evolution into erythrocyte, platelet, granulocyte/macrophage, or lymphocyte lines. The multipotential capacity of single cells has been demonstrated by injecting cells from a normal rat into a genetically identical rat whose bone marrow has been destroyed by radiation. After a brief period, many of the injected cells die, but a few cells lodge in the bone marrow and spleen and begin producing hematopoietic colonies. After a period of cell division, colonies of blood cells can be observed in the spleen of the recipient rat. Stem cells within these colonies restore not only the circulating blood cells but also the immune system. Stem cells capable of differentiation into all cell lines are called colony-forming units–spleen abbreviated **CFU-S** (Fig. 5–3). The differentiated daughter cells acquire properties unique for each hematopoietic cell line. Erythroid precursors grow in bursts rather than colonies and are called erythroid burst-forming units **(BFU-E).** Megakaryocyte precursors are called **CFU-M;** the partially differentiated cell with granulocyte and monocyte potential is the **CFU-GM.** No single lymphoid cell has been cultured with simultaneous T-cell and B-cell offspring, but it is clear that all lymphocytes derive from a common precursor **(CFU-L).**

Stem cells differentiate under the influence of a host of various hormones, growth factors, and locally produced cytokines. Genes for several of these factors have been isolated, and, with recombinant DNA techniques, these factors can be produced by microorganisms and used therapeutically. **Granulocyte-macrophage colony-stimulating factor (GM-CSF)** promotes growth of neutrophils and mono-

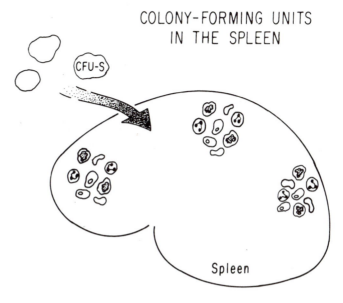

COLONY-FORMING UNITS
IN THE SPLEEN

FIGURE 5-3. The multipotential capacity of individual hematopoietic stem cells (see Fig. 1-3) is shown when single cells introduced into the spleen of an irradiated experimental animal develop into colonies that contain many different cell types. Cells capable of establishing these multicellular splenic colonies are called *colony-forming units—spleen* (CFU−S).

cytes. **Erythropoietin (EPO)** promotes the growth of erythrocytes. Hematopoietic stem cells, lymphoid stem cells, and lymphocytes can be grown in tissue culture if provided with appropriate growth factors. Human hematopoietic stem cells can be harvested from marrow or circulating blood and used for tissue transplantation to reconstitute the blood and immune systems of patients treated for malignant diseases.

Early Lymphoid Features

The idiotypically unique receptor molecules that typify lymphocytes are synthesized through the action of genes at known locations. Cells that have undergone DNA rearrangement at these sites are the earliest differentiated forms in each cell line. Rearrangement of chromsome 14 characterizes B-cell precursors; rearrangement of chromosome 7 or 14, T-cell precursors. Activation of genes results in production of distinctive CD markers, enzymes, and many cytoplasmic proteins characteristic of lymphocytes at different stages of maturation. B-cell and T-cell precursors can be identified by these various products. Some cells with lymphocyte morphology and function lack identifiable membrane receptors for specific antigens. Cells called **natural killer** or **NK cells** (see later section) and described as **large granular lymphocytes** do not have idiotypic specificity. Nonetheless, they display some of the genetic rearrangements characteristic of T cells and are thought to be descended from the common lymphoid precursor. Another feature of very early lymphoid differentiation is the presence of the nuclear enzyme **terminal deoxynucleotidyl transferase (TdT),** which facilitates genetic rearrangements associated with synthesis of surface receptors. TdT disappears as cells become more mature, but it persists longer in developing T cells than in B cells. By the time cells display distinctive B-cell features, TdT has usually disappeared. By contrast, early T cells retain TdT until the last stages of full functional capability.

DEVELOPMENT OF T LYMPHOCYTES

The Thymus

The **thymus** is a lobulated mass of lymphoid tissue in the upper anterior portion of the chest. At birth it weighs 12 to 15 g, proportionately very large in the small body of the newborn. Its largest absolute weight, 30 to 40 g, is achieved just before puberty. The thymus is most active during fetal and early childhood development, when immunologic activity is expanding. The importance of this organ in an adult is not completely known. Thymectomy can be performed on an adult with no ill effects and is sometimes used therapeutically for the treatment of an autoimmune disease such as myasthenia gravis. Developing lymphocytes assume the properties of T cells as they pass through the thymus. This process generates enough committed precursor cells adequate to maintain normal T-cell levels for life, long after the organ atrophies.

The thymus is composed of loosely packed epithelial cells covered by a connective tissue capsule. Connective tissue extends from the capsule into the interior of the thymus, dividing it into lobules. The outer portion of the thymus, the **cortex,** contains densely packed lymphocytes undergoing continuous cell division and proliferation. In the inner portion of the thymus, the **medulla,** there are fewer developing lymphocytes with epithelial cells clearly visible. Blood vessels entering the thymus have unusually thick basement membranes and an outer layer of epithelial cells that prevents circulating antigen from entering the thymus. In the thymus, developing T cells are formed that can tolerate self antigen and respond against foreign antigen. The presence of foreign antigen in the thymus may cause T cells to become tolerant of these antigens as well.

Precursor T cells leave the bone marrow and are attracted to the thymus, where they enter the cortex. Developing lymphocytes in the thymus are called **thymocytes** and are immature cells. The thymocytes become more mature as they move centripetally through the thymus, from cortex to medulla. The outer cortex contains about 10 to 20 percent of all thymocytes. Rapid proliferation and also a tremendous amount of cell death occur in the cortex. Only a small number of survivors migrate to the medulla, where they undergo further maturation and eventually leave as mature peripheral T cells.

The thymus "programs" T cells. Mature T cells must be able to tolerate all the antigens of the normal body, but still recognize and respond to foreign antigen. Thymic epithelial cells carry all the normal body antigens. Thymocytes that respond to body antigen are destroyed. Therefore, the large amount of cell death that occurs in the thymus is the result of a careful selection process. The supporting epithelial cells along with dendritic cells and macrophages are considered thymic stromal cells and are in intimate contact with the thymocytes. These cells secrete substances that promote cellular differentiation. Some of the known substances are thymosin, thymopoietin, thymulin and the cytokines, tumor necrosis factor-alpha (TNF-α) and interleukin-1α (IL-1α). Thymic stromal cells also express high levels of major histocompatibility complex I (MHC I) and MHC II molecules. Functional T cells recognize antigen only when associated with MHC. Developing T cells that form antigen-MHC recognition receptors for MHC present on the thymic stromal cells are selected and allowed to mature. Thymocytes that are inappropriately programmed and unable to recognize MHC will die. Thymic stromal cells likely induce this process of cell death called **apoptosis.** Figure 5–4 summarizes these relationships.

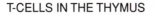

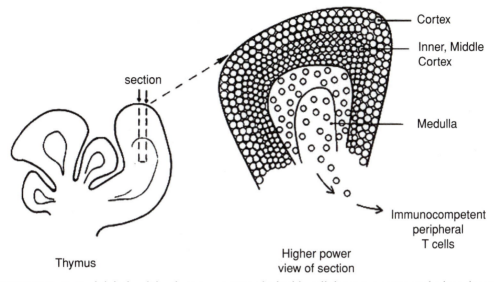

FIGURE 5–4. Each lobule of the thymus consists of a highly cellular outer cortex and a less dense inner medulla. Prothymocytes enter the thymus at the periphery and immediately begin acquiring T-cell properties. Differentiation with positive and negative selection of immunocompetent thymocytes increases as the cells move toward the center. Thymocytes in the middle and inner cortex exhibit tremendous proliferation and subsequent destruction. Only a few cells emerge as immunocompetent peripheral T lymphocytes.

Acquisition of Surface Antigens

As cells progress through the thymus, they acquire membrane antigens; some antigens persist and others disappear. The first membrane marker to develop identifies immature thymocytes in the outermost cortex and remains as a thymus-associated feature through every maturational stage, including circulating peripheral cells. This molecule, now designated CD2 was the first cytologic feature found to distinguish T cells from B cells. It was originally known as the E-rosette receptor because cells possessing this antigen formed rosettes of adherent cells when they were incubated with sheep red blood cells (RBCs). Until more sophisticated tests became available, the only way to identify T cells in a blood sample was to induce rosettes by incubating the lymphocytes with sheep cells. The CD2 molecule is now seen as an adhesion molecule and receptor for intercellular communication and signal transduction. Subsequent acquisition of other CD markers and a functional T-cell receptor is characteristic of normal T-cell maturation. Identification of membrane antigens and the gene rearrangements that must occur to produce functional T-cell receptors can be studied with monoclonal antibodies and restriction endonuclease analysis of genomic DNA. Table 5–2 provides a description of some of the T-cell antigens.

The T-Cell Receptor

T lymphocytes recognize their specific antigens through a complex membrane protein called the **T-cell receptor (TCR),** which is composed of two glycoproteins.

TABLE 5–2. **Selected CD Antigens of T Cells***

Antigen	T- Cell Population	Non–T Cells Sharing Antigen	Comments
CD1	Thymocytes with both CD4 and CD8	Langerhans' cells of epidermis, some B cells	Molecule is associated with B_2-microglobulin; disappears with evolving immunocompetence
CD2	Earliest T-specific antigen, persists through full maturation	None	Receptor for rosetting with sheep red cells; adhesion molecule, participates in signal transduction
CD3	All T cells	None	Associated with T-cell receptor (TCR), necessary for signal transduction
CD4	Thymocytes and 55–70% of peripheral T cells with helper-inducer function	Some monocytes	TCR accessory molecule; binds to MHC II; participates in signal transduction
CD5	All T cells	Some B cells	Ligand for CD72; involved in cell activation/adhesion
CD8	Thymocytes and 25–40% of peripheral T cells with cytotoxic, suppressor function	None	TCR accessory molecule; binds to MHC I; participates in signal transduction
CD11a/ CD18 (LFA-11)	All T cells	B cells, NK cells, granulocytes, monocytes/ macrophages	Adhesion molecule; binds to ICAM-1 and ICAM-2
CD25	T cells	Activated B cells responding to IL-2	Receptor for IL-2; with cell activation, receptor expression increases
CD28	Helper and cytotoxic T cells	None	Binds to B7-2 on antigen-presenting cells
CTLA4	CD4+ T cells	None	Binds to B7-2 and GL-1 on B cells
CD4 0-L	CD4+ T cells	None	Binds to CD40 on B cells; increases growth and antibody production

*All these surface molecules are glycoproteins, identifiable by polyclonal antibodies or monoclonal antibodies.

These glycoproteins are different from each other and therefore are referred to as **heterodimers.** Two major classes of TCRs exist. Most T cells carry alpha/beta (α/β) heterodimers and a much smaller minority of T cells (1 to 3%) carry gamma/delta (γ/δ) heterodimers. Each of the glycoproteins consist of four domains similar to the MHC molecule: two extracellular domains, a transmembrane, and a cytoplasmic domain. The extracellular domains have structural similarities to immunoglobulin and therefore are considered members of the immunoglobulin supergene family. The extracellular domain farthest from the cell membrane has the greatest amount of amino acid variability compared with the rest of the TCR domains. The amino acid variability occurs in distinct regions of this domain and makes up the antigen recognition site. The other domains of the TCR have a more constant amino acid composition and function to anchor the molecule in the membrane, interact with other membrane-bound molecules, and promote signal transduction from the cell surface to the interior of the cell.

γ/δ TCRs are mainly found on immature T cells and are characteristic of the first cells to colonize the embryonic thymus. Mature γ/δ-bearing T cells leave the thymus and migrate to other tissues. It has been proposed that γ/δ TCRs have direct cytotoxic function and can lyse target cells. In the mouse, γ/δ T cells are a major T-cell population in the skin and intestinal and pulmonary epithelium, where they may protect epithelial cell surfaces (Fig. 5–5).

T-Cell Receptor Accessory Molecules

In addition to the TCR that recognizes antigen carried by MHC I or II glycoproteins, a host of other molecules (both membrane-bound and cytoplasmic) are necessary to optimally activate T cells.

CD3

CD3 is a complex of four polypeptides or two dimers. The dimers are referred to as gamma/epsilon (γ/ε) and delta/epsilon (δ/ε). These dimers flank either side of the TCR. γ/ε is linked to the alpha chain of the TCR. δ/ε is linked to the beta chain of the TCR. The cytoplasmic tail portion of the TCR is too short to effectively transmit a signal when the TCR binds to antigen. Therefore, the CD3 complex can transmit the antigen-binding signal to cytoplasmic enzyme systems, which eventually lead to gene activation and response by the T cell (Fig. 5–6).

T-CELL RECEPTOR (TCR)

FIGURE 5–5. The T-cell receptor (TCR) is composed of alpha/beta (α/β) or gamma/delta (γ/δ) heterodimers. Binding to antigen and MHC occurs through the variable regions of the outermost extracellular domains. Other domains of the TCR have a more constant amino acid composition and aid in maintaining structure, anchoring the molecule in the surface membrane, interacting with other membrane molecules, and promoting signal transduction from the cell surface to the interior.

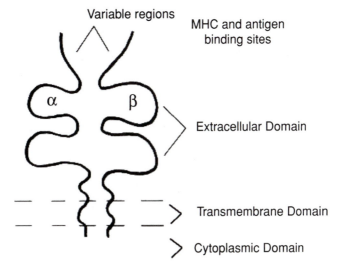

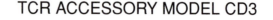

TCR ACCESSORY MODEL CD3

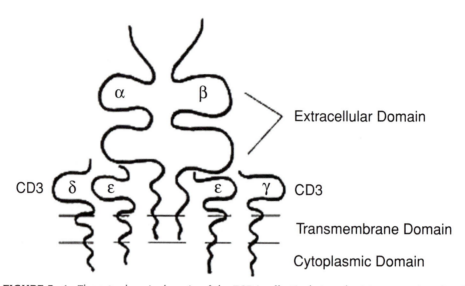

FIGURE 5–6. The cytoplasmic domain of the TCR is effectively too short to transmit a signal upon antigen binding. Therefore, CD3 aids in transmission of the antigen-binding signal to cytoplasmic enzyme systems that eventually lead to gene activation and T-cell responses.

CD4 and CD8

Mature T cells possess either of the membrane molecules, CD4 and CD8. The presence of either of these two molecules divide T cells into two major T-cell populations: CD4-positive (CD4+) or CD8+. CD4 is a single-chain glycoprotein of 55 kD. It is present on approximately 65 percent of human T cells circulating in the blood. T cells with CD4 molecules recognize antigen only in association with MHC II glycoproteins and function to enhance and promote actions of other immune cells. Antibody formation to many types of antigen is dependent on recognition by CD4+ cells. CD4+ cells are therefore also known as helper T cells.

CD8 is a disulfide-linked heterodimer composed of subunits of 34 kD each and is found on approximately 30 percent of blood T cells. Both CD4 and CD8 are members of the immunoglobulin supergene family. CD8 recognizes antigen in association with MHC I molecules. Binding of CD8 to MHC I is necessary for T cells to respond to endogenous antigen fragments. Recognition of an endogenous antigen by the TCR and CD8 can result in direct killing of a virus-infected cell or other altered cells. CD8+ cells are therefore called cytotoxic T cells or suppressor cells for their immune-suppressive effects.

CD4 and CD8 are associated with the TCR and migrate with the TCR-CD3 complex. CD4 and CD8 function as adhesion molecules. By binding to MHC I or II, the strength of the interaction between the TCR and the antigen is greatly increased, and concomitantly the sensitivity of the TCR to very low levels of antigen and MHC is increased. CD4 and CD8 function not only to increase adhesion and interaction of specific T cells with antigen-presenting cells, but also to aid in signal transduction. The cytoplasmic domains of CD4 and CD8 are associated with an enzyme called **lck**

tyrosine kinase. This enzyme is one of the first of the signal-transducing enzymes necessary for T-cell activation (Fig. 5–7).

The ratio of CD4+ cells to CD8+ cells may be used as an indicator of normal immune function. The CD4 molecule is also the receptor for attachment and cellular invasion by the retrovirus called human immunodeficiency virus (HIV), which is the virus that causes AIDS. As the symptoms of AIDS become progressively more severe, a loss of CD4+ cells occurs. Normally, the number of CD4+ cells in the blood is greater than the number of CD8+ cells (approximately 2:1). With disease progression, this ratio becomes reversed and immune activity becomes progressively deficient.

Costimulatory Signals

In addition to CD4 and CD8, other cell adhesion molecules participate in T-cell and antigen-presenting-cell interactions (Fig. 5–8). By themselves, these molecules will not activate the T cell; however, they do help to stabilize and strengthen the TCR-antigen bond. When a T cell with a TCR capable of binding to antigen and MHC come together, CD28 on the T cell binds to B7-2 on the antigen-presenting cell. **B7-2** is a membrane glycoprotein expressed on activated macrophages, activated B cells, and dendritic cells. With binding of antigen, CD28, and other costimulatory signals, the T cell becomes activated. Once activated, another receptor for B7-2 is expressed by the T cell. CTLA-4 has a greater affinity for B7-2 than CD28 and also binds a B-cell marker called **GL-1.** Expression and binding of these receptors and ligands by activated macrophages, helper T cells, and B cells ensure a successful immune response. Other signals are necessary, however, this communication pathway is known to be significant because blockage of these reactions results in tolerance to an antigen rather than immune reactivity. Binding of monoclonal

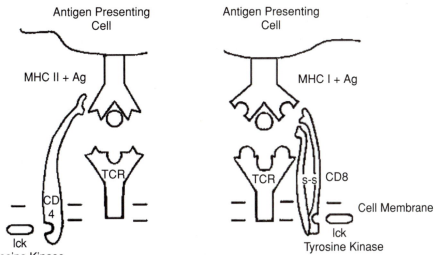

FIGURE 5–7. TCR on a CD4+ T-cell recognizes (is restricted) to MHC II. Likewise, the TCR of a CD8+ cell recognizes (is restricted to) MHC I. CD4 and CD8 aid in adhesion to the antigen-presenting cell and signal transduction in the T cell via tyrosine kinases.

COSTIMULATORY MOLECULES

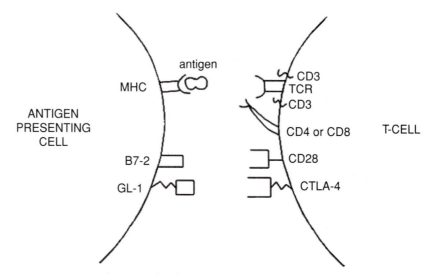

FIGURE 5–8. Costimulatory molecules (some of which are shown above) help strengthen and stabilize the TCR-antigen bond.

antibodies to CD28 or CTLA-4 heightens the T-cell response to antigen. These antibodies induce increased production of the cytokines IL-2, IL-3, and IL-4, interferon-gamma (IFN-γ), TNF, and GM-CSF and increased expression of receptors for IL-2 (IL2-R).

Identification of receptors and ligands that heighten immune reactivity can have clinical applications and significance. The gene for B7-2 can be transferred into tumor cells. Expression of this membrane molecule by the tumor cells increases recognition by immune cells and may aid in destruction of the tumor. Injection of monoclonal antibody to CD28 or CTLA-4 may also be useful for enhancing immune reactivity to tumors.

CD40-ligand (CD40-L) is closely related to CD28. Antigen binding to the TCR will induce the T cell to make CD40-L. CD40-L is a membrane glycoprotein expressed on CD4+ T cells; upon activation by antigen, CD40-L–bearing T cells bind to CD40. CD40 is also a membrane glycoprotein, but is expressed on B cells, dendritic cells, and thymic epithelial cells. Binding of CD40-L to CD40 induces B-cell growth and antibody production. It also stimulates T cells to divide in the presence of IL-2, and thus the expansion of a clone of responsive T cells and B cells occurs.

Signal Transduction

To activate T cells, antigen must bind to the TCR, costimulatory molecules must interact, and all this surface activity must be transmitted through the cytoplasm to the nucleus and to appropriate genes. This is a multistep, multilinked process called **signal transduction.** All the details and enzyme systems involved have not been elucidated. However, it is known that the alpha and beta chains of the TCR are linked to CD3 chains that have cytoplasmic tails that can activate tyrosine kinases. Tyrosine kinases are cytoplasmic enzymes that add phosphate ($-PO_4$) groups to the amino acid tyrosine present in other cytoplasmic proteins. Addition of PO_4 modifies the structure of the target protein and therefore activates the protein. Tyrosine kinases that are activated by surface molecules include lck, fyn, and a protein called ZAP-70. The lck tyrosine kinase is a unique kinase expressed only in T cells and NK cells.

These activated kinases can phosphorylate an enzyme called **phospholipase C (PLC).** Phosphorylated PLC subsequently hydrolyzes a cytoplasmic component called **phosphatidyl inositol biphosphate (PIP)** into two messenger molecules: inositol triphosphate **(IP)** and diacylglycerol **(DAG).** IP causes the release of calcium from intracellular organelles and opens calcium channels in the cell membrane. This results in an increase in cytoplasmic calcium concentration, which is necessary for cell activation. DAG activates another kinase called **protein kinase C.** Activated protein kinase C in turn causes the release of DNA-binding proteins called **transcription factors.** Transcription factors can enter the nucleus and bind to specific sites on genes that turn on mRNA transcription and protein synthesis. An example of a transcription factor is **NF-κB** and **NF-AT**. NF-κB is important for activating genes necessary for antibody production. NF-AT aids in the activation of IL-2 genes in T cells (Fig. 5–9).

T-Cell Maturation

Now that the TCR and other surface-signaling molecules have been introduced, T-cell maturation can be explained in more detail. Progenitor T cells (prothymocytes) from the bone marrow enter the thymus, where they undergo maturation and selection. During the maturational process, rearrangement of genes encoding the TCR, which enables recognition of specific antigen and production of accessory molecules, occurs. Immunocompetent helper and cytotoxic T cells that produce high-affinity receptors for antigen and self MHC are selected. Immature thymocytes express specific TCR-CD3 complexes and both CD4 and CD8.

The microenvironment of the thymus (cells and chemical messengers) is selective for only thymocytes that bind antigen and self MHC molecules. Nonproductive gene rearrangements that result in thymocytes with TCRs that do not bind antigen and self MHC or recognize self MHC molecules alone or self antigen alone are eliminated. It is estimated that more than 95 percent of thymocytes die without maturing. This is a highly selective "weeding-out" process to ensure that immunocompetent T cells exiting the thymus recognize foreign antigen in association with MHC and can appropriately stimulate humoral or cell-mediated responses and *do not* respond to self antigen. The selection of T cells with appropriate TCRs involves two processes: first, a **positive selection** for thymocytes bearing receptors capable of binding to self MHC I or MHC II molecules (MHC restriction); second, a **negative selection** process to eliminate thymocytes with high-affinity receptors for self MHC alone or self MHC presenting self antigen.

Thymic stromal cells (epithelial cells, macrophages, and dendritic cells) have an important role in T-cell maturation. Thymocytes interact closely with thymic stromal cells that have high levels of MHC I and II on their cell membranes. It has been

SIGNAL TRANSDUCTION

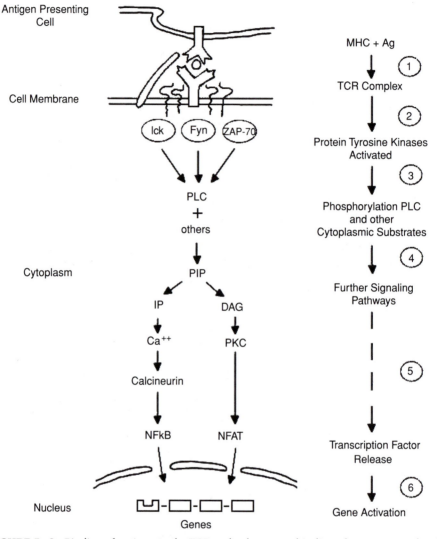

FIGURE 5–9. Binding of antigen to the TCR and subsequent binding of accessory molecules results in signal transduction. Signal transduction involves a sequence of cytoplasmic events and proposed biochemical pathways as outlined in this figure so that the antigen-binding signal from the TCR is transmitted to the nucleus for cell activation. PLC, phospholipase C; PIP, phosphatidyl inositol biphosphate; IP, inositol triphosphate; DAG, diacylglycerol; PKC, protein kinase C.

proposed that those thymocytes with correct receptors are somehow protected by binding to the stromal cells. The thymocytes not binding are induced to undergo apoptosis. Likewise, self-reactive cells are destroyed. Those selected thymocytes with appropriate TCRs become positive for either CD4 and CD8 and leave the thymus as mature cells (see Table 5–2).

DEVELOPMENT OF B LYMPHOCYTES

B lymphocytes undergo instruction and differentiation in the bone marrow and possibly also in the fetal liver. Birds possess a distinct organ, called the **bursa of Fabricius,** which provides instruction to B cells comparable to that of the thymus for T cells. Mammals have no single organ comparable to the avian bursa, but their cells obviously experience effective instruction. The "B" in B lymphocytes originally meant "bursa equivalent"; it now seems reasonable to consider B to mean "bone marrow."

Clonal Selection of B Cells

The response of B cells to antigen is clonal. Lymphoid stem cells committed to B-cell maturation differentiate randomly to produce clones of B cells. Each clone is committed to respond to a single epitope. The antigen receptor for B cells **(BCR)** is specific membrane-bound antibody. The antibody is positioned so that the antigen-binding portion of the molecule extends to the exterior of the cell and the "tail" section is embedded in the cell membrane. Early events in B-cell maturation involve rearrangement of genetic sequences responsible for immunoglobulin production and the production of antibody with specific antigen-binding capabilities. Mature B cells with their specific antigen receptors populate the cortex of lymph nodes, white pulp of the spleen, Peyer's patches, and lymphoid tissue throughout the body. Only a small number of B cells circulate in the peripheral blood.

Mature B cells interact with macrophages or other antigen-presenting cells carrying MHC II molecules and antigen and helper T cells with a TCR capable of recognizing this particular antigen. Antigen-activated macrophages and helper T cells secrete cytokines that activate B cells. B cells with appropriate antibody receptors then undergo division. The clone is enlarged and further differentiation into B-memory cells and antibody-secreting plasma cells occurs (see Fig. 4–8). The antibody that is produced is identical in specificity with the B cell's membrane-bound antibody.

B cells can also act as antigen-presenting cells because they carry MHC II and can also bind antigen via their antibody receptors. Unlike macrophages, which phagocytose and process any antigen, B cells are capable of greater specificity and through clonal selection become even more specific. The BCR is similar to the TCR with a cytoplasmic domain too short to effectively transduce an antigen-binding signal to the nucleus, and therefore accessory membrane molecules are required. The heterodimers Ig α and Ig β, which are also members of the immunoglobulin supergene family, are linked to the tail portion of the BCR. The antigen-binding signal is then relayed via protein kinases and transcription factors similar to T cells.

Further enhancing signals to promote B-cell proliferation include binding of helper T cells via CD adhesion molecules and the production of lymphokines such as IL-2 and IL-4. The BCR can bind free, intact circulating antigen, unlike the TCR, which binds only antigen presented on MHC. Intact antigen attached to the BCR may be endocytosed, processed, and presented on B-cell MHC II to T cells and memory cells. The ability of the B cell to bind and present antigen increases the repertoire of antigen that may be recognized by the immune system.

Changes with Maturation

Very early B cells, like early T cells, have the enzyme (TdT) in the nucleus. This enzyme is necessary for rearrangement of immunoglobulin genes. TdT is no longer present in B cells once antibody specificity is established.

Immature B cells carry IgM (immunoglobulin mu) on their cell membranes. Mature B cells have IgM and IgD class immunoglobulin as antigen receptors, and after antigenic stimulation B cells may also express any of the other immunoglobulin classes (IgA, IgE, IgG) (Fig. 5–10).

Another transient marker for early B cells is the membrane glycoprotein called **CALLA,** or **CD10.** This protein was first identified as a leukemia marker. It was found on cells of nearly all those with acute lymphoblastic leukemias (ALL), most of which could not be assigned to either T-cell or B-cell origin (see pp. 225–226). The antigen, present on these undifferentiated leukemia cells, came to be called the **common ALL antigen,** or CALLA. Increasingly sensitive cell-typing techniques reveal that most CD10+ leukemias have rearrangement of chromosome 14 in the leukemic cells, which indicates that they are of B-cell lineage. Normal B-cell precursors are CD10+, and CD10 can be found on certain nonlymphoid cells as well. Presence of CD10 on circulating lymphoblasts, is abnormal and indicative of leukemia.

Receptors for Proteins

Several additional receptors appear as B cells acquire functional maturity. One of these interacts with a structural element of the immunoglobulin molecule, the **Fc** segment (see Chapter 6). Unstimulated B cells have relatively few Fc receptors. Contact with antigen generates strong Fc-combining capacity, allowing the activated B cell to interact with antibody molecules in the surrounding medium. Fully differentiated plasma cells engaged in antibody production do not have Fc receptors. Fc receptors are thought to mediate up and down regulation of antibody responses. Some T-cell populations also have Fc receptors, suggesting an additional aspect of mutual regulatory effects between T cells and B cells.

B cells also have membrane receptors for several proteins of the complement system (see Chapter 8). The complex interactions of the complement components generate an array of proteins and fragments. B cells express a complement receptor called CR1, which binds specific intermediate complement products, designated C3b and C4b. Complement receptors with various specificities are also present on macrophages and other accessory immune cells, on certain granulocytes, and on RBCs. The receptor for C3d, designated CD21 or CR2, is the target molecule whereby the Epstein-Barr virus (EBV) infects B lymphocytes. Although CD21 exists on certain antigen-presenting cells, B lymphocytes seem to be the only cells to experience EBV infection.

Evolution to Plasma Cell

The fully differentiated plasma cell loses most membrane markers characteristic of B cells and assumes an appearance and function very different from the parent lymphocyte. Plasma cells are specialized to manufacture and secrete immunoglobulin; they need no further environmental stimulation or regulation. Membrane immunoglobulin is no longer expressed; the MHC class II products disappear, as do receptors for immunoglobulin heavy chains and for complement proteins. After several days of manufacturing and releasing immunoglobulin molecules, the individual

MATURATION OF B CELLS

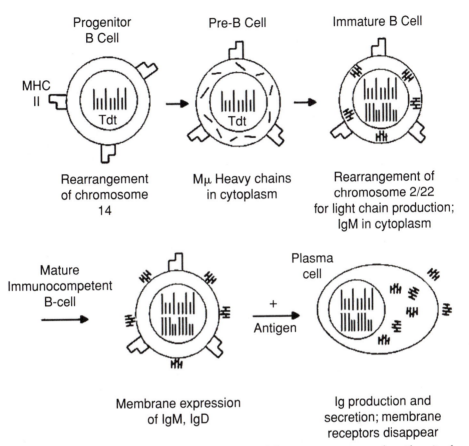

FIGURE 5–10. Irreversible commitment to B-cell differentiation occurs when the site for heavy-chain production on chromosome 14 undergoes rearrangement. Pre–B cells are identified by rearrangement of the heavy-chain site and synthesis of heavy chains in the cytoplasm. MHC II present on B cells at the earliest stages persists through all B-cell phases, but disappears from plasma cells (PC). The immature B cell has rearranged the light-chain gene and has immunoglobulin monomers in the cytoplasm, but not on the membrane. Presence of membrane IgM and IgD with the same antigenic specificity marks the cell as a mature, immunocompetent B cell. After activation, proliferation, and differentiation to a PC, immunoglobulin production increases; immunoglobulin is secreted to the exterior; and membrane characteristics necessary for communication with the environment disappear because the PC has a relatively short life span.

plasma cell dies without reproducing itself. Figure 5–10 summarizes aspects of B-cell maturation.

NATURAL KILLER CELLS

Approximately 5 percent of blood lymphocytes have neither the membrane immunoglobulin characteristic of B cells nor the surface markers characteristic of T cells. Originally called "null" cells, these cells are now known as **NK cells** (natural killer cells) because of their ability to lyse target cells, regardless of antigenic specificity, MHC expression, or previous exposure. NK cells are large granular lymphocytes with abundant cytoplasm and numerous enzyme-containing granules.

Identifying Features

NK cells originate in the bone marrow. Their development probably represents a differentiation event that occurs shortly after division into T-cell and B-cell lines. NK cells develop outside the thymus, as shown by the fact that "nude" mice (a specially bred strain of mice with no hair and no thymus) have NK cells. NK cells do not have CD4, immunoglobulin, or TCRs on their cell membranes. Although NK cells do not rosette when incubated with sheep cells, they do react with monoclonal antibodies specific for CD2. They also react with antibody to CD38, an antigen present not only on thymocytes but also on B cells at certain stages of differentiation and activation. Monoclonal antibodies have identified an antigen apparently unique to NK cells, designated HNK-1 (CD56). NK cells use CD11a/CD18 as adhesion molecules.

NK cells have on their membranes low-affinity receptors for the Fc portion of the IgG class. These receptors enable NK cells to recognize target cells coated with antibody and to aid in destruction of foreign cells with and without the presence of specific antibody.

Effector Functions

NK cells attack target cells with which they have had no previous experience. An important function of NK cells is their spontaneous participation in viral infections. Cells infected with a virus display viral antigens on their surfaces. NK cells are able to selectively kill these cells, even though they have not had previous exposure to these antigens. Viral infection also can result in reduced HLA expression, which serves to activate NK cells. NK activity increases under conditions of heightened immune activity. Immune reactions generate cytokines that enhance NK activity, especially gamma interferon (IFN-γ), a product of antigenically stimulated T cells, and IL-2, produced by T cells exposed to IL-1. NK cells themselves produce IFN-γ and can activate macrophages to participate in further cell killing.

Intimate contact with the cell membrane of a target cell is essential for NK-mediated cytolysis. The effect resembles a lethal injection. Cytotoxic T cells and NK cells contain proteins called **perforins.** Perforin forms tubular complexes that produce lesions in target cell membranes. Cytotoxic and proteolytic enzymes in the granules of NK cells are released and can enter through the perforins to cause apoptosis. NK cells can inflict a lethal "hit" on a target cell, disengage, and then repeat the process with the next target.

Laboratory Findings

Although NK cells act against a wide range of target cells, they display more discrimination than do macrophages and neutrophils, the totally nonspecific inflammatory cells. The surface properties of target cells with which NK cells react include HLA antigens of all allotypes, viral products, and membrane markers present on immature cells of various lines. The less mature the cell, the more susceptible it is to NK-mediated cytolysis. Thus, NK cells react strongly, *in vitro*, against such normally present cells as hematopoietic precursors, fetal cells, and the connective tissue cells that produce collagen. Their most conspicuous action in the laboratory is against abnormal populations such as tumor cells and virus-infected cells. Observations in patients with defective NK activity and with various tumors and infections invite the conclusion that NK cells defend against inappropriate cell proliferation and therefore have an important protective role in immunity.

SUMMARY

1. Lymphocytes are characterized by their microscopic appearance (size, shape, and staining characteristics), substances they secrete, mitotic activity, response to agents that selectively inhibit or enhance metabolic activity, and specific membrane markers. Membrane markers (antigens) can be identified with monoclonal antibodies, which are highly specific reagents produced by fusing B cells programmed to secrete a specific antibody with cancerous myeloma cells.

2. Membrane molecules characteristic for various cell types are referred to as cluster of differentiation markers or cluster determinants (CDs). CD terminology is assuming increasing prominence.

3. Other techniques for characterizing immune cells and their functions include enzymatic digestion of proteins to ascertain polypeptide sequences and structure of molecules. Restriction enzymes can be used to digest DNA into fragments. Nucleotide sequences of the "restriction fragments" can be inferred by pairing of single-stranded DNA with known DNA sequences called gene probes. An isolated gene can be copied innumerable times by a molecular technique called the polymerase chain reaction (PCR).

4. After a gene has been identified, it is possible to inject this gene into a fertilized egg of a mouse. If the gene is successfully incorporated and expressed by immune cells, a change in function should be detectable. This mouse is then referred to as a transgenic mouse. Inactivation of a specific gene results in a "knock-out" mouse. Through such genetic experimentation it is possible to define functions of specific membrane molecules, cytokines, intracellular enzymes, and so forth.

5. Lymphocytes are derived in the bone marrow from a multipotential stem cell referred to as a CFU-S. Under the influence of various hormones, growth factors, and locally produced cytokines, lymphoid precursor cells develop from the CFU-S and begin to express distinctive antigen receptors, CD markers, enzymes, and cytoplasmic proteins characteristic of lymphocytes at various stages of maturation.

Continued on following page

6. Early precursor T cells (prothymocytes) leave the bone marrow and migrate to the thymus. The thymus is most active during fetal and early childhood development and has a critical role in "programming" T cells so that mature competent T cells tolerate self antigens, but still recognize and respond to foreign antigen. Thymocytes that have antigen receptors to self antigens are induced to undergo apoptosis.

7. T cells recognize antigen through a complex membrane protein called the T-cell receptor (TCR), which is composed of either alpha and beta chains or gamma and delta chains. Antigen is bound by a hypervariable region of amino acids in the extracellular domain formed by interaction of both chains. Accessory and costimulatory membrane bound molecules such as CD3, CD4, and CD8 aid in stabilizing the antigen and TCR bond and transmitting this signal to cytoplasmic proteins for cell activation (signal transduction). CD4 and CD8 also bind to MHC II and I, respectively, to help stabilize the bond between antigen-presenting cells and T cells.

8. B lymphocytes are derived from lymphoid precursor cells in the bone marrow and remain in the bone marrow and possibly fetal liver to undergo differentiation. Early events in B-cell differentiation involve rearrangement of genetic sequences responsible for antibody production. This antibody is inserted into the cell membrane, where it serves as an antigen-binding receptor (BCR). Initially, IgM and IgD make up the BCR on mature B cells. With binding of specific antigen (clonal selection), the B cell undergoes proliferation and differentiation into antibody-secreting plasma cells and B memory cells. Similar to that which occurs with activation of T cells, B cells require accessory adhesion molecules and cytokines. B cells also carry MHC II on their cell membranes and can act as antigen-presenting cells to T cells.

9. Natural killer (NK) cells have neither the membrane immunoglobulin characteristic of B cells nor the surface markers characteristic of T cells. They do have large granules in their cytoplasm that contain cytotoxic and proteolytic enzymes. These granules are released into cancer cells and virally infected cells. Even though NK cells have not been previously exposed to antigen on these abnormal cells, NK cells can recognize and kill them.

REVIEW QUESTIONS

1. The multipotential hematopoietic stem cell is called a _____.
   a. CFU-M
   b. CFU-H
   c. CFU-S
   d. CFU-GM
   e. CFU-L

2. Inappropriately "programmed" thymocytes are induced to undergo _____.
   a. activation
   b. differentiation
   c. adhesion
   d. clonal selection
   e. apoptosis

3. The accessory molecule necessary for stabilizing the T-cell receptor to MHC I and antigen is _____.
   a. CD4
   b. CD8
   c. CD28
   d. CTLA-4
   e. CD40-L

4. Heterodimers that form the T-cell receptor are called _____.
   a. $\gamma\delta$
   b. $\alpha\beta$
   c. $\gamma\beta$
   d. $\alpha\delta$
   e. a and b

5. Monoclonal antibodies are produced from a hybridoma cell that results from the fusion of _____ and _____.
   a. T cell . . . myeloma cell
   b. B cell . . . myeloma cell
   c. monocyte . . . myeloma cell
   d. macrophage . . . myeloma cell
   e. Natural killer cell . . . myeloma cell

6. The BCR is linked to _____ for signal transduction.
   a. Ig $\alpha\beta$ heterodimers
   b. $\gamma\delta$ heterodimers
   c. κ light chains
   d.   J chain
   e. $\alpha\alpha$ homodimers

7. Immunoglobulin class(es) first expressed on mature, competent B cells is/are
   a. IgM
   b. IgD
   c. IgG
   d. IgA
   e. a and b

8. One of the first signal transducing enzymes necessary for T-cell activation is

   _____.
   a. CTLA-4
   b. terminal deoxynucleotidyl transferase (TdT)
   c. IL-2
   d. phospholipase C (PLC)
   e. lck tyrosine kinase

9. _____ is a transcription factor capable of binding to promoter sites on genes to stimulate mRNA production and antibody synthesis.
   a. Diacyl glycerol (DAG)
   b. NF-κB
   c. Tyrosine kinase
   d. Phospholipase C (PLC)
   e. *c-myc*

MATCHING QUESTIONS

Match the cell characteristics in Column I to the cells in Column 2.

Column 1

10. antibody used as an antigen receptor
11. Will differentiate into plasma cells
12. Require MHC for antigen recognition
13. CD4 present on the cell membrane
14. Spontaneously recognize and kill tumor cells

Column 2

a. T cells
b. B cells
c. a and b
d. Null cells
e. Natural killer cells

TRUE/FALSE

15. Thymectomy can be performed on an adult with no ill effects.
16. B cells can act as antigen-presenting cells.
17. More CD8+ cells than CD4+ cells normally circulate in the blood.

SUGGESTIONS FOR FURTHER READING

Clement LT: Isoforms of the CD45 common leukocyte antigen family: Markers for human T-cell differentiation. J. Clin Immunol 1992;12:1–10

Hemler ME: VLA proteins in the integrin family: Structure, functions and their role on leukocytes. Ann Rev Immunol 1990;8-365–400

Karre K: Express yourself or die: Peptides, MHC molecules and NK cells. Science 1995;267:978–979

Kipps TJ: The cluster of differentiation (CD) antigens. In: Beutler E, Lichtman MA, Collen S, Kipps TJ, eds: William's Hematology, 5th ed. New York: McGraw-Hill, 1995:113–140

Miller JFAP: The discovery of the immunological function of the thymus. Immunol Today 1991;12:42

Nunez C, et al: B-cells are generated throughout life in humans. J Immunol 1996;156:866–872

Trent RJ: Molecular medicine, an introductory text for students. London: Churchill Livingstone, 1993

Weissman IL, Cooper MD: How the immune system develops. Scientific Am 1993;269:65–71

REVIEW ANSWERS

1. c	8. e	15. True
2. e	9. b	16. True
3. b	10. b	17. False
4. b	11. b	
5. b	12. a	
6. a	13. a	
7. e	14. e	

6 Immunoglobulins

Antibodies are proteins that are further classified as **immunoglobulins.** Immunoglobulins are synthesized by B lymphocytes and their differentiated progeny, plasma cells. Immunoglobulin (Ig) molecules have a characteristic four-chain structure. Those for which a corresponding antigen can be identified are called **antibodies,** but millions of Ig molecules have not been matched with specific antigens. All antibodies are Igs, but not all Igs can be considered functional antibodies. Ig molecules inserted into the B-cell membrane serve as receptors through which B lymphocytes interact with antigen. Plasma cells do not have membrane-bound Ig, but secrete vast quantities of Ig that function as antibodies.

IMMUNOGLOBULIN STRUCTURE

The basic Ig molecule consists of two pairs of identical polypeptide chains, one longer set and one shorter set. The longer chains, called **heavy chains (H chains),** contain approximately 440 amino acids; the **light chains (L chains)** have approximately 220 amino acids. The four-chain unit is called an Ig **monomer** (Fig. 6–1). Molecules consisting of two or more monomers are called **polymers.** Some Igs are composed of two, three, or five monomers and are referred to as **dimers, trimers,** or **pentamers,** respectively.

Isotypes and Ig Classes

An Ig monomer is Y-shaped with the antigen-binding sites on the "arms" of the molecule. Each monomer therefore has two binding sites that are formed between the variable regions of the L and H chains (Fig. 6–1). The **variable regions** of the L and H chains have unique amino acid sequences that ensure binding or recognition of specific antigens. This recognition binding site is the **idiotype** of the molecule. The remaining portions of the L and H chains have amino acid sequences shared by a large number of Ig molecules and are referred to as **constant regions** or **domains.** Two different l-chain constant sequences exist and are designated **kappa** and

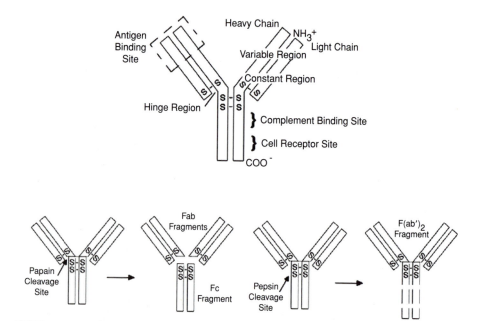

FIGURE 6–1. The generalized immunoglobulin monomer is composed of two identical heavy chains and two identical light chains. Each chain has a variable region and a constant region. The specificity of antigen binding or the idiotype resides in the variable regions of the light and heavy chains. Light and heavy chains are held together by disulfide bonds. Treatment with papain cleaves the heavy chains just above the hinge region, yielding two identical fragments (Fab) that contain the antigen-binding sites and one fragment (Fc) that contains the carboxy-terminal ends of both heavy chains. Pepsin cleavage yields a bivalent fragment called F(ab')$_2$.

lambda. There are five H-chain sequences, which are designated **alpha, delta, epsilon, gamma, and mu.** Igs are categorized into **classes,** according to the H chain expressed: **IgA, IgD, IgE, IgG,** and **IgM.** In all classes, approximately two-thirds of the molecules have two kappa L chains, and one-third have two lambda chains. Hybrids with one kappa and one lambda chain do not occur.

Regardless of the antigen they recognize, all IgM molecules have the same amino acid sequence in their mu-chain constant region, and this is different from the constant-region sequence in Igs of other classes. When characteristic features are present in all members of a molecular category and that category is distinguishable from groups with other characteristics, the category is called an **isotype** (Fig. 6−2). Minor differences in the amino acid sequences of the constant regions of the alpha and gamma chains occur, which lead to further classification of IgG and IgA into **subclasses.** Two subclasses of alpha H chains exist, which are designated alpha-1 and alpha-2. Four subclasses of gamma H chains exist, designated gamma-1, gamma-2, gamma-3, and gamma-4. Therefore, four IgG subclasses are produced and are present in healthy individuals: IgG1, IgG2, IgG3, and IgG4. The slight differences in amino acid sequences contribute to differences in structure and biologic activities of the Ig molecule. For example, IgG1, IgG3, and IgG4 can cross the placenta and have an important role in protecting the fetus. Most of the IgG subclasses can activate complement, although their effectiveness varies with the subclass (Fig. 6−3).

Domains and Intramolecular Bonds

Amino acids are joined by peptide bonds, which link the amino group of one amino acid with the carboxy group of the next in a head-to-toe fashion. No matter how

ISOTYPE vs. SPECIFICITY

FIGURE 6−2. Immunoglobulins are composed of variable and constant domains. The constant domains of the heavy chains determine the class or isotype of an antibody molecule. The unique amino acid sequences of the variable domains determine the idiotype, which gives the molecule specificity. The amino acid sequence for a single idiotype can be attached to different heavy chains, causing a single specificity to be present in different immunoglobulin classes. In this figure, both antibodies at the top identify a square-shaped antigen; on the bottom, both recognize a triangle. However, the individual molecules are of different classes. The two molecules on the left have gamma heavy chains and those on the right have mu heavy chains.

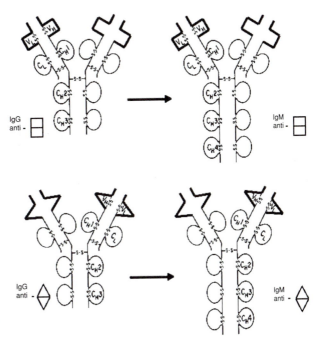

IgG SUBCLASSES

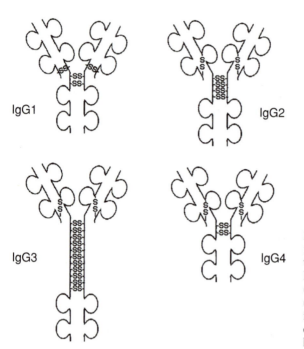

IgG1

IgG2

IgG3

IgG4

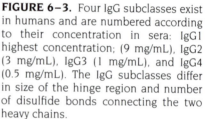

FIGURE 6–3. Four IgG subclasses exist in humans and are numbered according to their concentration in sera: IgG1 highest concentration; (9 mg/mL), IgG2 (3 mg/mL), IgG3 (1 mg/mL), and IgG4 (0.5 mg/mL). The IgG subclasses differ in size of the hinge region and number of disulfide bonds connecting the two heavy chains.

long the polypeptide chain is, there is always an amino group at one end and a carboxy group at the other. The H and L chains of the Ig monomer join so that all amino terminals are at one end and all carboxy groups are at the other. The variable portion involves approximately half of the L chain and one-fourth of the H chain that are at the amino-terminal end.

Each L chain is joined by a **disulfide bond (S-S bond)** to one H chain. One or more S-S bonds link the two H chains at approximately their midportions, in an area of considerable flexibility called the **hinge region.** Flexibility at this site allows the molecule to change shape while interacting with antigen epitopes located at irregular intervals or in awkwardly accessible sites. S-S bonds also join Ig monomers into polymers, but they are more easily broken than those in the hinge region or those joining L to H chains. IgM pentamers are easily dispersed into five monomers by treatment with reducing agents like dithiothreitol or 6-mercaptopurine, whereas breaking the S-S bonds that link chains within the monomer requires intense reducing techniques not used in routine immunologic testing.

Characteristics of Domains

Protein molecules do not exist in the body as two-dimensional strings of amino acids. They have complex three-dimensional configurations formed by attraction and repulsion among the amino acids and their attached side chains. The primary amino acid sequence defines the variability necessary for the specificity of the antigen-binding site and functional differences of Ig classes and subclasses. A functional protein must have a secondary, tertiary, and sometimes quaternary structure.

The extended polypeptide chain folds back and forth upon itself to form sheetlike structures that are stabilized by strategically localized intrachain S-S and hydrogen bonds. The sheets of amino acid chains are then folded into compact globular structures referred to as **domains** (see Fig. 6–2). L chains have two domains; H chains have either four or five domains. Antigen recognition involves the domains of the H and L chains that are nearest the amino-terminal end. These regions of the polypeptide chain are called **variable domains.** The other domains are the **constant domains.** Variable domains of H and L chains are denoted as V_H and V_L, respectively. L chains have only one constant domain, C_L. Alpha, delta, and gamma H chains have three constant domains, numbered C_H1, C_H2, and C_H3. Epsilon and mu chains have an additional domain, C_H4. C_H1 and C_L domains stabilize the antigen-binding site. C_H2 domains function as complement-activating sites and binding sites for complement receptors on phagocytic cells.

The physiologic and functional differences among the Ig classes are reflected in the properties of the constant domains characteristic of each class. The subclass differences within alpha, gamma, and mu isotypes result from differences in amino acid sequence in specific constant domains. Despite conspicuous differences among constant-domain sequences of isotypes and subclasses, many long amino acid sequences are common to segments of all Ig chains.

The Immunoglobulin Superfamily

Many other proteins exist that have structures similar to Ig domains. These proteins form a group called the **immunoglobulin superfamily.** Many of the proteins of the Ig superfamily are associated with surface membranes and have binding or adhesive functions. Because of the similarities in structure, deoxyribonucleic acid (DNA) sequences must also be similar. Proteins with Ig domains are thought to arise from a common ancestor gene because they share similar sequence homology. Eight families of glycoproteins with multiple Ig domains and 12 families of glycoproteins with single domains have been identified. Many of the cluster determinant (CD) markers have single Ig domains. The T-cell receptors, MHC I, and MHC II, have multiple Ig domains.

The Antigen-Binding Site

Antibody does not recognize and combine with antigen unless the molecule includes both H and L chains. The three-dimensional configuration that interacts with the epitope gets half of its shape from the variable domain of each chain. Only certain segments of the variable domain actually do vary; many sequences are exactly the same in molecules with different specificities. Invariant sequences within the variable domains provide the structural framework for the idiotypically unique amino acid sequences that recognize antigens. The portions of the variable domain that are unique for each idiotype and determine the shape of the antigen-binding site are called the **hypervariable** or **complementarity-determining regions;** three such segments occur in both H-chain and L-chain variable domains. The intervening amino acid sequences that are common to molecules of all specificities are called the **framework regions.** To have distinctive amino acid sequences in the hypervariable regions, each Ig-producing cell must have a unique DNA sequence at the loci that determines manufacture of H and L chains. The genetic events that produce these unique sequences are discussed in detail in a later section about Ig diversity.

Enzymatic Cleavage

Use of proteolytic enzymes to divide the molecules into constituent parts allows greater understanding of antibody structure and behavior. A useful technique is to separate the antigen-combining sites from the constant portions of the molecule. This must be done without breaking the S-S bond that joins H and L chains, because antigen recognition requires simultaneous presence of both chains. The enzyme **papain** breaks the H chain at a point just above the hinge, generating three separate fragments: two identical fragments consisting of an L chain linked to the amino-terminal half of the H chain and one fragment that contains the hinge region and the remaining H-chain constant domains. The two fragments that carry the antibody activity are called **Fab** fragments (for **f**ragment with **a**ntigen-**b**inding capacity). The linked H-chain fragment is called **Fc,** denoting that it can be crystallized. This is also the portion of Ig that reacts with complement. The Fc fragment contains the constant domains that determine the biologic and serologic characteristics of the Ig class or subclass.

Another enzyme sometimes used to cleave Igs is **pepsin,** which cleaves the H chain below the hinge to yield a large fragment that includes both combining sites. This fragment, which has two recognition sites, is called **F(ab)$'_2$** and is capable of uniting with two epitopes simultaneously. The remainder of the H chains is degraded into small fragments with no immunologic activity.

The J Chain

Ig monomers are composed of only H and L chains. Ig polymers characteristically include an additional chain, called the **J** (for joining) **chain.** This is a short polypeptide manufactured by the plasma cell and is added to the polymerized Ig just before it leaves the cell. IgM molecules that serve as antigen receptors on the B-cell membrane are monomers and do not express a J chain. Only secreted polymers include a J chain, and there is only one to a molecule, regardless of the number of monomers present.

Immunoglobulin Synthesis

Plasma cells have far more capacity to synthesize and secrete Ig than their parent lymphocytes. All proteins are assembled on **ribosomes,** which by transmission electron microscopy look like tiny spheres. Ribosomes serve as sites for translation of the genetic information carried by the mRNA into protein. Proteins made for export from the cell (such as immunoglobulin) are synthesized on ribosomes attached to a web of internal membranes called the **endoplasmic reticulum.** Polypeptides destined to leave the cell then enter the space enclosed by these membranes and travel to a specialized intracellular site, called the **Golgi apparatus,** in which proteins are processed for external secretion. The heavy concentration of ribosomes and endoplasmic reticulum necessary for protein synthesis and secretion is the reason for the abundant cytoplasm and dark-blue color seen in most stained microscopic preparations of plasma cells.

H and L chains are synthesized independently on different ribosomes. It takes about 30 seconds to assemble an L chain and 60 seconds to assemble an H chain. Constituent chains are linked through S-S bonds while traveling through the endoplasmic reticulum. In the Golgi apparatus, Ig monomers are packaged into membrane-bound units that traverse the cytoplasm, merge with the cell membrane, and discharge their contents to the exterior. Polymerization of IgA and IgM occurs late in the process, shortly before the protein leaves the cell. Ig polymers are not secreted until the J chain is attached.

Techniques for Study

There are several ways to characterize Ig classes. Detailed amino acid sequences can be determined, but most investigations observe the behavioral characteristics of the molecules. Igs migrate in an electrical field with other globulins with gamma immunoglobulin migration being the slowest (Fig. 6–4). Antibodies are sometimes described collectively as **gamma globulins,** because IgG molecules are the most abundant antibody class and because they migrate in the gamma range. The term is

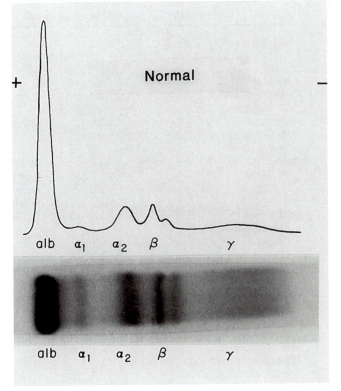

FIGURE 6–4. The strip at the bottom of this figure shows migration of serum proteins through an electrophoretic gel. Molecules move at rates determined by their individual characteristics; concentration is reflected in the density of stain, which is graphically rendered in the tracing above the strip. At pH 8.6, large numbers of homogeneous albumin molecules move rapidly toward the anode, at left. The remaining bands are less sharply defined because molecules within these groups show greater diversity. Globulins designated gamma move toward the cathode (at right) at this pH. The gamma category includes so many different proteins that the migration band is indistinct. The aggregate concentration of gamma globulins in this specimen is almost the same as that of the less heterogeneous β- and α_2-globulin categories.

somewhat misleading because some Ig classes migrate more rapidly, in the beta portion of the electrophoretic tracing.

When subjected to analytic ultracentrifugation, Igs sediment at characteristic rates that reflect molecular size and shape. The unit of measurement is the **Svedberg unit** (abbreviated **S**), and molecules are described by their **sedimentation constant.** IgM molecules are sometimes called 19S antibodies and IgG are 7S, properties that describe the entire class without regard to antigenic specificity.

Some Definitions

The different Ig classes express a variety of physiologic functions, which will be discussed in Chapters 9 through 14. These activities have been evaluated by observations of healthy individuals and patients with absent or abnormal Ig and by *in vitro* manipulation. The H-chain constant domains carry the configurations that determine these activities. The study of antibodies in serum or other body fluids is called **serology;** observations demonstrate the **serologic** properties of immunoglobulins. The earliest serologic activities to be characterized were clumping of particles, called **agglutination,** and dissolution of red blood cells (RBCs), called **hemolysis.** These and other ways to demonstrate Ig activities are described in Chapters 15 through 19.

TABLE 6–1. **Characteristics of Immunoglobulins**

	IgM	IgG	IgA	IgE	IgD
Heavy (H) chain class	μ	γ	α	ξ	δ
H-chain subclasses		γ1, γ2, γ3, γ4	α1, α2	None	None
Constant domains on H chain	4	3	3	4	3
Approximate molecular weight (in kD)	900	150	160	190	180
Polymerization	Pentamer	No	Mostly dimers in secretions; Monomers in serum	No	No
Serum concentration (mg/dL)	120–150	1000–1500	100–300	1–3	0.003–0.005
% of serum Ig	8–12%	70–75%	10–20%	<1%	Trace
Serum half-life (days)	5	23–25	6	1–5	2–8
Complement fixation (classical pathway)	4+	1–3+	No	No	No
Crosses placenta	No	Yes	No	No	No
Skin sensitization	No	?Minimal	No	Yes	No
Transported across epithelium	Occasionally	No	Yes	No	No

SPECIFIC IMMUNOGLOBULINS

Immunoglobulins constitute approximately 20 percent of plasma proteins and are present at varying concentrations in other body fluids. Wide differences in distribution and properties exist among Ig classes. These are summarized in Table 6–1.

IgM

It is logical to discuss IgM first because it is the first class of Ig produced by the maturing B cell, the first class to appear in the serum of maturing infants, and the first class of antibody detected in primary immune responses. In body fluids, IgM is a pentamer, but on the B-cell membrane monomeric IgM serves as an antigen receptor. This section will consider only the pentameric secreted form, which is the largest of the Ig molecules. It has a molecular weight of 900 kD and a diameter of approximately 100 nm. The five monomers form a star-shaped molecule (Fig. 6–5), which can combine simultaneously with antigenic determinants widely separated from one another. Although the 5 monomers include 10 combining sites, only 5 are available for combination with most antigens. All 10 sites can react with very small, soluble haptens.

IMMUNOGLOBULIN CLASSES

IgG

Greatest concentrations in serum
Crosses the placenta

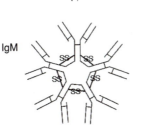

IgM

Effectively binds complement
Causes cell lysis
Does not cross the placenta
Is produced by the fetus

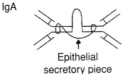

IgA

Secreted onto
internal surfaces

Epithelial
secretory piece

IgE

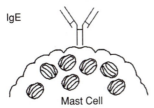

Mast Cell

IgD

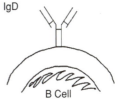

B Cell

FIGURE 6–5. The various immunoglobulin classes are defined by distinctive heavy chains, association into dimers and pentamers with accompanying proteins, and insertion into specific cell membranes.

IgM as Agglutinin

Large molecular size has several consequences. Nearly all secreted IgM is found in the bloodstream. Very little IgM is in tissue or in other body fluids unless vessels become abnormally permeable or there is actual rupture of capillaries or other vessels. The presence of the J chain promotes binding of IgM to receptors on secretory cells, which then transport the IgM to mucosal surfaces, where it aids IgA in protecting the more vulnerable internal surfaces of the body.

Because of their large diameter, IgM antibodies readily combine with antigens on the surface of dispersed particles, agglutinating them into easily observed clumps. IgM antibodies are effective agglutinins because of their size and multiple combining sites. Although many laboratory tests use agglutination as an end point, agglutination is relatively insignificant in physiologic events. More important in the living host is the ability of IgM antibodies to initiate the classical pathway of complement activity (see Chapters 8 and 9). Complement activation is a function of the Fc portion of the Ig monomer. Because IgM is composed of five monomers, the multiple Fc portions ensure that ample complement activity occurs. Another important function of *in vivo* IgM antibody reactions is enhancement of macrophage activity. Macrophages have membrane receptors for complement components.

Appearance and Disappearance

IgM antibodies appear earlier than IgG in the primary immune response, but synthesis continues only while antigen remains in the system. As antigen molecules are degraded or eliminated, IgM production declines and no memory cells develop for IgM secretion. On subsequent exposure to the same antigen, the interval before IgM antibodies become detectable is the same as in the primary response (see Fig. 4–10). Like all proteins, IgM molecules are metabolized at a predictable rate. The disappearance of molecules from the circulation is often expressed as the **half-life,** the time required for half of the molecules originally present to be degraded. IgM antibodies in the bloodstream have a half-life of 5 days.

IgG

IgG is the most abundant Ig in serum, constituting 70 to 80 percent of circulating Igs and 20 to 25 percent of total serum proteins. Quantities of IgG accumulate for two reasons: individual molecules have a long half-life (23 to 25 days), and there is continuous high-level stimulation for IgG production. After an individual develops immunity to antigens in the environment, there is frequent opportunity for repeated contact and anamnestic stimulation; anamnestic antibodies are IgG. As shown in Table 6–2, the four IgG subclasses differ substantially in biologic behavior and half-life; most generalized statements about IgG refer to IgG1, which constitutes 60 to 70 percent of serum IgG. IgG is always a monomer, with a molecular weight of approximately 150 kD and a diameter of 25 nm. As the smallest Ig, IgG easily enters tissues and plays a major role in antibody-mediated defense mechanisms.

Effects on Cells and Proteins

IgG antibodies unite with antigens on particle surfaces but seldom cause agglutination. Attachment of IgG antibodies to antigenically reactive cells or organisms has

TABLE 6–2. **Characteristics of IgG Subclasses**

	IgG1	IgG2	IgG3	IgG4
Percent of total IgG	60–70	15–25	4–8	2–5
Serum half-life (days)	23	23	8	23
Fixes complement	2+	1+	3+	0
Crosses placenta	Yes	No	Yes	Yes
Macrophages have receptors for this Fc	Yes	No	Yes	No
Neutrophils have receptors for this Fc	Yes	Yes	Yes	±
Molecular weight of H chain (in kD)	51	51	60	51
Allotypic variation (Gm groups) present	Modest	Modest	Marked	Absent

two major consequences. The most important is that the Fc portion of the gamma chain remains accessible on the particle surface; antigen-antibody recognition involves the Fab portions, leaving the Fc portions extending outward. Macrophages and neutrophils have high-affinity receptors for gamma-chain Fc, so particles coated with IgG antibody are far more susceptible to cellular attack than cells or organisms in their native state. Enhancement of phagocytic activity by alteration of a surface is called **opsonization;** IgG antibodies are potent **opsonins,** as are some of the protein fragments generated by the complement sequence. All IgG subclasses except IgG4 activate complement by the classical pathway. However, IgG complement activation occurs less consistently and less intensely than with IgM.

Effects on the Fetus

IgG is the only class of antibody that crosses the placenta from mother to fetus. The fetus occupies a sealed, sterile environment and normally is not exposed to microorganisms in the environment. After birth and upon entering the world without maternal antibodies, normal newborns would have little or no immune protection against the world. Infants born with the mother's antibodies rarely suffer infections from common environmental bacteria and viruses. Protein degradation, however, occurs more rapidly than immune maturation, so antibody levels fall dramatically after 6 to 8 weeks of age and the infant becomes susceptible to infection. In rare cases, transmission of maternal antibodies has harmful effects. Transfusion, exposure to fetal antigens, or other stimuli may cause a woman to produce antibodies against antigens absent from her own cells but present on fetal cells. If these antibodies enter the fetus in high concentration, cell damage may ensue. The most conspicuous example of this is the condition called **hemolytic disease of the newborn (HDN),** which affects fetal RBCs.

IgA

More IgA is produced than any other class of Ig, but serum concentration is relatively low. Most IgA is in secreted fluids present on the epithelial surfaces of the alimentary, respiratory, and reproductive tracts and in urine, saliva, and milk. Serum IgA circulates as a monomer, but the secreted forms are largely dimers. Secreted IgA has, in addition to the J chain present in polymerized Igs, a glycoprotein chain called the **S** (for secretory) **component.** The S component derives from epithelial cells, not from the plasma cells that synthesize IgA. IgA is produced mainly by plasma cells in mucosa-associated lymphoid tissue beneath surface epithelium.

To enter secreted fluid, IgA must pass through the overlying epithelial cells. IgA dimers bind to receptors on the basal surfaces of mucosal epithelial cells. The IgA is taken into the epithelial cell by endocytosis and is transported to the luminal surface of the cell, where it is secreted. The receptor remains bound to the IgA as the secretory component (Fig. 6–6). The presence of the S component appears to protect the IgA polymers in secreted fluids from degradation by surface enzymes. IgA binds bacteria, viruses, and other microorganisms and prevents attachment of pathogens to mucosal cells. Fc receptors for IgA have also been found on phagocytic cells and therefore IgA may function as an opsonin.

IgE

Normal serum and body fluids contain very little IgE. Increased levels of IgE are found in persons who have allergies or are infected with certain parasites. IgE binds to the membrane of highly specialized tissue granulocytes called **mast cells;** some IgE is present on basophilic granulocytes in the blood. Basophils and mast cells have membrane receptors specific for the Fc of IgE; attachment occurs through the fourth constant domain of the epsilon heavy chain. Fab sites are not involved in this interaction, and cell-bound IgE antibodies remain capable of combining with antigen (Fig. 6–7). When the Fab sites unite with antigen, the change in molecular configuration signals the underlying cell to release substances stored in its granules.

Mast cells are heavily concentrated in the skin and the lining of the respiratory and alimentary tracts. Their densely basophilic cytoplasmic granules contain histamine, heparin, and other substances that affect smooth muscle contraction, vascular permeability, and inflammatory events. The physiologic consequences of antigen binding to IgE produces a sequence of events called **immediate hypersensitivity reactions,** which cause the symptoms seen in allergies, but are also a useful defense against parasites (see Chapter 12).

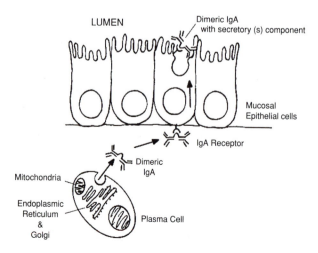

FIGURE 6–6. Dimeric IgA is secreted by plasma cells located beneath mucosal epithelial cells. IgA then binds to receptors on the basal surface of the epithelial cells. Epithelial cells endocytose and transport the IgA to the luminal surface where it is secreted. The receptor remains bound as the secretory component.

IgE on Basophils

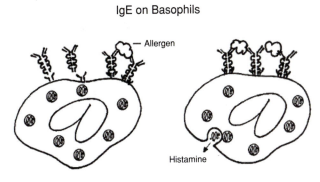

FIGURE 6–7. Basophils in blood and in tissue (where they are called **mast cells**) have membrane receptors that bind the fourth constant domain (CH4) of the epsilon chain. IgE molecules bound to the cell remain free to combine through their Fab sites with available antigen (allergen). Crosslinking of IgE with allergen triggers release of histamine and other mediators of hypersensitivity reactions.

IgE antibodies have several names that reflect their biologic characteristics. The term **cytophilic antibody** denotes their propensity to bind firmly to cells. **Skin-sensitizing antibody** reflects the effects of IgE in the skin, where mast cells are abundant. A potentially confusing term sometimes applied to IgE antibodies is **reagin.** The same name is also used for the anticardiolipin antibody that develops in conditions of immune dysfunction, especially syphilis. The two antibodies designated "reagin" are completely different in structure, function, and clinical significance.

IgD

Serum contains very small amounts of monomeric IgD molecules with a 2- or 3-day half-life. Most IgD is found on the surface of immunocompetent B lymphocytes that have not experienced primary stimulation. IgD is thought to function as a cell-membrane antigen receptor in association with IgM on the B cells.

GENETICS OF IMMUNOGLOBULIN DIVERSITY

All cells in an individual possess identical genetic information; yet vastly different cell types develop from this common genetic germ-line information. The process of cell maturation and the assumption of innumerable different cell properties is called **differentiation.** Differentiation is a result of selective gene expression. Cells in the immune system, with initially identical genes as any other cell type, differentiate into lymphocytes capable of recognizing and responding to millions of different antigens with an equal number of uniquely structured antibodies. How is this possible? Studies over the past decade have elucidated molecular events that offer a plausible explanation for such immunologic diversity.

Introns and Exons

Antibodies are proteins. Sequences of nucleotide triplets in the DNA called **codons** determine the selection of amino acids for polypeptide or protein chains. Each set of three bases codes for a specific amino acid. The first step in production of a new protein is **transcription** of the DNA chain into messenger RNA (mRNA), which can carry the encoded information to the ribosomes in cytoplasm. Ribosomes coordinate **translation** of mRNA. Within the ribosome, the nucleotide triplets of the mRNA are read by transfer RNA, which binds the respective amino acids together in the order dictated by the mRNA (Fig. 6–8). Many DNA segments do not code for peptides. These noncoding DNA segments are called **introns.** Expressed gene segments are called **exons.** Before mRNA leaves the nucleus, it is processed so that introns are removed and exons are spliced together. The removal and splicing of introns and exons are very important in the generation of Ig diversity.

Immunoglobulin Gene Construction

Immunoglobulins are composed of a variable region and constant region. Multiple genes contain codes for the variable region. A much smaller number of genes code for the constant region. Three gene families on three different chromosomes contain the genetic information for construction of Ig peptide chains. H-chain genes are on chromosome 14. Kappa- and lambda-chain genes are on chromosomes 2 and 22, respectively. Each gene family is composed of gene segments called **V genes** (variable), **C genes** (constant), and **J genes** (joining). H chains have in addition **D genes** (diversity). H- and L-chain genes also have **L genes** (leader), which encode peptides that guide H and L chains through the endoplasmic reticulum (ER) before they are

PROTEIN SYNTHESIS

Nucleus

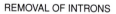

TRANSCRIPTION

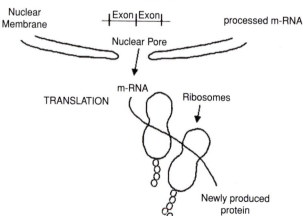

FIGURE 6–8. The basics of protein synthesis are diagrammed in this figure. Antibodies are proteins and therefore are produced in the same fashion as all proteins. Critical to the diversity of antibodies is the selection and recombination of gene segments from multigene families contained within the DNA.

joined together by S-S bonds. H and L chains are synthesized on separate ribosomes. Leader peptide sequences are cleaved after H and L chains enter the ER and therefore do not appear in the finished Ig product.

L chains (kappa and lambda) have a variable region and constant region. The information for the amino acid sequences of the variable and constant regions are found in separate gene segments. Genes for the variable region are called V-kappa or V-lambda and also include J-gene segments. The constant region is encoded in C-lambda or C-kappa gene segments. Humans have an estimated 100 V-lambda and 100 V-kappa gene segments, five to six J-kappa and lambda gene segments, six C-lambda genes, and a single C-kappa gene. Antibody diversity is generated by random selection of individual V-gene segments joined to individual J-gene segments, which are then connected to a C-gene segment (Fig. 6–9).

H-chain genes differ from L chains with the addition of another family of short gene segments called D genes. D genes provide additional nucleotide sequences between the V-heavy (V-H) and J-heavy (J-H) gene segments. As in L chains, V-H and J-H gene segments code for the variable region of the Ig, and therefore selection of D genes provides even more potential variability and diversity. There are approximately 100 to 300 V-H gene segments, which are divided into six families based on similarities in DNA sequences. Many of these V-H genes are **pseudogenes.** No functional proteins are made from these genes, but they can contribute short segments of DNA to other V-H genes to increase diversity. Nine J-H gene segments and at least five D-H segments have been identified as well as one C-H gene for each class of Ig that exists.

Generation of Antibody Diversity

Antibody diversity is generated by random selection of gene segments from the multigene family of V genes, J genes, and in H-chain synthesis from the D gene family. Variable-region gene selection and recombination occur in an ordered sequence during B-cell maturation in the bone marrow. The H-chain variable-region genes are combined first. Then the L-chain variable regions are arranged so that a functional antigen-binding site is formed. Each B cell will then contain a single functional vari-

GENE SEGMENT REARRANGEMENT

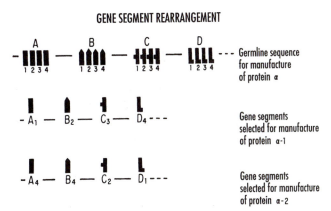

FIGURE 6–9. (*Top panel*) The germline sequence in which all alternative sequences in each gene family (A, B, C, and D) are available for selection. If one segment from each gene family is selected for expression, the two lower panels show rearrangements by which two cells can produce two different versions of the same protein. Immunoglobulin gene construction involves selection of gene segments from each multigene family. Gene segments are then spliced together to form a complete nucleotide sequence containing the information for the manufacture of a light chain and a heavy chain in each B cell.

able-region DNA for its H chain and a single functional variable region for its L chain. The cell is now committed to recognizing a single antigenic epitope and expresses membrane-bound antibody on its surface.

Junctional Events

In addition to random selection of variable genes from multiple gene families and recombination of V, J, and VDJ genes, **recombinational inaccuracies** occur, which result in further diversity. The process of cutting, rearranging, and rejoining DNA segments is subject to random error. When a V segment links with a J segment, a few nucleotides may be joined, which result in a new translation of amino acid. This can occur unpredictably at either end of either segment. Thus, even if the same V segment and the same J segment are selected in two different cells, slightly different final DNA sequences will be seen, expanding still further the number of possible sequences that can develop. The effects of imprecise joining are called **recombinatorial diversity,** which occurs only once in L-chain manufacture, because only a single splice between V and J takes place. For H chains, V combines with D and D combines with J, providing two opportunities for recombinatorial diversity.

Nucleotides are read as triplets. The nucleotides must be joined in a "correct reading frame." Inappropriate splicing may result in an out-of-phase reading frame and a nonproductive rearrangement. A mRNA is made, but a nonsense protein results. Immature B cells can attempt to salvage a nonproductive rearrangement of a H chain by switching to alternate kappa or lambda alleles until a functional L chain is produced, which results in a functional Ig. However, if no functional Ig is formed, the cell cannot be stimulated by antigen and will thus undergo apoptosis.

Further diversity is possible through the activities of the enzyme **terminal deoxynucleotidyl transferase (TdT).** At the V-D and D-J splice points, TdT can insert randomly selected nucleotides in a brief sequence called an **N region.** Thus, the DNA pattern for the H-chain variable domain has the sequence V-N-D-N-J. These N regions of unpredictable length and composition further increase the number of possible sequence combinations. TdT is present in the nucleus only at the very early maturational phase when the H-chain gene undergoes rearrangement. By the time L-chain genes rearrange, TdT has disappeared, and L-chain genes do not express N regions.

An Estimated Total

The potential number of different sequences available for Fab construction has been calculated from data obtained with mice, using rather conservative estimates for effects of recombinatorial diversity and insertion of N regions. These figures are 4×10^3 for L chains and 2.4×10^7 for H chains. Because any L chain can link to any H chain, the number of potential Ig molecules is the product of these two numbers. The staggering final figure is 10^{11} different Fab configurations—more than enough to recognize all the past, present, and future antigens an individual might encounter.

Somatic Mutation

The antibody diversity established by gene-segment rearrangement and base additions, and so on, which occur during lymphocyte differentiation still does not account for all the antibody variability seen *in vivo*. **Somatic mutation** is a process whereby individual nucleotides in the VJ and VDJ rearrangements can be replaced with other nucleotides, thus altering the specificity of antigen binding. Three areas of hypervariability are found in Ig V regions. These areas are called CDR1, CDR2, and CDR3. Variability in CDR3 can be explained by its location; it is located close to the VJ and VDJ splice site and therefore subject to gene recombination variability. CDR1 and CDR2 are located some distance away, and variability in these sites must occur by another mechanism. Monoclonal antibodies (Mabs) were produced against the hapten phosphoryl choline. When the amino acid sequence of the V-H region of 19 related Mabs was determined, it was found that 10 Mabs had identical amino acid sequences and 9 had numerous amino acid substitutions. The substitutions were the result of single-base changes in the CDR1 and CDR2 variable gene sites.

In the process of clonal selection, an antigen-responsive B cell is activated. This B cell has an IgM receptor capable of binding to the inciting antigen. As this clone of B cells undergoes proliferation, V-region genes (CDR1, CDR2) of responding B cells undergo random somatic mutation so that some B cells have enhanced antigen binding. These cells have increased **antigen affinity** or better-fitting antigen binding sites. Antigen binds better with the result that these cells will have an increased stimulus to divide. With time, antigen affinity of B cells improves. There is "selection of the fittest." The B cells that produce Ig receptors that do not bind antigen are not stimulated to divide and die off. Somatic mutation occurs in germinal centers as B lymphocytes undergo clonal expansion and in B cells undergoing H-chain class switching. Table 6–3 summarizes the various mechanisms for generating antibody diversity.

Diversity of Classes

These genetic "gymnastics" affect only the variable regions. All Ig molecules within an isotype have the same amino acid sequences in their constant portions, so gene rearrangement need not occur for the constant-region portion of the gene locus. Antibodies of a single specificity, however, often show diversity of Ig class (Fig. 6–10). The same Fab site can be found on antibody molecules with different H-chain isotypes. Immature B cells make IgM, so V regions are joined to C mu genes. Subsequently, a B cell will also make IgD, which involves V regions joined to C delta. With antigenic stimulation, Ig production switches to C gamma, C alpha, or C epsilon. The same antibody specificity is retained, but Ig function differs depending on H-chain isotype. This process is regulated by helper T-cell cytokine production (IL-4) and contact of B-cell CD40 membrane markers with CD40-L on helper T cells. Bind-

TABLE 6–3. **Mechanisms for Generating Antibody Diversity**

– Selection from multiple germ-line gene segments (V, D, and J)
– Possible multiple combinations of VJ and VDJ genes
– Recombinatorial diversity (effects of imprecise joining)
– N-region nucleotide addition
– Light- and heavy-chain recombination
– Somatic mutation

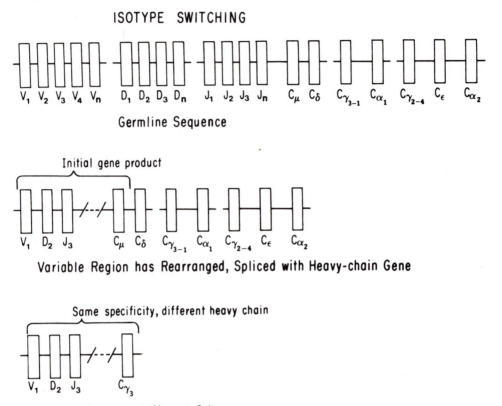

FIGURE 6–10. In the germline sequence for manufacturing immunoglobulin chains, multiple gene segments of the V, D, and J variable gene families lie adjacent to numerous sequences for the constant region (*top panel*) After selection of V, D, and J genes to determine the variable portion, the productive sequence then attaches to the constant-region segment for mu or delta heavy chains, (*middle panel*). Unstimulated B cells synthesize these isotypes. Heavy-chain constant-region segments can be deleted (*bottom panel*), allowing attachment of the variable region to the constant-region sequence for other Ig classes.

ing of CD40 to CD40 ligand (CD40-L) stimulates B-cell proliferation and switching of antibody isotypes to IgG. Binding of CD40 to CD40-L also promotes B-memory cell production.

The importance of CD40 is seen with the rare immunodeficiency disease, X-linked hyperimmunoglobulin M syndrome. Patients with this disease have a defect in their CD40-L membrane glycoprotein. Therefore, helper T cells fail to communicate effectively with B cells, and high levels of IgM are produced but very little of other classes (Fig. 6–11).

Allelic Exclusion and Failure to Rearrange

If the VJ or VDJ rearrangements result in a functional antibody, this is called a **productive rearrangement.** Gene segments may also be joined out of phase so that

HYPERIMMUNOGLOBULIN M SYNDROME (HIM)

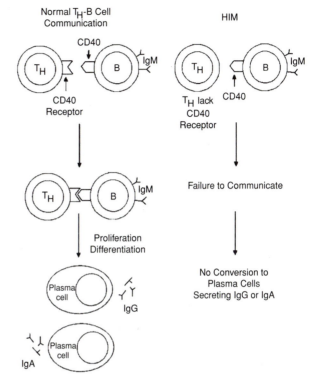

FIGURE 6–11. Normal switching of immunoglobulin isotype from IgM to IgG and IgA requires binding of CD40 on B cells to CD40 ligand (CD40L) on helper T cells (Th). Hyperimmunoglobulin M syndrome is a rare inherited immunodeficiency disease characterized by an inability to switch from IgM production to other isotypes. The cellular defect in these patients has been localized to CD40L on the Th cell.

translation results in a **nonproductive rearrangement.** B cells, like all cells in the body, contain two sets of chromosomes. If one allele undergoes a nonproductive rearrangement, the other allele can be rearranged and may result in a productive rearrangement.

Only one allele is expressed by the B cell. For many characteristics, such as blood group antigens and MHC products, genes on both chromosomes are active and direct the synthesis of a protein, a biologic phenomenon described as **codominance.** B cells, however, produce Igs from rearranged H-chain genes of only one chromosome and rearranged L-chain genes from only one chromosome. This process is called **allelic exclusion,** and it ensures that each B cell is specific for only one epitope. Once a functional VDJH gene combination is made, gene rearrangement of the other H-chain allele is turned off and rearrangement of kappa L-chain genes is turned on. Productive rearrangement of kappa L-chain genes results in a L chain that can pair with a H chain and form a complete antibody molecule. Formation of a productive L chain inhibits rearrangement of L-chain genes on the alternate allele. Nonproductive kappa rearrangement can induce lambda L chain gene rearrangement. Failure of both kappa and lambda rearrangements to produce a functional protein results in apoptosis.

Switching Isotypes

On chromosome 14, the DNA sequence for the variable region lies adjacent to the sequence that determines the constant-region sequence for the mu chain. After the variable-region sequence has been productively rearranged, it combines with the constant-region sequence for the mu chain. The Ig that contains this chain is IgM. DNA sequences for other H-chain isotypes are downstream from the mu-chain segment. If suitably stimulated, a daughter call can detach the entire variable-region sequence from one H-chain sequence and attach it to another (see Fig. 6–10). The signals controlling this switch are incompletely understood.

Unstimulated B lymphocytes can manufacture IgM and IgD simultaneously, and many naive B cells have as membrane receptors both IgM and I_8D molecules of a single idiotype. After activation and clonal expansion occur, only IgM is secreted. Daughter cells in a single clone subsequently encounter and respond to different regulatory messages; cells exposed to different cytokines subsequently secrete antibody of different classes. Memory cells seem to develop only from cells that have switched isotype away from mu-chain production; anamnestic stimulation does not provoke accelerated IgM synthesis.

IMMUNOGLOBULIN ALLOTYPES AND IDIOTYPES

It is not strictly correct to describe the constant regions of all antibodies in a single isotype as identical. Ig molecules produced by different individuals have short segments of amino acid sequences that differ from one person to another according to which alleles they possess. In a single individual, all IgG1 molecules have the same amino acid sequence, but IgG1 molecules from a different individual may have different amino acids in a limited segment of the chain. These amino acid configurations can elicit antibodies specific for one sequence if introduced into an individual whose Ig chains have a different sequence. The molecular feature defined by these antibodies is the **allotype** of the Ig.

Allotypes reside in the constant region of the Ig chain. They are not affected by antigen-binding specificity and do not seem to affect the biologic properties of the Ig molecule. Humans occasionally develop antibodies to Ig allotypes to which they have been exposed by transfusion or pregnancy, but such antibodies have no adverse clinical effects. Allotypes, as best as we know, are significant only as genetic traits that differentiate individuals from one another.

Allotypic distinctions are most prominent in gamma H chains and kappa L chains. Gamma chains of subclasses 1, 2, and 3 manifest allotypic differences named **Gm groups.** The allotypic distinctions on kappa chains were called **Inv groups** when first discovered, but are now called **Km groups.** The alpha2 chain exhibits **Am groups** and a recently discovered polymorphism in the epsilon chain is called **Em.**

Unique amino acid sequences in the VH and VL domain of an antibody form the antigen-binding site. These unique amino acid sequences are formed in response to antigens that are encountered after fetal development of the immune system. Therefore, these amino acid sequences can also be antigenic. Some of these unique amino acid sequences are located in the antigen-binding site, and some are located in non–antigen-binding areas of the V region. These amino acid sequences are referred to as **idiotypes,** and the sum of the individual idiotopes is called the

ALLOTYPES AND IDIOTYPES

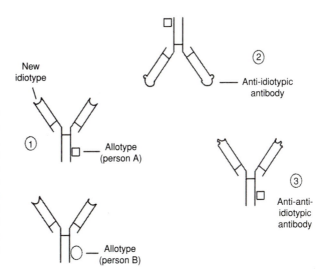

FIGURE 6-12. Allotypes differ slightly in the constant region of antibodies from different individuals. The idiotype refers to the unique amino acid sequences in the variable region of the antibody. The idiotype is foreign, and therefore a network of interacting anti-idiotype antibodies is formed upon antigenic stimulation of immune cells, which regulates further progression of the immune response.

idiotype of the antibody. The idiotype of an antibody defines the antigen with which it is capable of binding, and all antibodies that react with the same antigen have the same idiotype, regardless of class (isotype). During an immune response a large number of specific Igs carrying new idiotypes are produced. These idiotypes are recognized as being foreign by lymphocytes and **anti-idiotypic** antibodies are made. These anti-idiotypic antibodies also have new variable regions and can induce anti–anti-idiotypic antibodies. This process may continue to form a complex network of idiotype-anti-idiotype interactions. These interactions have been proposed to play an important role in regulating the immune response as anti-idiotypic antibodies may bind to B-cell and T-cell antigen receptors and suppress or enhance immune activities.

Figure 6-12 and Table 6-4 summarize the features that distinguish Ig molecules from one another.

TABLE 6-4. **Classification of Immunoglobulins**

Discriminator	Identifying Feature
Idiotype	The unique amino acid sequence in the variable regions of L and H chains, through which antibody interacts with a specific antigen. All antibodies that react with the same antigen have the same idiotype, regardless of class.
Isotype	The features of the antibody molecule determined by distinctive constant regions of H-chain class or subclass and L-chain class. All antibodies possessing those chains possess those features, regardless of antigenic specificity or the genome of the person producing the antibody.
Allotype	Genetically determined amino acid sequence at specific sites in constant regions, present in Ig molecules from individuals who possess that allele, regardless of idiotypic specificity of the antibody.

T-CELL RECEPTOR DIVERSITY

Genetic rearrangement occurs not only in B cells but also in T cells for the generation of diversity in the T-cell receptor (TCR). Most antigens are presented in combination with MHC and require recognition by the TCR. The amino acid variability in the antigenic binding regions of the TCR is generated by similar mechanisms as seen in B-cell antibody diversity. The B-cell antigen receptor is Ig of a single epitope specificity with a hydrophobic tail section for insertion into the B-cell membrane.

T-cell receptors likewise have single epitope specificity. TCRs are composed of alpha and beta or gamma and delta heterodimers with similar domain structures as Igs. TCRs have variable and constant domains. The variable domains are involved in antigen binding and are encoded in rearranged VDJ or VJ gene segments. All helper and cytotoxic T cells rearrange gene segments to form specific TCRs. Most T cells express alpha/beta chains. A small proportion express gamma/delta. Alpha and delta genes are on chromosome 14. Immature T cells make delta chains as part of their TCRs. Mature T cells make alpha chains. Alpha chains are formed from selection and rearrangements of VJ and C gene segments. About 50 V-alpha gene segments and 70 to 75 J-alpha genes are present in humans. Many more J-gene segments are available for TCR production than for Ig production. Delta chains are also made from VDJ- and C-gene segments.

Beta-chain genes are on chromosome 7. Fifty-seven V-beta gene segments have been identified in humans with two repeats of DJ and C segments. Each repeat of DJC segments has about six functional J gene segments. Any V-beta gene segment may be joined to either of the two DJC combinations. Gamma-chain genes are also on chromosome 7 and consist of 14 V-gamma gene segments, five J-gamma gene segments, and two C-gamma gene segments.

Diversity in TCRs is generated by mechanisms similar to Igs. Multiple germ-line genes exist. Gene segments are looped out and deleted, thus bringing selected V, D, and J gene segments together to form unique variable domains. In the process of forming VJ and VDJ combinations, gene segments can be inverted. Reading frames may be changed and result in productive rearrangements. Random bases may be inserted at V, D, and J junctions, resulting in new amino acid combinations. Any one or all of these mechanisms could occur in the formation of a functional TCR and therefore a functional T cell. DNA recombinase enzymes and TdT are also active in these T-cell genetic machinations.

Somatic mutation does *not* occur in TCR variable regions. It is essential that the TCRs recognize antigen in association with the presenting MHC molecule. Random somatic mutation could result in the generation of T cells that are unable to recognize antigen or are able to react with self antigen and therefore cause autoimmunity.

Obviously with the number of VJ and VDJ combinations and molecular modifications possible in the joining of gene segments, a huge diversity of TCRs is generated. This diversity is what allows for the ability of the immune system to recognize diverse antigens and respond to the multitude of different disease causing organisms today and in the future.

SUMMARY

1. Antibodies are proteins that are further classified as immunoglobulins (Igs). Immunoglobulins have a characteristic structure and are composed of two heavy (H) chains and two light (L) chains. The binding site for antigen is located at the amino-terminal ends of the H and L chains and constitute the variable region. The remaining portions of the H and L chains are referred to as the constant regions or domains. Two L chains with different constant regions exist and are designated kappa (κ) and lambda (λ). Five different H-chain constant sequences exist, and Igs are categorized into classes according to the type of H chain in the molecule. Ig domains can also be found in other proteins in the body. Therefore, all proteins sharing similar amino acid sequences and thus deoxyribonucleic acid (DNA), sequences form a group called the immunoglobulin superfamily.

2. The antigen-binding site (idiotype) is formed from the variable domains of both H and L chains. Portions of the variable domains are unique for each idiotype and affect the shape of the binding site. These portions are called hypervariable or complementarity-determining regions and require that unique DNA sequences be present in the gene loci determining these regions of the H and L chains.

3. The study of antibodies is called serology. Antibodies can be observed by their abilities to cause agglutination or hemolysis. Because of their characteristic shape, size, and associated electrical charge, Igs can be separated by electrophoresis or ultracentrifugation. Igs can be cleaved into fragments of characteristic size by the use of papain or pepsin.

4. The constant region of the H chain contributes to the different functions of the various Igs.

    a. IgM as a monomer is inserted into the B-cell membrane and serves as an antigen receptor. Secreted IgM is a pentamer and will have at least five antigen-binding sites. It is therefore very effective for agglutination of particulate antigen and for complement activation.

    b. IgG occurs strictly as a monomer and can be further subclassified according to the characteristic changes in the amino acid sequences of the constant region of the H chain. IgG is the most abundant isotype in the serum. It is an effective opsonin, and most IgG subclasses activate complement. Because of its small size, IgG easily enters tissues and plays a major role in antibody-mediated defense.

    c. Only small amounts of IgA are present in serum; however, more IgA is produced than any other class of Ig. IgA is the principal protective mechanism for mucosal surfaces and is present in almost all secreted fluids.

    d. Antigen binding to IgE produces a sequence of events called immediate hypersensitivity. Immediate-hypersensitivity reactions cause the symptoms obeserved with allergies, but are also a useful defense against parasites.

    e. IgD is mostly found on naive B lymphocytes and functions as an antigen receptor.

Continued on following page

5. The production of specific antibodies with unique amino acid sequences in the variable regions of the H and L chain entails the generation of unique DNA sequences. These sequences are generated by the random selection of gene segments from the VJ and D gene families. Many combinations are possible, and, in the process of joining the gene segments, recombinational inaccuracies occur, which result in further diversity. Terminal deoxynucleotidyl transferase (TdT) is a nuclear enzyme that can insert selected nucleotides at V-D and D-J splice points to increase possible sequence combinations in the H-chain variable regions. L and H chains both undergo this process of gene selection and recombination. After the variable regions are established, constant genes are added and can subsequently be switched, resulting in change of predominant isotype (e.g., from IgM to IgG).

6. Somatic mutation is a process whereby further specificity in the variable region of Igs is achieved. CDR1 and CDR2 are hypervariable regions within the Ig V region that are subject to single nucleotide base substitutions. As activated B cells undergo proliferation, somatic mutation occurs in CDR1 and CDR2 so that the B-cell receptor (BCR) of some B cells have enhanced antigen binding. Antigen binds better to these B cells; therefore, there is an increased stimulus to divide. With time, antigen affinity of B cells improves.

7. The constant regions of an Ig isotype differ slightly from one individual to another because of inheritance of different alleles. If Ig is injected into an individual with a different allotype, the slight difference in amino acid sequences can elicit antibodies. Allotypic differences in gamma H chains are called GM groups. Allotypic differences in kappa chains are called Km groups.

8. The unique, new amino acid sequences in an idiotype can induce the formation of anti-idiotypic antibodies. Anti-idiotypic and anti–anti-idiotypic antibodies can bind B-cell and T-cell antigen receptors and other molecules and thereby play a role in regulation of the immune response.

9. A process of genetic rearrangement similar to that seen in the production of the BCR occurs in the production of the T-cell receptor (TCR). TCRs have single epitope specificity, which lies in the variable domains of α and β or γ and δ heterodimers. VJ or VDJ gene segment selection and recombination occur in the formation of these variable regions. Somatic mutation does *not* occur because it is essential that the TCR recognize antigen in association with the major histocompatibility complex (MHC). Random somatic mutation could result in the generation of T cells that are unable to recognize antigen and MHC or that are capable of reacting to self antigen, thereby causing autoimmune disease.

REVIEW QUESTIONS

1. Immunoglobulin monomers are composed of _____ heavy chain(s) and light chain(s).
   a. 1,1
   b. 2,2
   c. 1,2

    d. 2,1
    e. 5,2

2. A Fab fragment is produced by cleavage with _____ and has
_____ antigen-binding site(s).
    a. papain . . . one
    b. pepsin . . . two
    c. trypsin . . . one
    d. neuraminidase . . . two
    e. lysozyme . . . one

3. Antibodies that specifically bind to the antigen-binding site of an immunoglobulin are called _____.
    a. anti-allotypic antibodies
    b. anti-isotypic antibodies
    c. anti-idiotypic antibodies
    d. anti-CDR antibodies
    e. anti-Kim antibodies

4. _____ is a technique for separating serum proteins based on electrical charge and migration rate through a gel.
    a. Electrophoresis
    b. Precipitation
    c. Sedimentation
    d. Sequencing
    e. Polymerase chain reaction (PCR)

5. Somatic mutation occurs in the hypervariable region(s) _____.
    a. CDR1
    b. CDR2
    c. CDR3
    d. a and b
    e. b and c

6. The only immunoglobulin isotypes that are expressed simultaneously on a B-cell membrane are _____.
    a. IgM and IgG
    b. IgA and IgG
    c. IgG and IgD
    d. IgM and IgD
    e. I_8D and IgE

7. Construction of the variable region of the Ig heavy chain requires _____.
    a. V genes
    b. J genes
    c. D genes
    d. a and b
    e. a, b, and c

8. Hyperimmunoglobulin M syndrome is caused by a lack of _____.
    a. CD40-L on T cells
    b. CD40 on B cells
    c. IL-1R on T cells
    d. CR1 on B cells
    e. B7-2 on B cells

TRUE/FALSE

9. A switch in immunoglobulin class involves both the variable and constant regions.

10. The affinity of IgG antibodies increases as an immune response progresses.

11. CDRs on each Fab region of an antibody are identical.

12. All immunoglobulin molecules on the surface of a given B cell have the same idiotype.

MATCHING QUESTIONS

Match the characteristic in Column I to the class of immunoglobulin in Column 2.

Column 1	*Column 2*
13. Primarily associated with mucosal surfaces	a. IgM
14. Primarily functions as a B-cell antigen receptor	b. IgA
15. Ig produced in greatest quantities in the body	c. IgG
16. Contains a J chain	d. IgD
	e. a and b

Column 1	*Column 2*
17. Is most effective at activating complement	a. IgM
18. Is a mediator of allergies	b. IgG
19. Is transported through the placenta	c. IgA
20. First Ig to be produced in a primary immune response	d. IgD
21. Most effective for bacterial agglutination	e. IgE

ESSAY QUESTIONS

1. Describe how somatic mutation contributes to antibody diversity and how it is related to clonal selection.

2. HIV enters primarily through mucosal surfaces. how would you design a vaccine for HIV? Include in your discussion how IgA is made and how it provides protection for mucosal surfaces.

SUGGESTIONS FOR FURTHER READING

Greenspan NS, Bona CA: Idiotypes: Structure and immunogenicity. FASEB J 1993;7:437–444

Kishimoto T, Hirano T: Molecular regulation of B lymphocyte response. Ann Rev Immunol 1988;6:485–51

Moss PAH, Rosenberg WMC, Bell JI: The human T-cell receptor in health and disease. Ann Rev Immunol 1993;10:71–76

Schatz DG, Oettinger MA, Schlissel MS: V(D)J recombination: Molecular biology and regulation. Ann Rev Immunol 1992;10:359–368

Williams AF, Barclay AN: The immunoglobulin superfamily domains for cell surface recognition. Ann Rev Imunol 1988;5:381–405

REVIEW ANSWERS

1.	b	12.	True
2.	a	13.	b
3.	c	14.	d
4.	a	15.	b
5.	d	16.	e
6.	d	17.	a
7.	e	18.	e
8.	a	19.	b
9.	False	20.	a
10.	True	21.	a
11.	True		

7 Cytokines, Cellular Cooperation, and Cell-Mediated Immunity

Previous chapters presented information about the various lymphocyte populations and their receptors for antigen and how specific antibody is made in response to antigen. Immune reactions, however, extend far beyond the interaction between antigen and a membrane receptor of complementary configuration. Many populations of cells interact to enhance, suppress, modulate, and otherwise orchestrate the events we identify as a detectable immune response. This chapter discusses some of the ways that cells and their products interact after antigenic exposure stimulates an immunocompetent host.

CELLULAR INTERACTIONS AND CYTOKINES

The cellular interactions that occur in an immune response involve macrophages, B cells or other antigen-presenting cells, helper T cells, cytotoxic or suppressor T cells, antibody-producing cells, and memory, and other effector cell types. Macrophages process and present antigen in association with major histocompatibility complex (MHC) II. B cells likewise can present antigen in association with MHC II. Unlike macrophages, B cells bind specific antigen because of their receptors. Antigen is presented to helper T cells, and those helper T cells with appropriate T-cell receptors (TCRs) capable of recognizing the foreign antigen will undergo activation. T-cell activation involves the process of antigen binding to membrane receptors, signal transduction, and subsequent clonal proliferation and secretion of proteins. Many of these proteins regulate the response of other cells. Helper T cells have a central role in the generation of humoral and cell-mediated immune responses (Fig. 7–1).

Cell products that influence activities of other cells are called **cytokines.** If synthesized by a lymphocyte, the product is also called a **lymphokine,** and if secreted by a monocyte/macrophage, it is sometimes referred to as a **monokine.** Cytokines are crucial for mediating or regulating immune cell activities. These signaling proteins can have effects on many different cell types and rarely is only one cytokine produced at a time. Activated macrophages are capable of secreting many different cytokines, and likewise activated T cells secrete mixtures of lymphokines. Different cytokines can have similar activities. Therefore, an immune response to a single antigen involves a complex interaction of cell types mediated by an even more complex network of cytokines.

This bewildering array of cytokines can be divided into five major categories:

1. **Interleukins** are cytokines that mediate interactions between lymphocytes, monocytes/macrophages and other leukocytes.
2. **Interferons** are primarily known for their viral inhibitory activities, although they also have immune regulatory activities.

CELL INTERACTIONS AND CENTRAL ROLE OF T-HELPER CELLS

FIGURE 7–1. The first step in an immune response is presentation of antigen. Macrophages secrete interleukin-1 (IL-1) and a host of other cytokines that activate helper (CD4+) T cells and other immune and inflammatory responses. Helper T cells, in response to antigen and IL-1, secrete IL-2, which promotes proliferation and differentiation of antigen-specific Th1 and Th2 cells. Cell-mediated and humoral responses are then generated toward the same antigen. With an antigen such as a virus, a cell-mediated response predominates. Both cell-mediated and humoral activities are necessary for a successful immune response. Th, helper T cells; Th1 and Th2, helper T cell subtypes; B, B cell; PC, plasma cell; IL-1, interleukin-1; IL-2, interleukin-2; IL-2R, receptor for IL-2; IFN-γ, interferon-γ; TC, cytotoxic T cell.

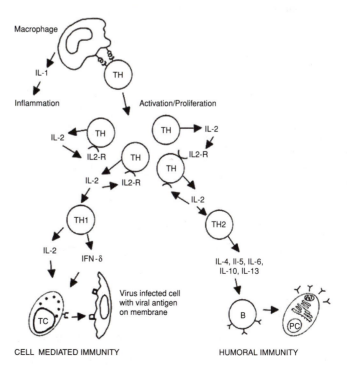

3. **Tumor necrosis factors,** as their name suggests, are cytotoxic to tumor cells but also have many other activities.
4. Various **growth factors** are considered cytokines. These growth factors have roles in the healing process, which may follow inflammation and an immune response. They also ensure that an adequate supply of the various blood cells are always present to meet the next invasive challenge.
5. **Chemokines** are chemotactic. They cause the selective migration of immune and inflammatory cells to a site of microbial invasion or any kind of cellular damage.

A complete discussion of every cytokine so far identified is beyond the scope of this text. However, it is important to have some understanding of how cytokines work in promoting inflammatory and immune responses. Understanding of cytokines also has significance because cytokines may be used therapeutically in the treatment of inflammatory and immune diseases.

Interleukin-1

Macrophages, as antigen-presenting cells, phagocytose microbes or other foreign material. This foreign material is destroyed by enzymatic degradation (lysosomal enzymes) and production of highly reactive bactericidal oxidative products: superoxide anion (O_2^-), hydrogen peroxide (H_2O_2), and hypochlorite (HOCl, bleach). Macrophages also produce toxic nitrogen oxides: nitric oxide (NO), nitrosamines, nitrosothiols, and other reactive oxides.

Besides their degradative activities, macrophages participate in inflammation and immune regulation through secretion of cytokines. One broadly reactive cytokine is **interleukin-1 (IL-1).** When first discovered in the late 1970s, this substance was seen to affect lymphocyte proliferation and reactivity and was called **lymphocyte activating factor (LAF).** Further investigation has revealed numerous additional functions of IL-1.

Almost anything that perturbs its cell membrane stimulates the macrophage to produce IL-1. The most potent stimulating event is incorporation of antigenic material, with subsequent processing and presentation. IL-1 has both local and systemic effects on many different cells, affecting metabolic and neurophysiologic events as well as immune and inflammatory reactions. Table 7–1 lists the major actions of IL-1. Systemic effects occur only when a large-scale stimulus induces secretion of IL-1 into the bloodstream. Local effects, especially those on nearby lymphocytes, can occur after limited macrophage activity. IL-1 provokes membrane changes in B cells, T cells, and natural killer (NK) cells, leading to enhanced sensitivity to other immunostimulating events. IL-1 causes T cells to produce the lymphokine, IL-2, and to express receptors for IL-2. B cells display increased levels of membrane immunoglobulin (mIg) and express receptors for IL-2. Macrophages produce IL-1 without regard to antigenic specificity, and the effects of IL-1 on target cells are not antigen-restricted. IL-1, however, induces conditions that increase the immunogenicity of any antigen that is present.

Interleukin-6

Interleukin-6 (IL-6) is produced not only by activated macrophages, but by many other cell types (lymphocytes, endothelial cells, fibroblasts, keratinocytes, and

TABLE 7–1. **Actions of IL-1**

On lymphocytes
    Induces IL-2 production and IL-2 receptor expression on T cells
    Influences suppressor cell activity
    Increases mIg expression in pre–B cells
    Promotes proliferation and differentiation of B cells
    Enhances natural killer cell activity
On inflammatory events
    Mobilizes neutrophils from marrow into circulation
    Attracts neutrophils, lymphocytes, monocytes to affected sites
    Increases systemic breakdown of proteins
    Stimulates hepatic production of C-reactive protein, "acute-phase reactants," amyloid A,
        metal-binding proteins, and so forth
    Reduces hepatic synthesis of albumin
On other cellular events
    Increases bone resorption by osteoclasts
    Increases production of proteolytic enzymes by cells of cartilage, synovium, and many
        epithelial sites
On central nervous system
    Leads to elevated body temperature
    Depresses appetite
    Promotes slow-wave sleep

mesangial cells of the kidney). IL-6 acts as a cofactor with IL-1 to promote IgM synthesis by B cells and production of IL-2 and receptors for IL-2 on T cells. IL-6 and IL-1 are needed for optimum proliferation of CD4-positive (CD+) cells. IL-6 has similar actions to those of IL-1 in infection and inflammation. It acts together with IL-1 to stimulate release of acute-phase inflammatory proteins from hepatocytes. It causes fever and stimulates hematopoiesis in the bone marrow.

Interleukin-12

Interleukin-12 (IL-12) is produced by monocytes, macrophages, neutrophils and dendritic cells, as well as by antibody-producing B cells. IL-12 activates NK cells and the production of another cytokine **interferon-γ (IFN-γ)** by T cells (Table 7–2). IL-12 and IFN-γ are potent stimulators for a subclass of helper T cells called T_H1. Th1 cells help cell-mediated immune responses. T_H2 cells aid B cells in antibody production and humoral immune responses. IL-4, IL-5, IL-6, Il-10, and IL-13 are secreted by Th2 cells. These interleukins stimulate growth and differentiation of B cells, regulate Ig class production, expression of MHC class II and other receptors on B cells, T cells, and macrophages, and can have both inductive and suppressive effects.

Tumor Necrosis Factor-α

Another important cytokine of macrophages is **tumor necrosis factor-α (TNF-α).** This cytokine causes necrosis and cell death of some tumor cell lines. It is also responsible for the weight loss seen in persons suffering from cancer, AIDS, and

TABLE 7−2. **Human Interferons**

	IFN-α	IFN-β	IFN-γ
Major producing cells	B lymphocytes, macrophages, large granular lymphocytes	Fibroblasts	T lymphocytes (T_H1, cytotoxic)
Major inducing stimulus	Viruses, RNA (double-stranded), B-cell mitogens, allogenic cells	Viruses, RNA (double-stranded), B-cell mitogens, allogenic cells	Specific antigens, tumor cells, T-cell mitogens

chronic bacterial and parasitic infections. Similar to IL-1, TNF-α affects the temperature-regulating center of the hypothalamus to cause fever and also affects hepatocytes to release acute-phase inflammatory proteins. Because of its ability to enhance inflammation, it is the primary cause of septic shock. Immune-mediating effects of TNF-α include the proliferation of B cells and T cells and the regulation of cytotoxic T cells. TNF-α will also enhance the effects of IL-2 on NK cells and monocytes.

Interleukin-2

On contact with antigenic material, a macrophage releases IL-1 at the same time that its MHC-II molecules are presenting the antigen. IL-1 stimulates T_H1 cells to produce IL-2 and modifies the T-cell membrane to enhance its reactivity with antigen. New receptors for IL-2 that stimulate clonal proliferation are made. IL-2 is a potent activator for helper and cytotoxic T cells, B cells, NK cells, and macrophages. It enhances NK activity of large granular lymphocytes, which express IL-2 receptors after stimulation by IL-1. Antigen specificity does not restrict the targets that NK cells attack, but specific antigens stimulate T cells to generate IL-2, which enhances the activity of nonspecific NK cells. IL-2 enhances proliferation of B cells that have undergone activation and immunoblast transformation, but B-cell stimulation requires much higher concentrations of IL-2 than does T-cell proliferation. With very high concentrations of IL-2, macrophages already in an activated state may acquire tumor-killing capacity. Table 7−3 lists the major actions of IL-2.

Other Lymphokines

Activated T cells and macrophages produce an impressive array of cytokines (Fig. 7−2). These products were initially identified by effects observed on target cells, and they were named for these activities. Lymphokines and cytokines have subsequently been intensively characterized, and some have been prepared in pure form by recombinant genetic techniques. A bewildering array of initials and numbers is used to identify cytokines. Table 7−4 lists some of the more important functions of cytokines.

TABLE 7–3. **Actions of IL-2**

On T cells
    Induces IL-2 receptor expression
    Enhances clonal expansion of antigen-stimulated cells
    Promotes production of IL-2
    Increases production of interferon and other lymphokines
    Increases cytotoxicity of antigen-stimulated CD8+ cells
On non–T cells
    Enhances proliferation and differentiation of antigen-stimulated B cells
    Promotes tumoricidal properties of large granular lymphocytes
    Increases cytotoxic actions of natural killer cells and macrophages

Cytokine Effects on B Cells

B cells also present antigen. T_H1 cells respond better to antigen presented by B cells. Binding of CD40 ligand (CD40-L) on activated T cells with CD40 on B cells and the presence of IL-2 promotes B cell proliferation and Ig class switching (Fig. 7–3). Quiescent B cells in G_0 of the cell cycle are stimulated by antigen and IL-1 to enter

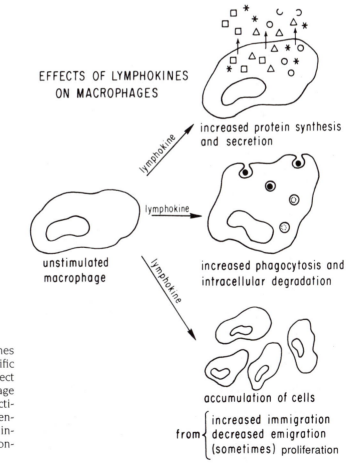

FIGURE 7–2. Lymphokines produced after antigen-specific stimulation of T cells affect many aspects of macrophage function and replication. Activation of only a few antigen-restricted lymphocytes can influence large numbers of nonspecific effector cells.

EFFECTS OF LYMPHOKINES
ON MACROPHAGES

increased protein synthesis
and secretion

lymphokine

lymphokine

unstimulated
macrophage

increased phagocytosis and
intracellular degradation

lymphokine

accumulation of cells

from { increased immigration
       decreased emigration
       (sometimes) proliferation

TABLE 7−4. **Major Categories of Lymphokine Activity**

Attraction of Cells (Chemotaxis)
Macrophages
Granulocytes
  Neutrophil
  Eosinophil
  Basophil
Lymphocytes
  B cells
  T cells
Fibroblasts

Inhibition of Cell Movement (Prevention of wandering of immune and inflammatory cells from a localized site)
Macrophages
Endothelial cells
Leukocytes

Promotion of Inflammation
Fever
Acute phase proteins
Adhesion molecules
MHC expression
Platelet aggregation
Procoagulants

Promotion of Cell Growth and Differentiation
Interleukin-2 (IL-2): T cells, some effect on B cells
Interleukin-3 (IL-3): T cells, B cells, multiple hematopoietic cell lines
Interleukin-4 (IL-4): T cells, B cells, mast cells
Interleukin-5 (IL-5): Eosinophils, activated B cells
Colony-stimulating factors for various cell lines

Enhancement of Cellular Activities
Macrophage activation
Interleukin, interferon secretion
Apoptosis
Healing
Cell-mediated, humoral immunity

CYTOKINE EFFECTS ON B CELLS

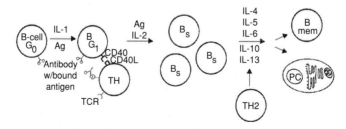

FIGURE 7−3. Interleukin-1 plus antigen stimulates quiescent B cells to enter G_1 of the cell cycle. Activated helper T cells secrete IL-2 and bind CD40-L with CD40 to promote cell proliferation and immunoglobulin (Ig) class switching from IgD to IgM and IgG. Th2 cells with secretion of additional lymphokines promote B-memory and plasma cell formation with secretion of additional Ig and Ig types. The cell cycle consists of G_0, resting phase; G_1, gene activation phase; S, DNA synthesis; G_2, preparation for mitosis; and M, mitotic phase.

G_1. B cells have receptors for IL-2 and, with binding of IL-2, undergo DNA synthesis and division. T_H2 cells promote the differentiation of B cells into plasma cells and B-memory cells with the secretion of IL-4, IL-5, IL-6, IL-10, and IL-13. In the presence of antigen and cytokines, newly matured B cells originally displaying IgD and IgM on their membranes will lose their IgD and switch to IgM production. Subsequently under the influence of cytokines, B cells switch Ig class from IgM to IgG, IgA and IgE.

The specificity of the binding site is retained and, because of clonal selection, the specificity of the binding site and secreted antibody is improved over time. B-memory cells resulting from this encounter with antigen will have a higher affinity for subsequent exposures to this antigen. Therefore, B-memory cells can be activated by lower levels of antigen. Each exposure to antigen results in production of a larger pool of B-memory cells, increased production of antibody, and increased production of IgG. Activation of memory cells is called a secondary immune response or an **anamnestic response** and is the reason booster shots are given for vaccinations.

T-independent antigens are antigens that can induce antibody formation by B cells without helper T-cell participation. These antigens are usually simple repeating polymers (e.g., lipopolysaccharides, pneumococcal polysaccharides, and dextran), which can crosslink B-cell antigen receptors (BCRs). Crosslinkage of BCRs activates the cell, and IgM is produced. However, because helper T cells are not involved, there is no cytokine production, and class switching from IgM to IgG does not occur.

HUMORAL IMMUNE RESPONSE

The cellular and cytokine interactions necessary for humoral immune responses can now be summarized. B cells arise from pluripotent stem cells in the bone marrow under the influence of growth factors and cytokines. IL-7 derived from bone marrow and thymic stromal cells induces proliferation of pre–B cells, thymocytes, and T cells. Progenitor B cells then undergo the process of gene rearrangement for productive antibody formation. Newly matured B cells bearing IgM and IgD on their cell surfaces migrate to and localize in immune tissue. Large concentrations of B cells are located in lymph nodes where antigen likewise becomes concentrated because of drainage by afferent lymphatics.

As antigen percolates through a lymph node, it is phagocytosed or retained by follicular dendritic cells, which form beaded structures called **iccosomes.** Iccosomes contain antigen-antibody complexes that are shed and may be endocytosed by B cells. The antigen is subsequently processed and presented to T cells. Lymphocytes capable of responding to antigen may enter via afferent lymphatics or may migrate from the bloodstream into lymphoid tissue across specialized endothelium called **high-endothelial venules (HEV).** The endothelium in HEV consists of extremely tall cells with unique cell adhesion molecules on their membrane called **addressins.** Lymphocyte surface-membrane markers include ligands of these addressins called **homing receptors.**

Binding of homing receptors to addressins and interaction of other cell adhesion molecules induces lymphocyte migration through the HEV. HEV are prevalent in the paracortical zone of lymph nodes where T cells and antigen-presenting cells are also located. On presentation of antigen, helper T cells in this area undergo activation, proliferation, and migration to primary lymphoid follicles, where they come into contact with B cells. With secretion of lymphokines by activated T cells, activated B cells form a dense zone of proliferative cells called the **germinal center.** Within the germinal center, differentiation into antibody-secreting plasma cells and memory cells occurs. Memory B cells may remain in a node, leave via efferent lymphatics to populate other lymphoid tissue, or recirculate as part of the surveillance function of the immune system.

CELL-MEDIATED IMMUNITY

Unlike humoral immunity in which antigens are eliminated by antibody, the cell-mediated branch of the immune system provides immunity by the actions of effector immune cells. Antibody may be involved in cell-mediated immunity (CMI), but it plays a secondary role. CMI helps to clear intracellular pathogens (e.g., virus-infected cells, tumor cells). Humoral immunity is more useful for clearance of extracellular pathogens (e.g., bacteria or bacterial toxins). A normal immune response involves both humoral immunity and CMI, although one or the other immune process is usually more prevalent.

Intracellular antigens are antigens synthesized within cells. Viral antigens are intracellularly produced and are processed and presented in association with MHC I on the host cell membrane. T cells with appropriate TCRs recognize antigen plus MHC I and induce a CMI response for elimination of the virus-infected cell. A mechanism by which some viruses may persist and evade CMI is suppression of MHC I in the host cell.

Super Antigens

Some antigens are not MHC-restricted (not recognized in the context of MHC I or MHC II). These antigens can form tight bonds between the V-beta chain of the TCR and the MHC of the antigen-presenting cell. A particularly powerful T-cell response is generated, and therefore these antigens are referred to as **super antigens.** An example of a super antigen is the toxin from *Staphylococcus aureus*, which can induce toxic shock syndrome. As a result of the toxin acting as a super antigen, massive amounts of IL-1 and TNF-α are released, causing fever, rash, kidney and liver damage, drop in blood pressure, and, in some cases, shock and death.

Types of Cell-Mediated Immunity

Cell-mediated immune responses can take several forms. Any activity that requires viable cell interactions and is targeted to specific antigens can be considered CMI. This contrasts with the humoral response, in which antibody molecules exert serologic and biologic effects independent of the Ig-producing cells, and also does not include the actions of macrophages and NK cells, which do not exhibit specific antigenic recognition. The major types of cell-mediated immune reactions are (1) **delayed (or tuberculin) type hypersensitivity (DTH),** (2) the effects of **cytotoxic T lymphocytes (CTL),** and (3) a combined cellular and humoral event called **antibody-dependent cell-mediated cytotoxicity (ADCC).** Delayed, tuberculin-type hypersensitivity was the first form of CMI recognized. In DTH responses, antigen-restricted T cells interact with their specific antigen and produce lymphokines, which activate effector macrophages and other cells that are not antigen-restricted. In T-cell cytotoxicity, the CD8+ effector T cells exert direct cell-to-cell effects on targets that display the appropriate antigen specificity. In antibody-dependent, cell-mediated cytotoxicity, antigenic specificity resides in antibody, which is synthesized by cells of B lineage. Antibody attaches to the antigen-bearing target cell. The effector cytotoxic cell interacts with the Fc of attached antibody; it does not respond to characteristics of the underlying cell. The actions of NK cells and of lymphokine-activated killer (LAK) cells are not antigen-directed and must be considered separately.

Delayed Hypersensitivity

In delayed-type hypersensitivity (DTH), antigen-specific T cells encounter an antigen, undergo activation and clonal expansion, and acquire memory for the antigen. A subsequent contact with the same antigen results in the release of lymphokines that affect other cells and tissues (Fig. 7–4). Major effects are accumulation of macrophages and enhancement of macrophage activity, increased blood flow and increased permeability of small blood vessels, and initiation of the coagulation and contact-activation kinin cascades. Tissue undergoing a DTH reaction is often somewhat swollen because increased fluid and protein accumulate in the interstitium. Early in the reaction, vascular congestion causes reddening, but if tissue changes are intense, necrosis and later scarring render the tissue pale or grayish white. Some of the protein that accumulates is fibrin, generated by the coagulation cascade. Other proteins include antibodies, complement components, albumin from the plasma, and some proteins synthesized by activated macrophages. The most conspicuous tissue change is accumulation of macrophages, often manifesting the altered appearance characteristic of heightened activation. The reaction is called "delayed" hypersensitivity because many hours elapse between contact of sensitized

TUBERCULIN REACTION

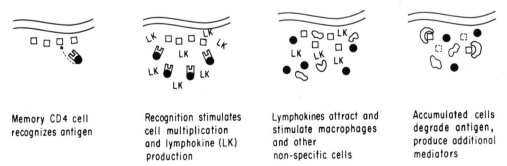

| Memory CD4 cell recognizes antigen | Recognition stimulates cell multiplication and lymphokine (LK) production | Lymphokines attract and stimulate macrophages and other non-specific cells | Accumulated cells degrade antigen, produce additional mediators |

FIGURE 7–4. The event that initiates delayed-type hypersensitivity or the tuberculin reaction is contact between injected antigen and antigen-specific CD4 cells with memory of previous activation. The anamnestic response stimulated by injected antigen promotes clonal expansion and subsequent production of lymphokines, which induce vascular changes and cellular accumulation. An individual who has never encountered the antigen will have no memory cells capable of promoting these changes.

T cells with antigen and the development of these vascular, protein, and cellular changes.

DTH-Activated Macrophages

The antigen-specific cells responsible for DTH are CD4+, primarily T_H1 cells. Delayed hypersensitivity develops only when MHC II+ cells present antigen initially and when sensitized memory cells encounter later examples of antigen in the context of MHC II products. Effective stimulants of delayed hypersensitivity include antigens from cells and complex organisms that are ingested but not immediately destroyed by macrophages. *Mycobacterium tuberculosis*, the etiologic agent of tuberculosis, is the most familiar organism that provokes this form of immunity. Other organisms that elicit DTH are *Mycobacterium leprae*, which causes leprosy; many fungi that elicit a macrophage response, such as *Candida*, *Histoplasma*, and *Blastomyces*; the protozoal invaders *Toxoplasma gondii* and several *Leishmania* species; and bacteria such as *Listeria monocytogenes* and certain salmonellae.

When T cells secrete lymphokines after stimulation by specific organisms, there is activation of macrophages that are not specific for antigens from these same organisms. The CD4+ cells that recognize and respond to the organism are highly specific; cells sensitized to M. *tuberculosis*, for example, will not respond to the presence of L. *monocytogenes*. Lymphokines provoked by the presence of M. *tuberculosis*, however, activate macrophages that exhibit heightened activity against other invaders. In experimental settings, macrophages stimulated after exposure to M. *tuberculosis* are more than normally effective in killing L. *monocytogenes* or any other intracellular invader. This phenomenon has been used in the development of immunotherapies for cancer. Preparations of microorganisms have been used to induce DTH of tumor cells.

The Tuberculin Test

The tuberculin skin test is a familiar example of DTH, which will determine whether previous immunizing exposure to the tubercle bacillus (M. *tuberculosis*) has occurred. A positive result is seen if memory cells are present for antigens of this organism. A small amount of antigenic material, called the **tuberculin antigen** or **purified protein derivative (PPD),** is introduced into an easily observed skin site. No viable organisms are present, so there is no danger of causing infection, and the quantity of antigen is too small to elicit primary immunization. If sensitized memory cells are present, tissue changes develop at the injection site. Within 48 hours, the skin becomes reddened, firm, and somewhat swollen, owing to vascular changes and macrophage accumulation induced by the lymphokines. The tissue events act to degrade the antigen within a few days, eliminating the immune stimulus and allowing the tissue to return to normal (see Fig. 7–4). If the individual does not have immune memory for the organism, no tissue changes occur at the injection site.

The tuberculin skin test is used to demonstrate DTH to various antigens in a variety of circumstances. It is used to diagnose previous or present infection with various fungi, to demonstrate memory-cell function against commonly encountered environmental antigens, and to investigate whether a patient has sufficient cell-mediated immune capability to mount a response after deliberate exposure to an unfamiliar antigen.

Cytotoxic T Lymphocytes

Cytotoxic T cells (CTLs) eliminate foreign cells and altered self cells. Examples of foreign cells or altered self cells include cells from organ or tissue transplants, virus-infected cells or tumor cells. These cells, if under attack by CTLs, will undergo direct lysis or apoptosis. Lysis can also be induced by NK cells (see Chapter 5) and macrophages.

Several populations of lymphocytes express the CD8 antigen. CD8+ cells are sometimes described as the **suppressor/cytotoxic population,** but different populations exist, performing different functions although sharing expression of the CD8 antigen. **Suppressor T cells** are immunoregulatory cells that inhibit or down-regulate effector actions of B cells or other T cells. The CTLs engage in lethal membrane interactions with target cells that express specific antigen.

CTLs recognize antigen that is presented in association with MHC I. An example of cytotoxic action is lysis of virus-infected cells. In a cell that harbors virus, the membrane often expresses viral antigens in addition to intrinsic cellular characteristics. Almost all cells express MHC I products, so any cell displaying viral antigens can be attacked by CD8 cells specific for the viral antigens.

Activation of CTLs requires specific TCRs plus CD8 that interacts with MHC I and antigen. The principal cytokine involved is IL-2; however, IL-4, IL-6, and interferon-gamma (IFN-γ) are also needed. Activated CTLs express more receptors for IL-2 (IL-2R), which then induces clonal expansion of antigen-specific CTLs. These cells become effector cells and cytotoxic T-memory cells. With elimination of antigen, IL-2 levels decrease and CMI subsides (Fig.7–5).

ACTION OF CYTOTOXIC T CELL

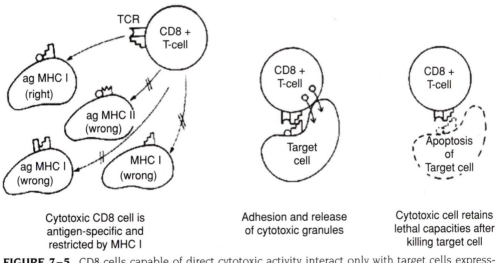

Cytotoxic CD8 cell is antigen-specific and restricted by MHC I

Adhesion and release of cytotoxic granules

Cytotoxic cell retains lethal capacities after killing target cell

FIGURE 7–5. CD8 cells capable of direct cytotoxic activity interact only with target cells expressing both antigen and the major histocompatibility complex (MHC) class I product. MHC restriction is significant only in experimental settings because in an intact individual, all cells have the host's MHC I products. The CD8 cell lethally damages the target cell without damaging itself and can move on to additional cells that express the right combination of membrane attributes.

Cell Adhesion

CMI involves binding of the CTL to the target cell and introduction of lethal material through the membrane. Similar adherence molecules essential for interaction of helper T cells and antigen-presenting cells are used in binding of CTLs to target cells. TCRs, CD3, CD8, and other costimulatory molecules bind to MHC I and antigen. In addition, CD11a, also known as **leukocyte function antigen I (LFA-1)** binds to **intracellular adhesion molecule I (ICAM-1)** on the target cell membrane. ICAM-1 is normally present on dendritic cells and B cells. With inflammation or an immune response, secretion of cytokines such as IL-1, TNFα or IFNγ causes the appearance of ICAM-1 on other cells. Expression of ICAM-1 on endothelial cells promotes binding and migration of lymphocytes and monocytes and other leukocytes into inflamed tissues. In the case of CMI, expression of ICAM-1 ensures adhesion of CTLs to target cells.

Another important cell adhesion molecule is CD28. It is expressed on almost all T cells. The ligand for CD28 is B7-2. Binding of CD28 to B7-2 rapidly causes activation of the CTL. Tumors or virus-infected cells that express B7-2 are killed much more rapidly by CTLs than by target cells that do not have B7-2 on their membranes. Experiments to use this phenomenon in cancer treatment have been attempted. Cancer cells are removed from a patient and genetically manipulated to increase expression of B7-2. These cells are then injected back into the patient to stimulate a greater CMI response to the genetically altered cells and naive cancer cells.

Killing of Target Cells

After CTLs have adhered to target cells, the next step is cell killing. Transmission electron microscopy of CTLs shows the presence of electron-dense storage granules. Within the storage granules are cytotoxic molecules that include perforin, granzymes, and lymphotoxin. These molecules are also present in NK cells (see Chapter 5). Perforins form tubular complexes that cause lesions in the target cell membrane similar to the lytic actions of complement (see Chapter 8). Through these lesions, granzymes and lymphotoxins can enter and induce apoptosis. Granzymes are esterases and have proteolytic actions. Lymphotoxin, also known as TNFβ kills tumor cells and other target cells.

Apoptosis is a process characterized by a rapid increase in intracellular calcium, which in turn activates intracellular enzymes that mediate cellular changes. Chromatin condensation and nuclear fragmentation occur. The cell shrinks with blebbing and cytoplasmic fragmentation. The CTL is not destroyed and can lethally engage several successive targets. The lethal effects need not be immediate. Target cell death has been observed at intervals ranging from 10 minutes to 3 hours after contact (Figs. 7–5 and 7–6).

Antibody-Dependent Cell-Mediated Cytotoxicity

Antibody-dependent cell-mediated cytotoxicity (ADCC) differs from other forms of CMI in that the effector cell does not recognize antigen. The effector cell does

APOPTOSIS

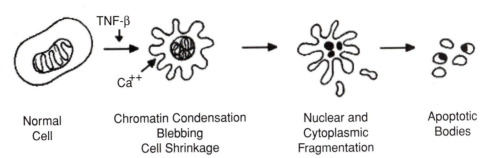

| Normal
Cell | Chromatin Condensation
Blebbing
Cell Shrinkage | Nuclear and
Cytoplasmic
Fragmentation | Apoptotic
Bodies |

FIGURE 7-6. The process of apoptosis occurs in a predictable pattern and involves an apoptotic signal followed by an increase in intracellular calcium and activation of intracellular enzyme systems. As a result, the apoptotic cell undergoes cell shrinkage, nuclear condensation, and blebbing with nuclear and cytoplasmic fragmentation. Apoptotic bodies are phagocytosed with no inflammation and thus no damage to adjacent cells or tissues. Cell death due to apoptosis is a normal process important to immunity as well as development of the immune system and probably other organ systems in the body.

have receptors for the Fc portion (FcR) of an antibody. The Fc portion of the antibody bound to a target cell extends from the surface membrane. Effector cells bind to the Fc portion through their FcRs and cause lysis of the target cell. Macrophages, monocytes, neutrophils, eosinophils, and NK cells all have FcRs and are capable of nonspecific cytotoxicity. Antibody directs these cells to the target cell with the antigenic specificity residing in the interaction between antibody and target cell membrane antigen. Complement is not involved. The effector cell does not phagocytose the coated cell; it exerts lethal injury after cell-to-cell binding occurs.

Large granular lymphocytes, which have virtually no phagocytic capability, are the cells most conspicuous in ADCC, although macrophages and granulocytes sometimes destroy an antibody-coated target rather than engulf it. The large granular lymphocytes recognize the target cell through the immunoglobulin Fc and bind to it through the LFA-1/ICAM-1 combination. Once bound, the effector lymphocyte releases lethal materials from its cytoplasmic granules.

Role of Antibody

The antigen-specific immune event in ADCC is interaction between antibody and cell-surface antigen. Before ADCC can occur, primary immunization must generate plasma cells that secrete specific antibody, and antibody molecules in body fluids must combine with antigen molecules on the target cell (Fig. 7–7). Targets of ADCC include bacteria, autologous cells coated with autoantibodies, and allogeneic cells introduced through transplantation. ADCC is restricted by Ig isotype. Macrophages, granulocytes, lymphocytes, and other antibody-directed cells express FcRs that recognize individual Ig classes. FcRs for the gamma chain of IgG are most often involved in ADCC. On mucosal surfaces, IgA antibodies and Fc-α receptors may be significant.

ANTIBODY-DEPENDENT CELL-MEDIATED CYTOTOXICITY

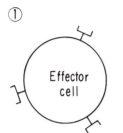

① Killer cell has Fc receptors

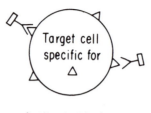

② Antibody binds to surface antigen

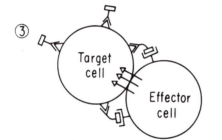

③ Fc receptor brings Killer cell into intense interaction with cell coated by specific antibody

FIGURE 7–7. The large granular lymphocytes that perform antibody-dependent cell-mediated cytotoxicity do not recognize specific antigens. They have membrane receptors with high affinity for the Fc of immunoglobulin molecules, as shown in 1. When the Fab sites of antibody combine with cell-surface antigen, the Fc portion remains accessible, as shown in 2, offering a ligand through which the effector cell can bind to the target cell and lethally damage it, as shown in 3. These effector cells will not react with target cells that have not first been coated with antibody.

SUMMARY

1. Cellular interactions necessary in immune responses involve antigen-presenting cells, helper T cells, cytotoxic/suppressor cells, and B cells. Antigen must be presented in association with major histocompatibility complex (MHC) I or MHC II for the most efficient immune response. Antigen binding to the T-cell receptor (TCR) results in signal transduction, clonal proliferation, and production of cytokines, which will regulate the response of other cells.

2. The many known cytokines can be divided into five categories: interleukins (IL), interferons (IFN), tumor necrosis factors (TNF), growth factors, and chemokines. Each of these cytokines has numerous overlapping roles, is produced by many different cell types, and may influence many cell types.

   a. IL-1 has local and systemic effects in immune responses and inflammation. As a result of IL-1 secretion, T cells produce IL-2, which activates other helper and cytotoxic T cells, B cells, natural killer (NK) cells, and macrophages.

   b. IL-6 acts as a cofactor with IL-1.

   c. IL-12 and IFN-γ are potent stimulators of a subclass of helper T cells (T_H1 cells), which aid in stimulating cell-mediated immune responses.

Another set of cytokines stimulates T_H2 cells, which aid B cells in humoral responses.

d. TNF-α causes necrosis of tumor cells and is a mediator of inflammation and immune responses.

e. Chemokines are small chemotactic molecules.

Many other cytokines have been characterized, and their participation is essential in ensuring an effective immune defense. The cell interactions and cytokine effects might be thought of as an orchestral composition, which, under most conditions, is flawlessly performed.

3. Activation of B cells for humoral immune responses requires the presence of cytokines and usually T cells. Direct binding of T cells to B cells occurs via CD40-L and CD40. IL-1 and antigen stimulates B cells to enter the cell cycle. IL-2 promotes proliferation and immunoglobulin (Ig) class switching. T_H2 cells with IL-4, IL-5, IL-6, IL-10, and IL-13 promotes differentiation of B cells into plasma cells and B-memory cells.

4. Because of clonal selection, specificity of the B-cell receptor (BCR) is improved over time, and B-memory cells can be activated by lower levels of antigen. Subsequent exposure to antigen results in a larger pool of B-memory cells and an increased antibody production with improved antibody specificity—an anamnestic response.

5. T-independent antigens induce antibody formation by B cells without helper T-cell participation. However, no isotype switching occurs and therefore only IgM is made.

6. Antigen-specific lymphocytes migrate to lymph nodes via high-endothelial venules (HEV). Lymphocytes have homing receptors capable of binding to addressins on HEV. Once within a lymph node, antigen-activated cells become organized into a dense zone called a germinal center. Within the germinal center, proliferation, differentiation, and antibody secretion occur.

7. Cell-mediated immunity (CMI) is the major mechanism for elimination of intracellular pathogens and abnormal cells. CMI requires antigen and MHC I presentation to appropriate T cells with resultant formation of cytotoxic T cells (CTLs) directly capable of killing a target cell.

8. Super antigens are antigens capable of forming a bond between the V-beta chain of the TCR and the MHC of the antigen-presenting cell. These antigens are therefore capable of stimulating a particularly powerful T-cell response and can cause such conditions as toxic shock syndrome.

9. Major types of CMI includes delayed-type hypersensitivity (DTH), effects of CTLs, and antibody-dependent cell-mediated cytotoxicity (ADCC).

a. DTH responses to antigen results in lymphokine secretion with accumulation of macrophages and localized inflammation. Many microorganisms besides *Mycobacterium* can cause DTH.

b. CTLs are CD8+ lymphocytes that recognize antigen and MHC I. Binding to a target cell requires the TCR and other costimulating and adhesion molecules. Subsequently, cytotoxic molecules are injected into the target cell resulting in apoptosis.

c. ADCC involves binding of antibody to a target cell. The effector cell capable of killing the target cell has receptors for the Fc portion of the bound antibody.

REVIEW QUESTIONS

1. Macrophages produce _____.
   a. interleukin-1 (IL-1)
   b. interleukin-6 (IL-6)
   c. interleukin-12 (IL-12)
   d. Nitric oxide (NO)
   e. All of the above

2. Which is *not* characteristic of T-independent antigens?
   a. Simple repeating units
   b. Bacterial in origin
   c. Dextran—a good example
   d. No T_H2 cytokine production
   e. Excellent stimulant for IgG production

3. Where are plasma cells primarily located?
   a. In the paracortical zone of lymph nodes
   b. In primary follicles
   c. In the germinal center
   d. In efferent lymphatics
   e. In the bloodstream

4. T_H1 cells _____ and are stimulated by _____.
   a. help CMI responses . . . IL-12, IFN-γ
   b. help humoral responses . . . IL-4, IL-5
   c. help CMI responses . . . IL-4, IL-5
   d. help humoral responses . . . IL-12, IFN-γ

5. Cell types affected by IL-1 include _____.
   a. PMNs
   b. hepatocytes
   c. neurons
   d. a and b
   e. a, b, and c

6. Binding of a cytotoxic T cell (CTL) to a tumor cell will result in _____.
   a. necrosis
   b. apoptosis
   c. cytolysis
   d. dysostosis
   e. dysmorphosis

7. For a CTL to bind to a tumor cell, _____ is necessary.
   a. tumor antigen
   b. MHC I
   c. B7-2
   d. a and b
   e. a, b, and c

8. For a CTL to kill a tumor cell, _____ is(are) necessary.
   a. perforins
   b. granzymes
   c. TNF-α
   d. a and b
   e. a, b, and c

9. Antibody-dependent cell-mediated cytotoxicity (ADCC) requires _____.
   a. Fab
   b. FcR
   c. ICAM
   d. a and b
   e. b and c

10. Activation of memory lymphocytes is called _____ and requires _____ antigen.
    a. anamnestic response . . . T-dependent
    b. anamnestic response . . . T-independent
    c. direct cytotoxicity . . . intracellular
    d. direct cytotoxicity . . . extracellular

MATCHING QUESTIONS

Match the surface structures in Column I to the cell type in Column 2.

Column 1	Column 2
11. IL-2R	a. B cells
12. Iccosomes	b. T cells
13. Addressins	c. Dendritic cells
14. Homing receptors	d. HEV
	e. a and b

ESSAY QUESTIONS

1. Describe a positive tuberculin skin test result and the tissue events that produce the symptoms

2. Summarize the activation process of naive B cells in a lymph node when presented with iccosomes. What cytokines are necessary for differentiation into antibody-secreting plasma cells?

SUGGESTIONS FOR FURTHER READING

Akira S, Hiramo T, Taga T, Kishimoto T, et al: Biology of multifunctional cytokines: IL-6 and related molecules (IL-1 and TNF). FASEB J 1990;4:2360–2867

Armitage RJ, Maliszewski CR, Alderson MR, et al: CD40L: A multifunctional ligand. Semin Immunol 1993;5:401–412

Barr PJ, Tomei LD: Apoptosis and its role in human disease. Biotechnology 1994;12:487–494

Clark EA, Ledbetter JA: How B and T cells talk to each other. Nature 1994;367:425–428

Dalton DK, Pitts-Meek S, Keshaw S, et al: Multiple defects of immune cell function in mice with disrupted interferon-γ genes. Science 1993;259: 1739–1742

Glauser MP, Zanetti G, Baumgartner JD, et al: Septic shock: Pathogenesis. Lancet 1991;338:732–736

Kagi D, Ledermann B, Burki K, et al: Cytotoxicity mediated by T cells and natural killer cells is greatly impaired in perforin-deficient mice. Nature 1994;369:31–37

Romagnani S: Human Th1 and Th2 subsets: Doubt no more. Immunol Today 1991;12:256–257

Taga T, Kishimoto T: Cytokine receptors and signal transduction. FASEB J 1993;7:3387–3396

Taniguchi T, Minami Y: The IL-2/IL-2 receptor system: A current overview. Cell 1993;79:5–8

Townsend SE, Allison JP: Tumor rejection after direct costimulation of CD8+ T cells by B7-transfected melanoma cells. Science 1993;259:368–370

REVIEW ANSWERS

1. e	8. e
2. e	9. e
3. c	10. a
4. a	11. e
5. e	12. c
6. b	13. d
7. e	14. e

8 The Complement System

Complement is a family of proteins circulating in the blood that interacts with antibodies and cells to generate reaction products that aid in antigen clearance and inflammatory responses. As far back as the 1890s, serologists observed that adding normal, nonimmune serum changed the consequences of many antigen-antibody reactions. This effect, which disappeared if the serum was heated, came to be known as **complement,** because it complemented immune activity that had developed independently. Complement activity evolves only after the constituent proteins interact in an obligatory sequence; antigen-antibody reactions often initiate the sequence, but other stimuli can also promote these interactions. Antigen-antibody reactions trigger the **classical pathway** of complement activation; other substances and events can initiate the **alternative pathway** of complement activation (Fig. 8–1). Biologic systems that require a stringent sequence of interactions are often described as **cascades.** Other physiologic cascades include the reactions that

145

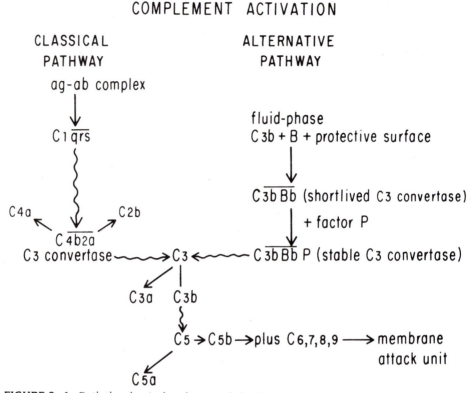

FIGURE 8–1. Both the classical pathway and the alternative pathway induce cleavage of C3, and the late-stage consequences are the same for both routes of activation. These consequences are generation of anaphylatoxic cleavage fragments, promotion of opsonic activity through attachment of C3b to surfaces, and generation of the membrane attack unit.

lead to coagulation activity, and the kinin system, which mediates many vascular events.

GENERAL PROPERTIES OF COMPLEMENT

Complement was first discovered in experiments with antibacterial antibodies. Native antibody would agglutinate suspended microorganisms into coarse clumps, but in the presence of complement, the antibody caused dissolution, or **lysis,** of the organisms. Antibodies against a variety of antigen-bearing cells may lyse their target when active complement is present. Lysis is especially conspicuous when the target is the red blood cell (RBC), because hemoglobin escapes from the cytoplasm and discolors the suspending medium.

Major Actions

Lysis is a commonly used end point for laboratory observations but is probably not the major role that complement plays in the human body. As the cascade progresses, enzyme activities evolve, proteins are cleaved, and polypeptide fragments accumulate. The major physiologic consequences of complement activation are opsonization, immune adherence, and anaphylatoxic activity, which influences inflammatory events.

Interaction With Cells

Fragments of complement molecules adhere to the surface of cells or particles at sites where activation occurs. Macrophages and neutrophils, the principal phagocytic inflammatory cells, have receptors for complement fragments; therefore, complemented coated cells or particles are engulfed and attacked much more effectively than uncoated targets. Enhancement of phagocytosis by the addition of materials onto the cell surface is called **opsonization.** Opsonization also results from attachment of immunoglobulin G (IgG) antibodies to surfaces. Phagocytic cells have receptors for the Fc portion of the IgG; these receptors are completely different from those for complement fragments.

Nonphagocytic cells also have receptors for complement fragments. B lymphocytes, RBCs, and many endothelial and epithelial cells express receptors for various complement fragments. In a process called **immune adherence,** protein aggregates that include complement or particles coated with complement may bind to receptors on cell membranes. This interaction intensifies the contact between a reactive cell and the antigen, particle, cell, or immune complex that provokes the reaction. Complement-mediated immune adherence can affect B-cell responses to antigen, the degradation of cells and proteins, and the regulation of inflammation and cell regeneration.

Effects on Inflammation

Complement exerts potent actions in enhancing inflammation. Several fragments generated by the complement sequence are called **anaphylatoxins;** these mediators promote vascular and cellular events in acute inflammation and stimulate basophilic and eosinophilic granulocytes and platelet granules to release stored materials that exert powerful effects on blood vessels, cellular synthetic processes, and coagulation sequences. Complement-derived anaphylatoxins attract neutrophils and macrophages, an action called **chemotaxis,** and affect endothelial cells and the permeability of small blood vessels. Complement products directly affect actions of macrophages, which are, in addition, secondarily stimulated by a variety of inflammatory and immune events.

Enzyme Activity

During sequential activation, many complement proteins acquire enzyme activity of the type described as **serine protease.** Serine proteases active in other contexts include trypsin, plasmin, thrombin, and elastase. All these proteins function as serine proteases and are powerful enzymes essential in restricted reactions but highly destructive if they manifest excessive, inappropriate, or misplaced activity. Serine proteases that evolve during the complement cascade generally lose their activity within a short time. While active, they may cleave protein substrates additional to those targeted in the complement sequence.

Terminology

Combination of antibody with antigen initiates the first step in the classical complement pathway. Contact of complement with protein aggregates or with materials of appropriate surface characteristics initiates the alternative pathway. The classical and alternative pathways converge and share a final common pathway (Fig. 8–1). Proteins of the classical pathway and of the later common phase are called **components** and are identified by numbers. Proteins of the alternative pathway are described as **factors** and are identified by letters. As interactions occur and inactive precursors become active, the state of activation is sometimes denoted by a bar above the letter or number. In the early activation phases, inactive precursor proteins are cleaved into **fragments** with various activities. The fragments are identified by lower-case letters. The "a" fragment is the small soluble molecule that enters the fluid medium, and the "b" and later fragments accumulate at the site of activation and participate in the cascade. The one exception to this nomenclature is C2. C2a is the larger fragment bound to the cell surface. As enzyme activity is generated, the active protein complex is called a **convertase,** because it converts the next protein in the sequence into the active form.

Cleavage of C3, the Pivotal Event

The most abundant complement component is C3; 1200 to 1600 μg is present in the serum. Both the classical and the alternative pathways have the same end point, namely, cleavage of C3 into C3a and C3b. This event has three major consequences: (1) the small, free C3a fragment has significant anaphylatoxic effect; (2) C3b and several of its evolutionary products have potent activity as opsonins and in immune adherence; and (3) suitably complexed C3b is the convertase necessary to perpetuate the cascade. Not every activation event precipitates the entire complement cascade; many physiologic effects occur following cleavage of C3, whether or not the later steps proceed. The liver is the site of most C3 synthesis, although activated macrophages may elaborate this and other complement components under localized conditions.

Consequences of C3 Cleavage

C3b perpetuates the complement cascade by serving as a C5 **convertase,** cleaving native C5 into C5a and C5b. C5a is a potent anaphylatoxin, with particularly striking effects on neutrophils. Accumulated C5a attracts neutrophils and causes increased enzyme activity and intracellular bacterial killing. C5b participates in the cascade, assembling the later-numbered components into the **membrane attack unit,** which lethally damages cell membranes. C5 cleavage is the last protein-splitting event in the complement cascade.

Later steps involve association and rearrangement of proteins. C5b causes C6 and C7 to form a stable C5b67 complex. This, in turn, attracts and gives structure to C8 and C9, the elements that actually penetrate the membrane. Association of C5b, C6, C7, C8, and C9 initiates the membrane attack unit without generating any independently active fragments. The classical and alternative pathways are identical in their effects on C5 and later assembly of the membrane attack unit.

THE CLASSICAL PATHWAY

Unfortunately, components of the classical pathway do not interact in the order in which they are numbered. Numbers were assigned as the proteins were identified, before clarification of their interaction sequence. The two phases of the classical pathway that lead to cleavage of C3 are called **recognition** and **activation.** C1 is involved in the recognition phase; C4 and C2 participate, in that order, in the activation phase that initiates C3 convertase activity.

Recognition

The recognition phase of the classical pathway requires the association of antibody with specific antigen. Once an antigen-antibody complex is formed, C1 binds if the antibody possesses a complement-binding domain in its heavy chain. Only after antibody has combined with antigen does complement activation begin, a process that takes place only at the site of antigen-antibody interaction. At least two Fc sites on adjacent bound IgG molecules are necessary for complement activation. IgM antibodies are more effective than any IgG subclass in activating the classical pathway because of their pentamer configuration and multiple Fc sites. Of the IgG subclasses, IgG1 and IgG3 are moderately effective, IgG2 is weakly active, and IgG4 is ineffective.

Physiologic Consequences

The greater efficiency of IgM has beneficial physiologic consequences. IgM antibodies, which develop early in the primary immune response, do not promote opsonization because phagocytic cells lack receptors for the mu chain. The combination of IgM with antigen, however, serves to attract and stimulate inflammatory cells by generating anaphylatoxic complement fragments and by promoting immune adherence and phagocytosis through deposition of C3b. Immune adherence brings the complement-coated antigenic material into contact with macrophages, the cells most capable of presenting it to additional antibody-producing cells. Antibodies that develop later in the immune response tend to have greater affinity for antigen than early appearing Igs and often express specificity against additional epitopes. As the immune response progresses, IgG antibodies predominate; these promote opsonization and immune adherence through their own properties, with less need for complement.

When Ig attaches to antigen through its Fab sites, a change in shape occurs that exposes the complement-binding site in the region. Complement does not bind to Ig molecules that have not first combined with antigen. Complement binds only when constant domains from two separate monomers lie close to one another; it does not unite with the symmetric parts of a single Fc portion.

The C1 Complex

C1 consists of three separable proteins that remain associated only in the presence of ionized calcium. The three proteins are called **C1q, C1r,** and **C1s.** It is C1q that attaches to the Ig heavy chain. After C1q binds to two Ig monomers. C1r and C1s undergo a configurational change that generates enzyme activity. C1q is a remarkable protein, consisting of 18 polypeptide chains and 6 globular protein masses (Fig.

8–2). Each globular mass is attached to three chains that twine into a triple helix; the complex resembles a bunch of flowers, with six blossoms, each supported by a triple-helical stem. The "six blossoms" are grouped into three pairs by disulfide bonds that link adjacent stems. Combination with Ig occurs through the globular heads; the stalks form a central support around which C1r and C1s enfold (Fig. 8–3).

Protein Interactions

At least two globular C1q heads must interact with constant domains of separate Ig monomers. A single bound IgG molecule will not initiate the process; there must be at least two IgG monomers sufficiently close together that two heads of a single C1q molecule can attach. IgM antibodies activate complement more effectively than IgG antibodies, because the IgM pentamer presents a simultaneous array of five different sites for C1q attachment. When IgM reacts with surface antigens, a single antigen-antibody event can initiate the complement cascade. If IgG is to activate complement, antigen sites must be spaced closely enough that two different antibody molecules can react independently within a small area. It has been estimated that at least 800 IgG molecules must attach to an RBC membrane before complement-mediated lysis will occur.

After C1q attaches, C1r undergoes a change in shape that uncovers serine protease activity. Active C1r̄ is an enzyme of exquisite specificity. Its only known substrate is C1s, which it cleaves to reveal another serine protease (Fig. 8–4). Activated C1s̄ also has highly restricted activity. Its only substrates are the next two components in the cascade, C4 and C2. The recognition phase of classical-pathway activation generates the C1q̄r̄s complex, which then initiates later events.

Inhibitory Actions

Factors that limit or modify the recognition phase are the specificity of antibody for antigen, the presence of appropriate domains on the Ig heavy (H) chain, the density of Ig monomers present, and the absence of interference with the actions of C1r̄ on C1s and of C1s̄ on other proteins. An inhibitor called **C1-INH**, interrupts this

STRUCTURE OF C1q

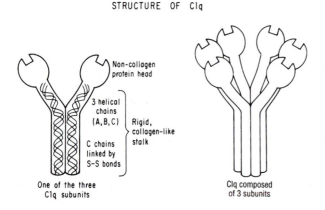

One of the three
C1q subunits

C1q composed
of 3 subunits

FIGURE 8–2. C1q consists of six globular masses of noncollagen protein plus strands of collagen-like protein twined into 18 helical chains. Each globular "head" has a "stalk" of three entwined chains, designated A, B, and C. Disulfide bonds link adjacent C chains to form paired units. Interaction with the heavy chain of bound immunoglobulin occurs through the globular protein heads. The collagen-like stalks provide the structural framework on which C1r and C1s interact.

STRUCTURE OF C1qrs

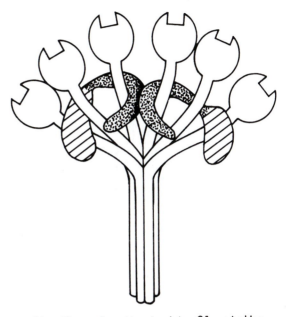

FIGURE 8–3. C1r and C1s are dimeric polypeptides that require the presence of ionized calcium to associate with one another and with the stalks of C1q. If ionized calcium is removed, C1r and C1s dissociate from C1q, and the classical-pathway cascade cannot occur.

C1r dimer is attached to C1q stalks.
C1s dimer is attached to C1r.

process if only small amounts are present, but massive accumulation of activated C1$\overline{\text{qrs}}$ overcomes the inhibitory effects. Absence of ionized calcium causes C1r and C1s to dissociate from C1q, so plasma anticoagulated with chelating agents like citrate or oxalate cannot manifest complement activity. Heating serum to 56°C will inactivate all elements of the C1 complex.

The Activation Phase

C1$\overline{\text{s}}$ exerts proteolytic action on the next protein, the large β_1-globulin called **C4.** C4 is the second most abundant complement protein, with a serum concentration of approximately 600 μg/mL, compared with approximately 1600 μg/mL for C3 and concentrations below 100 μg/mL for the other classical-pathway components (Table 8–1). Cleavage by C1$\overline{\text{s}}$ generates a small free-floating fragment, C4a, which has modest anaphylatoxic effect and a larger C4$\overline{\text{b}}$ fragment that possesses a highly reactive binding site (Fig. 8–5). This binding site is short-lived. Unless C4$\overline{\text{b}}$ binds to a substrate within a few seconds, it loses its ability to do so.

One C1$\overline{\text{s}}$ unit cleaves many molecules of C4, generating many activated C4b fragments, of which only a few actually attach to substrate. The rest are inactivated by a control protein **factor I,** formerly called C3bINA. C4$\overline{\text{b}}$ does not bind to the C1$\overline{\text{qrs}}$ complex or to the Ig molecule; it attaches to the cell membrane or bacterial wall at a separate site near the antigen-antibody reaction. C1 is the only complement protein that reacts directly with the Ig molecule.

ACTIVATION OF C1q̄r̄s̄

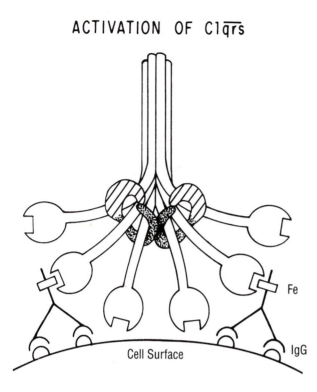

Attachment of C1q changes molecular shape, allows activation of C1rs.

FIGURE 8–4. When two or more globular heads of C1q attach to bound immunoglobulin molecules, the collagen-like stalks change their configuration. The resulting shape change causes C1r to evolve into a serine protease, which cleaves a small fragment off C1s. This uncovers the C1s serine protease, whose sole targets are C4 and C2.

C2 and Its Actions

Besides its action on C4, C1s also cleaves **C2,** a single-chain protein present at low serum concentration. Cleavage generates a small free fragment that enters the fluid phase and a larger fragment that adheres to the active surface. The nomenclature for the C2 fragments is anomalous; the large fragment that perpetuates the cascade is called "a" and the small fluid-phase fragment is 2b. C1s̄ has only weak action against free C2 molecules. However, C2 that has united with C4b is more suscepti-ble to C1s̄ cleavage. C1s̄ thus promotes accumulation of C4b2a on the antigen-bear-ing surface. C4b2a possesses potent but short-lived convertase activity against free C3 molecules (Fig. 8–6). If it does not encounter its substrate, C4b2a decays within a few minutes.

C4b2a divides the C3 molecule into the small, fluid-phase C3a, which has ana-phylatoxic activity, and the much larger C3b, which expresses an active binding site (Fig. 8–7). Each C4b2a complex cleaves many C3 molecules, generating many ana-phylatoxic C3a fragments and many C3b residues that must either bind promptly to a surface or be degraded by factor I. When C3b combines with C4b2a, the resulting C4b2a3b complex is a potent C5 convertase. Many C3b molecules bind indepen-

TABLE 8–1. **Proteins of the Complement System**

Designation	Molecular Weight (kD)	Electrophoretic Mobility	Inactivated by 56°C Incubation	Approximate Serum Concentration (μg/mL)
Classical Pathway				
C1q	385–400	γ2	Yes	70
C1r	190	β	Yes	34
C1s	87	α	Yes	31
C4	206–209	β1	No	450–600
C2	117	β1	Yes	25–30
C3	180–185	β1	No	1300–1600
Alternative Pathway				
Factor B	93–100	β2		200–240
Factor D	23–24	β2		1–2
Factor P (properdin)	220	γ2		25
C3	180–185	β1		1300–1600
Terminal Sequence				
C5	190–206	β1	Yes	70–75
C6	120–128	β2	No	60–65
C7	110–121	β2	No	55
C8	150–153	γ1	Yes	55–80
C9	71–79	α	Yes	60–160

CLEAVAGE OF C4

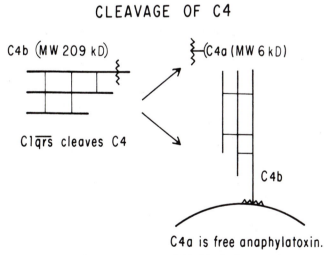

C4a is free anaphylatoxin.
C4b binds to membrane.

FIGURE 8–5. C4 is a large protein with three chains. The C1s protease cleaves a small fragment from the longest chain, uncovering a short-lived binding site through which the large fragment can attach to a membrane or surface. The small cleavage fragment C4a remains in the fluid phase and has anaphylatoxic activity.

CLEAVAGE OF C2

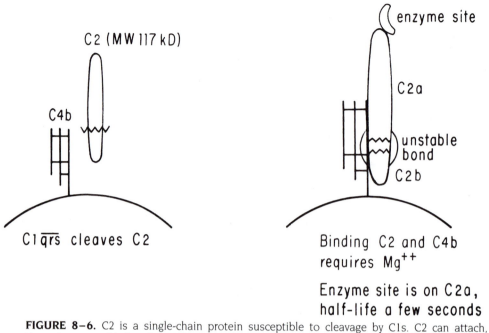

FIGURE 8–6. C2 is a single-chain protein susceptible to cleavage by C1s. C2 can attach, through an unstable bond, to C4b present on a membrane. C1s has stronger proteolytic activity against C2 molecules associated with C4b than against free C2. Cleavage of C2 by C1s generates a small fluid-phase fragment, designated C2b, and a large fragment, designated C2a, which joins the C4b complex and expresses an enzyme site capable of perpetuating the cascade.

dently to the membrane surface; these fragments do not propagate the complement cascade, but they do promote the immune adherence and opsonizing effects described previously.

Effects of Activation

Activation of the classical pathway results in an antigen-bearing surface that exhibits numerous attached C3b molecules. In the C$\overline{4b2a3b}$ complex is potent C5 convertase activity. Activation also generates moderate numbers of C4a fragments and larger numbers of C3a fragments free in the surrounding medium. After C$\overline{4b2a}$ forms, the Ig molecules and attached C1 are no longer necessary for cell lysis. Antibody can elute from the antigen-bearing surface without affecting later complement-mediated events.

Mannose-Binding Protein

Low levels of **mannose-binding protein (MBP)** are found in normal serum and have a role in activating the classical-complement pathway. MBP is a lectin, which is a protein that binds to sugars. Mannose is a sugar found in the cell wall of many bacteria. Binding of MBP to bacteria activates a proteolytic enzyme complex that

CLEAVAGE OF C3

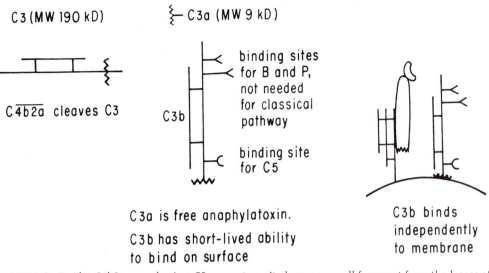

FIGURE 8-7. The C4b2a complex is a C3 convertase. It cleaves a small fragment from the larger of the two C3 chains; the small C3a fragment remains in the fluid phase as an anaphylatoxin. The large C3b fragment binds to the membrane near, but not in, the C4b2a complex. One C4b2a complex can generate large numbers of C3b units, which exert powerful opsonic effects. Membrane-bound C3b also serves as the C5 convertase, which perpetuates the cascade.

cleaves C4 and C2 to initiate the classical-complement cascade. Macrophages are also involved because activation of these cells induces the secretion of interleukin-1 (IL-1), IL-6, and tumor necrosis factors-α (TNF-α). These cytokines stimulate hepatocytes to secrete MBP. MBP is also a potent opsonin and therefore enhances phagocytosis and by means of complement activation, enhances the inflammatory response.

THE ALTERNATIVE PATHWAY

Like the classical pathway, the alternative pathway generates fluid-phase C3a and surface-bound C3b, which eventually results in formation of C5 convertase activity, but the initiating events are very different. Alternative-pathway activation is surface-dependent. The plasma proteins interact and accumulate exclusively on surfaces displaying the required characteristics. No antigen-antibody reaction is necessary, and no previous host exposure to foreign material or pathogenic microorganisms is necessary. Required proteins are already present in plasma. The critical element is a surface that permits accumulation.

Proteins Involved

Proteins of the alternative pathway perform activities approximately comparable to those in the classical pathway. **Factor D,** a small protein present in very low concentration, corresponds to C1s; **factor B,** present at approximately 240 μ/mL, is analogous to C2. C3 participates in the early interactions of the alternative pathway as well as in the later C5 convertase complex. Another major participant is **properdin (factor P),** a large molecule present in serum at approximately 25 μ/mL, which serves to stabilize the evolving molecular complex. The alternative pathway was originally called the **properdin system,** based on the enhancing effects of this large serum protein (Table 8–1).

It is important to understand that plasma proteins continually undergo low-level cleavage. Precursor proteins in many mediator systems spontaneously evolve into activated forms, but unless they accumulate to a critical concentration, the randomly activated molecules have no biologic effect. Alternative-pathway activation results from this continuous generation of C3b in normal body fluids and plasma.

Interactions in Fluid

The major C3 convertase of the alternative pathway is the $\overline{C3bBb}$ complex, of which small amounts accumulate through spontaneous cleavage events. C3 is cleaved to C3b, which generates slight activity as a C3 convertase and modest proteolytic action against the alternative-pathway protein called **factor B.** The enzyme principally responsible for cleaving factor B into Bb is not C3b, however, but **factor D.** Factor D circulates as an active protease in normal plasma, but at very low concentrations. It does not degrade plasma proteins in an uncontrolled fashion because it is highly restricted as to substrate. Factor D's only target is factor B, specifically factor B that has bound to C3b (Fig. 8–8). Factor B binds in a random fashion to available C3b and thus becomes subject to factor D action, but very little $\overline{C3bBb}$ accumulates. Under normal conditions, only small amounts of C3b are available because most normal cells have high levels of sialic acid, which inactivates bound C3b. C3b is also degraded by the control protein, **factor I.** Furthermore, interaction of factor B with C3b is inhibited by another control protein, **factor H** (see later section). Consequently, there is little C3bB complex on which factor D can act.

Interactions on Surfaces

The limiting conditions of described previously change if the plasma proteins interact on certain surfaces with appropriate properties. These include cell-wall polysaccharides of yeasts and some bacteria, aggregated protein complexes, bacterial endotoxins, and products of trypsin and other enzymes. The effect of these surfaces is to shelter C3b, factor B, and $\overline{C3bBb}$ complexes from the dissociative effect of factor H and the degradative actions of factor I (Fig. 8–9). This protection allows factor B to bind to C3b in quantities sufficient for factor D to generate abundant $\overline{C3bBb}$. Accumulating $\overline{C3bBb}$ serves as a C3 convertase that generates additional C3b, which attracts and cleaves additional factor B. Accumulating $\overline{C3bBb}$ is the target of additional factor D activity, and so on. This autocatalytic process does not exhaust serum C3 because C3 is present at serum concentrations more than adequate to perpetuate the process (see Table 8–1).

The $\overline{C3bBb}$ complex has a short half-life—approximately 5 minutes. The function of **properdin** is to bind to $\overline{C3bBb}$ and to prolong its half-life to 30 minutes,

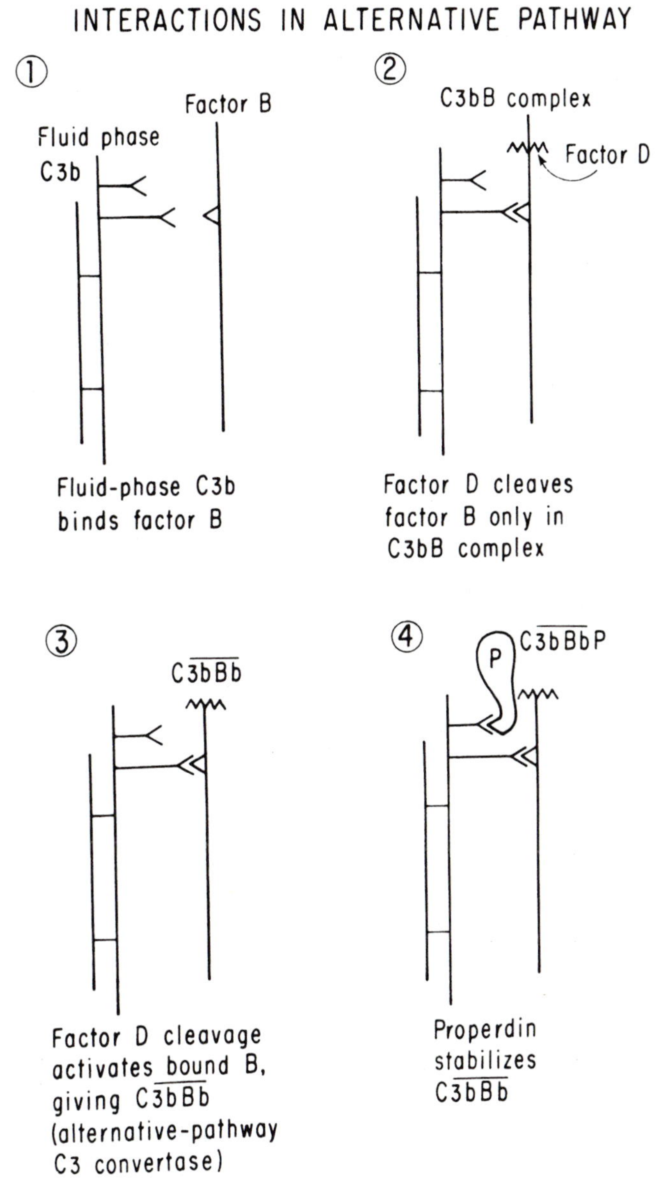

INTERACTIONS IN ALTERNATIVE PATHWAY

FIGURE 8–8. The alternative pathway involves four interactions. Small amounts of C3b form spontaneously in the fluid phase and bind factor B, shown in 1. Bound factor B is the target for cleavage by factor D, as shown in 2, leaving the large Bb fragment bound to C3b. The C3bBb complex is a C3 convertase, cleaving additional C3 molecules to generate additional C3b, which can bind additional factor B, as shown in 3. The C3bBb complex retains C3 convertase activity for only a short time, unless stabilized by combination with properdin (factor P), as shown in 4. Factors I and H, in the plasma, inhibit fluid-phase interactions among C3b, factor B, and factor D.

thereby amplifying its physiologic effects. Properdin does not initiate the sequence, but it enhances the accumulation and reactivity of $\overline{C3bBb}$ (see Fig. 8–8).

C5 is cleaved by molecular complexes that contain C3b. Surface-bound C3b generated by the alternative pathway has the same convertase effect as C3b produced by the classical pathway (Fig. 8–10). Both pathways achieve the same effects: (1) coating of the cell, particle, bacterium, or aggregate by opsonic C3b; (2) generation of the anaphylatoxins C3a and C5a; and (3) generation of C5b, which mobilizes C6, C7, C8, and C9 into the membrane attack unit.

ROLE OF SURFACE
IN ALTERNATIVE PATHWAY

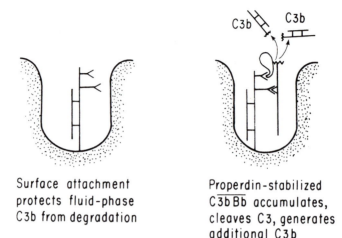

Surface attachment
protects fluid-phase
C3b from degradation

Properdin-stabilized
C$\overline{3b}$ $\overline{Bb}$ accumulates,
cleaves C3, generates
additional C3b

FIGURE 8–9. Effective generation of alternative-pathway activity requires a protective surface so that protein interactions can occur without inhibition by factors I and H. Alternative-pathway surfaces provide a sheltered location on which the C3bB complex can accumulate, allowing cleavage by factor D into the C3bBb complex, which then promotes additional C3b accumulation. Stabilization of the evolving C3bBb complexes by properdin enhances the capacity to cleave C3 and to generate activated products.

C3b IS C5 CONVERTASE

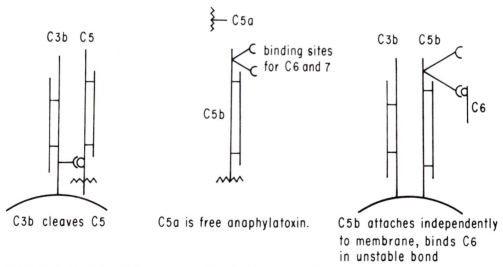

C3b cleaves C5.

C5a is free anaphylatoxin.

C5b attaches independently
to membrane, binds C6
in unstable bond

FIGURE 8–10. C3b, whether generated by the classical or the alternative pathway, acts as a C5 convertase. It cleaves a small fragment from the larger of the two C5 chains, generating fluid-phase C5a, which is a potent anaphylatoxin. The larger C5b fragment binds to membranes and interacts with C6 to form a loosely bound, unstable complex.

THE MEMBRANE ATTACK UNIT

Cleavage of **C5** generates the small fluid-phase C5a fragment and the larger residual molecule, C5b. C5a is a potent anaphylatoxin. C5b is a highly active molecule with a very short life. It decays spontaneously in 0.1 second if binding does not occur. C5b can interact with soluble complement proteins or can bind to nearly any membrane or surface. Its does not cleave other proteins; its effect on later components is one of steric rearrangement (see Fig. 8–10). C5b attracts **C6,** which forms a soluble C5b6 complex to which C7 subsequently attaches. C5b67, during its period of reactivity, will cling tightly to any cell membrane it touches. Fluid-phase C5b67 complex can deposit on any nearby cell or membrane, independent of the nature or location of the initial activating event. This is called the **innocent bystander phenomenon,** because the site on which the complex settles may be totally uninvolved in ongoing immune or inflammatory activities. Instead of attaching to membrane, the C5b67 complex may cohere into a free-floating spherical unit called a **micelle,** which can exert an independent destructive effect on viral proteins.

Association of C6 and C7 with C5b is followed by gradual attachment of **C8** and later of **C9.** When C8 combines with C5b67 on a membrane, it disturbs the membrane in a way that slowly damages osmotic regulation and gradually destroys the cell. Attached C8 provides a site on which C9 units can polymerize; polymerized C9 generates a discrete tubular structure that penetrates the membrane and causes rapid osmotic disruption of the cell (Fig. 8–11). Complement-mediated membrane dissolution lyses the target cell. The process may be activated by the cell in ques-

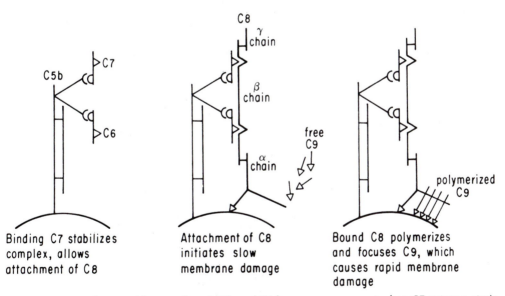

EVOLUTION OF MEMBRANE ATTACK UNIT

Binding C7 stabilizes complex, allows attachment of C8

Attachment of C8 initiates slow membrane damage

Bound C8 polymerizes and focuses C9, which causes rapid membrane damage

FIGURE 8–11. The unstable complex of C5b and C6 becomes permanent when C7 enters a steric bond with C5b. The C5b67 complex enters a steric interaction with the three-chain C8 molecule. The C5b678 complex initiates a slow attack on membrane integrity and also provides a setting on which individual C9 molecules can polymerize. Polymerized C9 rapidly generates a discrete "hole" in the cell membrane.

tion or can involve surrounding cells that are innocent-bystanders. Table 8–2 lists the numbered complement components and summarizes their interactions.

CONTROL OVER THE SYSTEM

Ordinarily, complement activity remains at the site of the initiating event, so only the antigen-bearing surface or the localized fluid environment sustains the potent biologic consequences. Uncontrolled or widespread complement activity could cause dangerous inflammatory and cytolytic effects. Two control mechanisms exist: (1) individual protein molecules have a relatively short half-life, and (2) numerous control proteins—some free in plasma and others on cell membranes—prevent excessive accumulation of activated elements. Every 24 hours, approximately half the plasma complement molecules undergo replacement. Although macrophages and other cells are capable of synthesizing many complement proteins, most of the circulating elements are derived from the liver. Plasma complement levels rise if systemic events enhance hepatic protein synthesis (e.g., acute inflammation). In severe liver disease, complement levels fall because reduced protein production cannot compensate for continuous degradation.

C1 Inhibitor

The control protein that acts earliest is C1 inhibitor, also called α_2-neuraminoglycoprotein or **C1-INH,** which interferes with activation of C1r and C1s. The C1 inhibitor combines irreversibly with C1q that has bound to Ig, forcing C1r and C1s to dissociate. C1q remains bound to the Ig, but no C1s esterase activity evolves to cleave C4. C1-INH has other targets besides C1r and C1s; it inhibits the actions of the pro-

TABLE 8–2. **Evolution of Complement Activities**

Original Protein	Active Protein	Physiologic Activities
C1q	Bound C1q	Binds to Ig heavy chain, activates C1r
C1r	C1r̄	Cleaves C1s
C1s	C1s̄	Cleaves C4 and C2 (more effective on C2 bound to C4b than free C2)
C4	C4a	Anaphylatoxin; provokes histamine release
	C4b̄	Binds to C2; has weak opsonic effect
C2	C2a	When bound to C4b, cleaves C3
C3	C3a	Anaphylatoxin; provokes histamine release
	C3b	Bound monomers are opsonic
		When bound to C4b2a complex, cleaves C5
C5	C5a	Potent anaphylatoxin; attracts and activates PMNs; promotes release of oxygen species, inflammatory mediators (also provokes histamine release)
	C5b	Promotes association of C6–9
		Binds to any available membrane
C6, 7	C5b67	Forms micelles; promotes attachment of C8 and C9
C8	C8	In C5b678 complex, causes slow membrane leak
C9	Polymerized C9	In C5b6789 complex, produces transmembrane tubule, acute osmotic lysis

PMNs, polymorphonuclear leukocytes.

teases: plasmin, kallikrein, activated factor XII (Hageman factor), and activated factor XI. Normal activity of the coagulation and inflammation systems depends on precisely adjusted concentrations of active materials. These proteases are intimately interrelated in maintaining suitably balanced levels of activated proteins. C1-INH, which is widely distributed in plasma, helps regulate these proteases and maintain adequate but not excessive levels of active products. In C1-INH deficiency, a relatively rare genetic abnormality, these complex interactions are significantly distorted.

Congenital Deficiency

C1-INH is the only material that inhibits activation of C1qrs. With deficiency of C1-INH, excessive C1s accumulates, large amounts of C2 are cleaved, and excessive levels of C2b develop. After contact with plasmin and other enzymes of the inflammatory and coagulation systems, C2b is converted into a protein that is inactive in the complement cascade but has massive effects on vascular permeability. Patients with C1-INH deficiency suffer from excessive and inappropriate enhancement of vascular permeability, in a condition called **hereditary angioedema.** Complement dysfunction is not conspicuous in this condition, presumably because the alternative pathway compensates for defective classical-pathway activation.

Factor I

The most broadly reactive control protein is **factor I,** formerly called C3b inactivator or C3bINA. Because it modifies the reactive portions of both C4b and C3b, it affects both the classical and the alternative pathways. Factor I cleaves the large C4b and C3b proteins into small, biologically inert free fragments designated "c" and residual large fragments called "d," which remain bound to the membrane but have no effect on other proteins. Generation of C4d aborts the classical pathway. Generation of C3d leaves cells coated with a protein that has little opsonic effect. Granulocytes and macrophages have receptors for C3b but not for C3d, and cells coated with C3d are not more rapidly phagocytized than noncoated cells or particles. B lymphocytes express C3d receptors, but the immunologic significance of this potential for interaction between C3d-coated material and resting B lymphocytes remains unclear.

Alternative-Pathway Effects

Factor I also affects the alternative pathway. When it interacts with C3b, it occupies the molecular site to which factor B would otherwise attach. During spontaneous evolution of C3b, factor B and factor I compete for this binding site. Attachment of factor I prevents accumulation of the C3bBb complex that initiates the alternative pathway. When the unbound proteins interact in fluid, factor I attaches more effectively than factor B. If C3b accumulates on an activating surface, the equilibrium shifts to favor factor B. Alternative-pathway activators provide a sheltered location in which C3bBb can evolve, allowing accumulation of active elements and protecting the bound C3b from cleavage by factor I.

Cofactor Proteins in Plasma

Several cofactors enhance factor I activity against its substrates C4b and C3b. Whereas accumulation on an activator surface shifts the C3b equilibrium toward

TABLE 8–3. **Plasma Proteins That Regulate Complement Interactions**

Designation	Other Terms Used	Molecular Weight (kd)	Approximate Serum Concentration (µg/mL)
C1 inhibitor	C1-INH, C1 esterase inhibitor	105	150–180
Factor I	C3b inactivator, C3bINA, KAF	88	35
Factor H	C3b inactivator accelerator, B1H	150	360–500
C4-binding protein	C4BP	500–590	400
Mannose-binding protein	C-type lectin	400–700	0.07–6.4

factor B attachment, combination with the control protein **factor H** gives factor I the competitive advantage. Factor H modifies one chain of fluid-phase C3b, rendering it more receptive to cleavage and degradation by factor I. When sheltered on an activator surface, C3b is not affected by factor H.

A separate protein enhances the interaction of factor I with C4b. Called **C4-binding protein (C4BP),** it acts on either fluid-phase or bound C4b, rendering it susceptible to attack by factor I. If C4BP and factor I predominate in the protein mix, classical-pathway activation will cease. If there is enough C4b to overcome the effects of C4BP, then C3b is generated in its bound form, and this circumvents the effect of factor H allowing the cascade to go on to completion. Table 8–3 lists the serum proteins that regulate complement activity.

Cell-Membrane Proteins

In addition to inhibitory proteins in serum, several cell-bound glycoproteins also restrict complement activity. A recently systematized group of proteins called **complement receptors (CR proteins)** have specificity for different fragments of C3 (Table 8–4).

CR1—The Receptor for C3b

The gene determining production of CR1 resides on chromosome 1 in a cluster that also contains genes for factor H and the C4-binding protein. CR1 glycoprotein acts as a cell-bound cofactor for factor I, affecting bound C3b in a manner comparable to the effect of factor H in the fluid phase. It also accelerates the decay of complexes that would generate more C3b. Cells exhibiting CR1 can form rosettes with cells coated with either C3b or C4b. Most blood cells, including RBCs, neutrophils, T and B lymphocytes, and monocyte/macrophages, express the CR1 glycoprotein.

CR1 can adsorb partially activated complement components or immune complexes (ICs) containing C3b that are in body fluids or on surfaces. The large numbers of RBCs with CR1 receptors may serve to remove ICs from the blood. Removal of ICs is important to prevent widespread tissue damage. Deficiency of CR1 receptors and C4, which affects binding of C3 to ICs, are among the most common predisposing defects of the autoimmune disease, systemic lupus erythematosus (SLE).

TABLE 8−4. **Complement Receptors on Cell Membrane**

Receptor	Ligand	Cellular Distribution	Function
CR1	C3b	RBCs, neutrophils, B lymphocytes, T lymphocytes (some), monocytes, macrophages, follicular dendritic cells, glomerular podocytes	Cofactor for degradation of immune complexes
CR2	C3d, C3dg*	B lymphocytes, follicular dendritic cells	Enhances B-cell response to antigen Acts as EBV receptor
CR3	iC3b*	Monocytes, macrophages, neutrophils, follicular dendritic cells	Involved in cell-adherence functions, antibody-mediated cellular cyto-toxicity Related to lymphocyte function-associated (LFA-1) antigen
CR4	C3dg*	Monocytes, neutrophils	Not clear
C5a receptor	C5a	Monocytes, macrophages, neutrophils, mast cells	Activates macrophage phagocytosis of complement-coated bacteria Mediator for anaphylatoxic effects of C5a on inflammatory cells
C1q receptor	C1q	Monocytes, macrophages, platelets, fibroblasts, neutrophils	Binds immune complexes; interacts with collagen-like portion of molecule

EBV, Epstein-Barr virus; RBCs, red blood cells. Intermediate cleavage fragments of C3.

Other Receptors

In contrast to CR1, the membrane protein called **decay-accelerating factor (DAF)** or CD55 affects only components on its own cell membrane. This glycoprotein, present predominantly on RBCs, protects the RBC from complement attack by enhancing the activity of factor I on either C3b or C4b. Patients with **paroxysmal nocturnal hemoglobinuria (PNH)** have RBCs that are excessively sensitive to complement-mediated hemolysis and have significantly reduced levels of DAF. The DAF deficiency, however, appears to develop as a consequence of the condition rather than existing as a constitutional abnormality that renders the person susceptible to PNH.

Another C3b-binding membrane glycoprotein is called **membrane cofactor protein (MCP),** This protein is present on macrophages, B cells and T cells, platelets, and endothelial cells. MCP acts as a cofactor for cleavage of C3b or C4b by factor I.

CD59 or **protectin** is another regulatory protein found on RBCs, endothelial cells, and white cells that acts late in the complement cascade. It blocks insertion of the C5b678 complex into the cell membrane and thus prevents polymerization of C9.

Table 8−5 summarizes the major controlling materials that affect the complement cascade.

TABLE 8–5. **Control Proteins in the Complement System**

Control Material	Target	Action
C1-INH	C1qrs Other serine proteases	Inhibits activation phase of classical pathway
Factor I (formerly C3bINH)	C4b and C3b, classical pathway	Generation of C4d and C3d, which have little physiologic function
	C3b, in alternative pathway	Prevents interaction with factor B, by occupying binding site
Factor H	C3b free in fluids	Renders protein more susceptible to cleavage by factor I
C4-binding protein (C4BP)	C4b, either bound or free in fluids	Renders protein more susceptible to cleavage by factor I
CR1	C3b bound to surfaces or complexes	Renders protein more susceptible to cleavage by factor I; inhibits C3 convertase action of complexes containing C3b
Decay-accelerating factor (DAF) (CD55)	C4b or C3b on same cell as DAF molecule	Renders protein more susceptible to cleavage by factor I
Membrane cofactor protein (CD46)	C3b, iC3b	Cofactor for cleavage of C3b or C4b by Factor I
Protectin (CD59)	C5b678	Blocks insertion of complex and polymerization of C9

SUMMARY

1. Complement is a family of proteins circulating in the blood, which interact in a sequential manner with antibodies (classical pathway) or surfaces of microorganisms (alternative pathway) to aid in clearance of antigens and the inflammatory response. Sequential activation of proteins is referred to as a cascade, and in the complement cascade enzyme activities evolve, proteins are cleaved, and polypeptide fragments accumulate. Complement fragments have anaphylatoxic activity, are opsonins, and are capable of immune adherence. Complement activation in its final stages results in lysis of cells.

2. Complement proteins are referred to as components in the classical pathway and factors in the alternative pathway. Each component in the classical pathway is indicated by a number, whereas alternative-pathway factors are indicated by letters. Fragments resulting from cleavage are identified by lowercase letters, with "a" usually indicating the smaller soluble fragment and "b" the larger fragment accumulating at the site of activation.

3. The pivotal event of either the classical or alternative cascade is cleavage of C3. Cleavage of C3 results in fragment C3a, which has significant anaphylatoxic activity, and C3b, which has opsonin and immune adherence activity and is a C5 convertase.

4. Initial phases of the classical pathway are recognition and activation.
   a. C1 is involved in the recognition phase. Antibody binding to antigen causes a structural modification of the Fc region, which exposes a complement-binding site. If two adjacent Fc complement-binding sites are present, the globular heads of C1q bind and associated C1r polypeptides gain serine protease activity. C1r then cleaves C1s.
   b. In the activation phase, C1s cleaves the next component in the cascade. Resulting fragments C4a have modest anaphylatoxic effects, and C4b is capable of binding to nearby cell membranes. C2 can attach through an unstable bond to C4b. Attached C2 is susceptible to cleavage by C1s. Formation of a C4b2a complex generates C3 protease activity.

5. Mannose-binding proteins (MBP) are found in normal serum and can bind to bacterial cell walls. Binding of MBP activates a proteolytic enzyme complex that cleaves C4 and C2 to initiate the classical complement cascade.

6. Alternative-pathway activation does not require antigen-antibody binding. Rather, plasma proteins interact and accumulate on appropriate surfaces. In the presence of surfaces such as cell-wall polysaccharides of yeast and some bacteria, C3b and factor B bind and can be cleaved by factor D to form C3bBb. Bacterial surfaces shelter the C3bBb complexes from degradation by factor I and the control protein factor H. C3bBb is a C3 convertase that generates more C3b, which in turn attracts and cleaves additional factor B. Properdin binds C3bBb, prolongs its half-life, and thereby amplifies its physiologic effects. The major physiologic effect of C3bBb complexes is to cleave C5.

7. The membrane attack unit is formed when C5b binds to nearby surfaces. C5b attracts C6 to which C7 subsequently attaches. C8 combines with C567 and provides a site for C9 polymerization. Polymerized C9 forms tubular structures that penetrate the membrane and cause rapid lysis. This process may occur on an appropriate target surface or may sometimes involve nearby normal cells that are "innocent bystanders."

8. Normally, complement activity is localized to an initiating site. Uncontrolled or widespread complement activity is inhibited by several control proteins. C1-INH interferes with activation of C1r and C1s. Factor I can cleave C4b and C3b, thus inhibiting the classical pathway. Factor I and factor B compete in fluid for binding with C3b. However, appropriate surfaces promote factor B interaction and therefore accumulation of C3bBb and subsequent cleavage of C5. Complement activity is also restricted by factor H. Various complement receptors on RBCs, neutrophils, lymphocytes, and monocytes bind complement fragments and thereby help to remove these fragments from the blood and aid in degradation.

REVIEW QUESTIONS

1. The most abundant complement component is _____.
   a. C1
   b. C2
   c. C3
   d. C4
   e. C5

2. _____ is the component necessary for initiating assembly of the membrane attack unit.
   a. C4b
   b. C5a
   c. C5b
   d. C6
   e. C7

3. Complement is formed by _____.
   a. hepatocytes
   b. macrophages
   c. neutrophils
   d. erythrocytes
   e. a and b

4. Activation of the classical pathway requires binding of at least _____.
   a. one IgG monomer or one IgM pentamer
   b. two adjacent IgG monomers or one IgM pentamer
   c. three adjacent IgG monomers or one IgA dimer
   d. two adjacent IgG monomers or two IgA dimers
   e. one IgM pentamer or one IgA dimer

5. The globular heads of _____ attach to _____ of antibody in the recognition phase of the classical pathway.
   a. C1q . . . the Fc region
   b. C1r . . . the Fc region
   c. C1s . . . the Fc region
   d. C1q . . . the Fab region
   e. C1r . . . the Fab region

6. Heating serum to _____ will inactivate complement components.
   a. 37°C
   b. 46°C
   c. 56°C
   d. 65°C
   e. 70°C

7. CR1 binds _____ and is present on _____.
   a. C3b . . . red blood cells
   b. C4b . . . monocytes
   c. C5b . . . epithelial cells
   d. a and b
   e. a, b, and c

MATCHING QUESTIONS

Match the descriptions in Column 1 to the components or factors in Column 2.

Column 1	Column 2
8. Have anaphylatoxic activities	a. C1, C4, C2, C3
9. Early components of the alternative pathway	b. C5, C6, C7, C8, C9

10. Component of the membrane attack complex

    c. C3bBbD

    d. C4b2a

    e. C3a, C5a

Column 1	*Column 2*
11. Will cleave B	a. D
12. Stabilizes C3bBb	b. C5a
	c. Properdin
	d. C1q
	e. C9

Column 1	*Column 2*
13. Has C3 convertase activity	a. C4b2a
14. Has C5 convertase activity	b. C3bBb
15. Reaction catalyzed by factor D	c. C4b2a3b
	d. a and b
	e. b and c

ESSAY QUESTIONS

16. Compare the activation steps for the alternative and classical-complement cascades. How are they different and how are they similar?
17. Uncontrolled complement activity can cause dangerous inflammatory and cytolytic effects in the body. Describe three control mechanisms and explain how they inhibit complement activity.

SUGGESTIONS FOR FURTHER READING

DiScipio R: The relationship between polymerization of complement component C9 and membrane channel formation. J Immunol 1991;147:4239–4247

Frank M, Fries LF: The role of complement in inflammation and phagocytosis. Immunol Today 1991;12: 322–326

Kinoshita T: Biology of complement: The overture. Immunol Today 1991;12:291–294

Matsushita M, Fujita T: Activation of the classical complement pathway by mannose binding proteins in association with a novel C1s-like serine protease. J Exp Med 1992;176:1497–1502.

Sim RB, Reid KBM: C1: Molecular interactions with activating systems. Immunol Today 1991;12:307–311

Terai I, Kobayashi K, Fujita T, Hagiwara K: Human serum mannose binding protein (MBP): Development of an enzyme-linked immunosorbent assay (ELISA) and determination of levels in serum from 1085 normal Japanese and in some body fluids. Biochem Med Metabol Biol 1993;50(1):111–119

REVIEW ANSWERS

1. c	6. c	11. a
2. c	7. d	12. c
3. e	8. e	13. d
4. b	9. a	14. e
5. a	10. b	15. b

PART
II
CLINICAL
APPLICATIONS

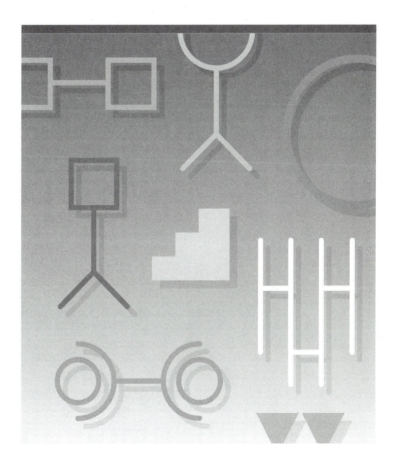

9 Protective Immunity

The immune mechanisms discussed in the preceding chapters serve protective functions against microbial invasion, and regulatory functions that affect generation, differentiation, and function of many cells and tissues. This chapter considers antimicrobial immune effects. The regulatory actions are distinguished most clearly through the consequences of malfunction; succeeding chapters consider immune deficiencies and dysfunctions.

Immunity can be acquired actively or passively. The transfer of protective material from an individual immune to a specific antigen to another individual with no established protection against that antigen is called **passive immunization. Active immunization** is the response made by an immunocompetent individual to microorganisms, their products, or other antigens. This chapter discusses the mechanisms of active and passive immunization and the protective effects of each type of immunity.

PASSIVE IMMUNITY

Passive immunization involves humoral immunity almost exclusively. Antibodies can be transferred from one individual to another easily, but transfer of viable cells is fraught with difficulties. In nature, the only route for passive immunization is transfer of maternal antibodies to the fetus. As a medical intervention, deliberate injection of specific antibodies is a useful therapeutic approach in selected circumstances.

Transfer Across the Placenta

The normal fetus develops in an immunologically protected environment. No infectious agents should penetrate the amniotic sac, and the intact placenta prevents maternal cells from entering the fetus. Small molecules, including some proteins, do cross the placenta, but these maternal molecules almost never provoke an immune response in the fetus. Having had little stimulus for immune activity, the newborn infant possesses little functionally mature immune tissue. The fetal bloodstream does contain antibodies. These are immunoglobulin-G1 (IgG1) and IgG3 molecules that have passed from mother to fetus across isotype-specific receptors on placental cells (Fig. 9–1).

There is no selection for antigenic specificity; IgG molecules of those subclasses are transferred indiscriminately from maternal to fetal bloodstream. This transfer may be deleterious if maternal antibodies have specificity for antigens present on fetal cells. **Hemolytic disease of the newborn (HDN),** discussed

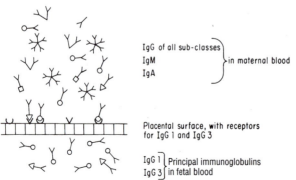

SELECTIVE TRANSFER OF IMMUNOGLOBULINS
ACROSS PLACENTA

IgG of all sub-classes
IgM   } in maternal blood
IgA

Placental surface, with receptors
for IgG 1 and IgG 3

IgG 1 } Principal immunoglobulins
IgG 3 } in fetal blood

FIGURE 9–1. Receptors on placental cells transfer IgG1 and IgG3 from maternal to fetal bloodstream. The receptors are specific for isotype, not for idiotype, so all antigenic specificities in the mother's IgG1 and IgG3 repertoire are present in the fetus.

more fully in Chapter 12, is an example of this event. With this exception, passively transferred maternal antibodies benefit the child. During a lifetime of exposure, the mother will have developed antibodies against a wide range of organisms. The newborn, who suddenly experiences all the pathogens present in the newly encountered environment, has the benefit of the mother's immune history. This protection is not, absolute. A large infecting dose can overwhelm available defenses, and the infant has no protection against organisms for which the mother had no antibodies.

Antibodies in Breast Milk

Along with the milk, the breast-fed infant ingests antibodies and many nonspecific protective materials such as complement proteins, interferons, the antibacterial enzyme called **lysozyme,** and an iron-binding protein **(lactoferrin)** that modifies bacterial multiplication. Milk contains antibacterial and antiviral antibodies of the IgA class. When adults ingest antibodies or other complex proteins, digestive enzymes rapidly degrade them, but the newborn alimentary tract has less proteolytic activity. Therefore, to a considerable extent, ingested proteins retain their function. Antibodies in breast milk neutralize bacterial toxins and prevent many viruses and bacteria from initiating infection. Breast-fed infants have significantly fewer intestinal infections than bottle-fed infants, especially where hygienic conditions are suboptimal. This partly reflects reduced opportunity for bacterial contamination of breast milk compared with bottle feeds, but part of the protection parallels the specificity and concentration of antibodies present in the milk. Some researchers believe that IgA antibodies in milk modify the ways in which proteins cross the infant's highly permeable intestinal mucosa. Therefore, presence of maternal IgA may explain why breast-fed infants seem to have fewer food allergies in later life; however, this view is not universally accepted.

Injection of Antibodies

Deliberate injection of antibody-containing serum has been used, both clinically and experimentally, since the turn of the century. Injecting antibodies is less significant as an antimicrobial therapy now than it was before widespread development of effective antimicrobial agents. However, in selected therapeutic circumstances passive protection remains extremely important.

After known exposure to a pathogenic organism, infection can sometimes be prevented or aborted by injecting antibodies against it. In the preantibiotic era, hyperimmune horse serum was used to protect against many infections. Once the infecting agent was identified, the patient could receive serum from animals with high-titered antibodies against the appropriate organism. Unfortunately, the equine protein often provoked an immune reaction, leading to the clinical syndrome called **serum sickness** (see Chapter 12).

Use of Globulin Preparations

Injected human antibodies rarely provoke immune reactions. Globulins can be concentrated from whole human serum or plasma to achieve very high levels of

TABLE 9–1. **Diseases in Which Passive Immunization is Useful**

Disease	Product	Source	Indications and Precautions
Botulism	Antibody to specific types of toxin	Horse	Patients known to have ingested toxins
Diphtheria	Antibody to bacterial toxin	Horse	To prevent systemic complications in those with established disease Adverse reactions common
Herpes zoster/varicella	IG* to zoster-varicella virus	Human	Postexposure to varicella (chickenpox) in immuno-suppressed children with no history of the disease
Hepatitis A	ISG† preparation containing multiple antibodies	Human	Protection after known specific exposure; prophy-laxis for endemic exposure risk
Hepatitis B	IG* specific for hepatitis B virus	Human	Protection after known needlestick or sexual ex-posure; infants born to mothers carrying hepatitis B virus
Hypogammaglobulinemia	ISG† preparation containing multiple antibodies	Human	Continuous prophylaxis for patients with humoral immunodeficiency
Measles	Antibody to rubeola virus	Human	After known specific ex-posure
Rabies	Antibody to rabies virus	Human	As soon as possible after bites, with part of dose directly around injured tissue; active immuniza-tion given at a different site
Rubella	Antibody to rubella virus	Human	Given after specific expo-sure, to modify symp-toms; does not prevent viremia
Snakebite	Antibody to venom of snake implicated	Horse	After exposure; polyvalent product effective against pit vipers, rattlesnakes, copperheads
Spider bite	Antibody to venom	Horse	After bite by black widow, related spiders
Tetanus	Antibody to neuro-toxin of *Clostridium tetani*	Human	Nonimmune individuals after potentially tetanus-contaminated injury; vaccine at separate site if immunization status un-certain

*IG: Immunoglobulin; concentrated preparation containing single antibody.
†ISG: Immune serum globulin; see text.

specific antibodies or groups of antibodies. Serum preparations with high levels of antibody against such viruses as varicella (cause of chickenpox and shingles) and hepatitis B are used to treat persons after episodes of known exposure. A concentrate of unselected antibodies, the product called **immune serum globulin (ISG),** can also be useful. ISG is prepared from alcohol fractionation of large pools of plasma and contains the wide range of antibodies present in the donor population. The broad-spectrum preparation can be given to individuals with defective humoral immunity. The unselected assortment of antibodies provides generalized immune protection that can be supplemented by antimicrobial agents or specific immunotherapy after episodes of known exposure. Passive immunization is short-lived. Antibody protection will decrease as transferred Ig undergoes normal protein degradation. Table 9–1 lists many conditions for which passive immunization may be useful.

Previously, ISG could be injected only into muscle because direct introduction into the bloodstream provoked potentially life-threatening problems of immune complex formation and stimulation of the complement and kinin systems. Human globulins are now available in a form suitable for intravascular use; intravenous ISG is used for an expanding list of immunodeficiency and immunodysfunctional conditions.

ACTIVE IMMUNITY

The natural way to acquire immunity is to experience either clinical or inapparent infection, which then stimulates cellular or humoral immune activity. Procedures for artificial induction of immunity originated from centuries of observations that persons who survived certain illnesses would never again experience those infections.

Exposure to Native Organisms

The earliest form of immunization was called variolation because the agent that causes smallpox is a virus called variola (see Chapter 1). Variolation involved introducing a small amount of material from a smallpox lesion into a healthy person. The healthy person would develop a mild case of smallpox and thereafter was protected from acquiring the disease. Unfortunately, the healthy person could also develop a much more severe case of smallpox that resulted in fatality. In the latter part of the eighteenth century with the introduction of cowpox or vaccinia in place of variola, vaccination against smallpox became much safer (see Chapter 1).

Cross-Reactive Immunity

The immunity to variola that follows exposure to vaccinia virus illustrates the principle of **cross-reactivity;** the two viruses have sufficiently similar antigenic composition that antibodies to the one prevent infection with the other (Fig. 9–2). Organisms that differ in clinical respects may share significant epitopes and thus elicit antibodies that react with an agent to which there has been no exposure. Cross-reactivity is not an unmitigated blessing. Antibodies to microbial antigens sometimes

PROTECTION AGAINST SMALLPOX
THROUGH CROSSREACTION WITH COWPOX

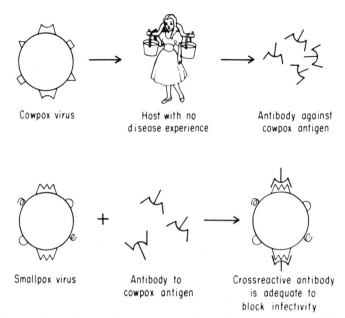

FIGURE 9–2. Certain antigens of the cowpox and smallpox viruses resemble one another. Infection with cowpox (*upper panel*) elicits antibodies for that virus. Because the antigenic configurations are so similar, antibodies to cowpox can block actions mediated by molecules of the smallpox virus (*lower panel*).

cross-react unexpectedly with host tissues or proteins. **Rheumatic fever** is a classic example; antibodies induced by infection with certain strains of β-hemolytic *streptococcus* or S. *pyrogenes* can react with antigens of human heart constituents and cause a destructive inflammatory process.

Exposure to Modified Antigens

Immunization attempts to achieve maximum protection with minimum risk to the patient. In the smallpox saga, variolation imposed excessive risk. Although unmodified cowpox virus carried less risk, it induced unpredictable protection. As outlined in Table 9–2, current strategies to induce immunity use a number of techniques to increase protection and to reduce risk. Immunity may develop after injection of **killed organisms,** which retain antigenicity as long as the appropriate epitopes are not denatured. Organisms express a wide range of antigens; antibodies that develop after natural infection react with microbial elements that may or may not participate in the pathologic process. If killed organisms induce antibodies against materials necessary for the organism to cause disease, then a killed preparation can be a safe

TABLE 9−2. **Preparation of Immunizing Materials**

Materials Used	Potential Problems
Killed organisms	May damage epitopes that elicit protective antibodies
	May fail to inactivate viable pathogens
Living attenuated organisms	During multiplication, nonpathogenic strain may recover virulence
	During multiplication, organisms may lose epitopes that induce protective antibodies
	Preparation containing viable organisms may be contaminated with other pathogens
Immunogenic fraction of pathogenic organisms	Difficulty in identifying the specific isolated epitopes that induce desired protective antibodies
	Difficulty in separating intact epitopes from whole organisms

and effective vaccine. Problems arise if the pathogens are not successfully inactivated or if significant antigens are damaged in processing.

Viable Organisms

Some strains of pathogenic organisms do not cause human disease but have the same antigens as their more dangerous counterparts. Such organisms, described as **attenuated,** remain capable of multiplying and of stimulating antibodies but lack properties that significantly damage tissue. Vaccines using attenuated organisms generally induce better immunity than do vaccines made of killed organisms. However, using living but attenuated organisms to induce immunity carries the risk that the organisms may revert to a more virulent state. An associated risk is that other unidentified infectious agents may lurk in a preparation of viable organisms that has not been subjected to inactivation or sterilization.

Antigenic Fractions

Another way to increase the safety of immunization is to identify epitopes that provoke protective antibodies and to inject only the part of the organism that exhibits the desired antigens. Successfully **fractionated material** induces protection but has no capacity to multiply or cause disease. This principle was exploited in developing vaccines against hepatitis B. The viral envelope material called **hepatitis B surface antigen (HBsAg)** elicits protective antibody, but purified HBsAg is not alive, does not cause disease, and can be processed to eliminate any other viable organisms. The most recent vaccines for hepatitis B use a HBsAg fraction synthesized by recombinant DNA technology. With this technique, the viral gene for HBsAg was isolated and transferred into a yeast. The altered yeast cells can be grown in huge vats and will produce large quantities of HBsAg, which is then purified and can be used in vaccines. Molecular genetic techniques can be used to modify a virus so that it becomes attenuated. A gene coding for a specific antigen may be transferred into the attenuated virus, and this virus is then used as a carrier in the production of a new vaccine. Table 9−3 lists many immunization preparations in current use.

TABLE 9–3. **Immunization Strategies for Specific Diseases**

Disease	Nature of Vaccine	Duration of Protection	Booster Schedule	Contraindications
Cholera	Inactivated bacteria	Modest protection for 3–6 months	Every 6 months, as needed	Severe reactions to previous dose
Diphtheria	Toxoid (denatured toxin)	Approx. 10 years	Repeat dose at age 4; every 10 years	Ongoing febrile illness; history of severe allergies
Hemophilus influenzae (b)	Purified capsular polysaccharide	Approx. 4 years	Varies with individual	Age under 18 months Allergy to vaccine constituents
Hepatitis B	Viral antigen, either fractionated from plasma or prepared by recombinant DNA technology	Approx. 5 years	Probably every 5 years	Allergy to vaccine constituents
Influenza	Killed virus, usually three different strains	One flu season	Yearly, with current strains	Anaphylactic allergy to egg; cancer chemotherapy
Measles	Attenuated live virus	$\geq$ 15 years	Not necessary	Ongoing pregnancy
Meningococcal infection	Purified capsular polysaccharide	3 years	Only if risk recurs	Allergy to vaccine constituents
Mumps	Attenuated live virus	$\geq$ 15 years	Not necessary	Ongoing pregnancy; anaphylactic allergy to eggs
Pertussis (whooping cough)	Killed bacteria	4–6 years	Contraindicated in adults	Age over 7 years; ongoing febrile illness; severe allergic history

Disease	Type	Duration of immunity	Booster schedule	Contraindications
Plague	Killed bacteria	Not fully characterized	Every 6 months to 1 year if risk persists	
Pneumococcal infection	Purified capsular polysaccharides of 23 strains	At least 5 years	Contraindicated	Ongoing pregnancy
Poliomyelitis	Attenuated live virus, given orally	Probably lifelong	Only if high risk is established	
Rabies	Inactivated virus, grown in human cells	Approx. 2 years	Every 2 years if risk continues	Severe allergic history
Rubella	Attenuated live virus	$\geqq$ 15 years	Not necessary	Ongoing pregnancy / Ongoing febrile illness
Smallpox	Attenuated live virus	3–10 years	Varies with risk state	Only indication is for laboratory personnel working with virus
Tetanus	Toxoid (denatured toxin)	Approx. 10 years	Every 10 years or after high-risk exposure	Ongoing febrile illness / Severe allergic history
Tuberculosis	Live attenuated organism (Bacillus of Calmette-Guerin—BCG)	Partial only; duration varies	Not used	Immunosuppressed state
Typhoid	Killed bacteria	$\geqq$ 3 years	Only if high risk exists	Severe reaction to previous dose
Yellow fever	Live attenuated virus	$\geqq$ 10 years	Every 10 years if risk persists	Immunosuppressed state / Anaphylactic allergy to egg

Anti-idiotype Vaccines

A potential new approach to immunization is the production of anti-idiotype vaccines. An anti-idiotype antibody mimics the image of the original stimulating antigen (see Chapter 6). Anti-idiotype antibodies can be made by producing a monoclonal antibody to the desired antigen. This monoclonal antibody is injected into an animal. The immunized animal then produces an anti-idiotype antibody. This antibody has as its idiotype the same shape as the original epitopes on the stimulating antigen. Injection of the anti-idiotype antibody as a vaccine circumvents use of any form of the original pathogen and promotes formation of highly specific anti–anti-idiotypic antibodies.

Problems With Active Immunity

Many circumstances conspire against effective immune protection. Some pathogenic organisms, especially viruses, continually change their antigenic features. Several different strains may produce clinically similar disease states, but antibody elicited by one strain may not confer protection against other variants. Some viruses have more variants and are more likely to change their characteristics than others. The influenza viruses and the many agents responsible for the "common cold" are highly heterogeneous and, in addition, mutate frequently into renewably infective strains. The smallpox and measles viruses, by contrast, are antigenically very stable, and successful vaccines have been produced against these pathogens.

Immunity provoked by infection with some organisms may not be protective. Besides the apparent lack of immunity that occurs when antigenically diverse strains all produce identical clinical events, there is the problem that antibodies provoked by some microorganisms genuinely have no effect on limiting disease or preventing subsequent infections. A prominent example is the antibody response to the human immunodeficiency virus (HIV-1); several of the antibodies that this virus elicits document the presence of HIV but do not protect against clinical illness.

Adverse Effects

Another problem in vaccine development is undesirable side effects. Microbial proteins can elicit localized or systemic reactions that are uncomfortable or, in some cases, dangerous. Soreness at the injection site is usually tolerable, but many patients consider malaise and fever acceptable only if the native disease is significantly more dangerous or unpleasant than the reaction to immunization. Still worse are dysfunctional immune reactions that occasionally occur after immunization, especially those that damage the central or peripheral nervous system.

Preparations of live organisms may pose a threat to nonimmunized persons. Attenuated agents that are harmless to healthy subjects can cause significant disease if they spread to immunologically compromised individuals. This can occur if a live virus given to a pregnant woman crosses the placenta or if a immunodeficient person acquires organisms excreted by recently immunized contacts.

EVENTS THAT PROVOKE IMMUNE RESPONSES

Immune activation requires exposure of a certain minimum intensity and duration. Immune responses may not occur to (1) very small doses of a microorganism, (2) very transient contact, (3) very superficial infection, or (4) multiplication in a nonaccessible body site. Conversely, otherwise normal hosts may fail to react if exposed to overwhelming quantities of a microorganism. Stimuli effective for healthy individuals may be insufficient for those with congenital or acquired immunodeficiency. The following discussion of developing immunity presupposes immunocompetence in the host and exposure to adequate but not lethal doses of a pathogen.

Intrauterine Exposure

The normal fetus inhabits a sterile environment. Although organisms may enter the amniotic sac under pathologic conditions, most maternal infections do not affect the fetus. In addition, some pathogens do not stimulate immune activity because their presence induces fetal death or premature delivery. An immune response is most likely to occur when a moderate dose of pathogen enters the fetal bloodstream weeks or months before delivery. Direct infection of amniotic fluid rarely elicits a response because the process is usually acute, terminating either in fetal death or accelerated delivery. When infecting agents cross the placenta, long-term contact between fetus and microorganism is established; intrauterine infections that develop shortly before full-term birth may have inadequate opportunity to exert immune effect.

Consequences to the Fetus

Exposure to microbial antigens stimulates precocious development of the fetal immune system. Because IgM of maternal origin does not cross the placenta, the presence of IgM antibody in fetal or cord blood indicates that there has been intrauterine infection to which the fetus has responded. IgM antibodies of fetal origin are diagnostic for intrauterine infection but are not protective. Despite circulating antibody, fetal tissues may contain viable microorganisms.

Intrauterine infections are more often viral than bacterial. Notorious examples are rubella virus and cytomegalovirus, which cause asymptomatic or trivial infection in the mother but may cause severe developmental anomalies in the fetus who survives transplacental infection. Premature delivery and persisting congenital infection are characteristic of many rubella or cytomegalovirus syndromes. Transplacental infection with syphilis spirochetes (*Treponema pallidum*) causes a variety of congenital anomalies. Other organisms that may provoke immune response in the fetus are species of M*ycobacterium*, *Toxoplasma gondii*, and P*lasmodium* (malarial organisms).

Subclinical Infection

An individual with no history of overt disease may nonetheless exhibit immunity to a pathogen because many environmental agents can multiply within the body without causing discernible illness. There are several ways in which the host may become aware that immunity exists. If the individual remains well when others exposed to a known pathogen develop illness, prior immunity may be inferred. However, many uncontrolled variables affect clinical disease, so that wellness hardly constitutes a reliable test for established immunity. Specific tests are available (see Chapters 15 through 18) to demonstrate antibodies, but demonstrating cell-mediated immunity is more difficult. For generations, skin testing for delayed hypersensitivity was the only way to document the presence of cellular immunity to particular antigens or organisms. The skin-test procedure is called the **tuberculin test** when mycobacterial antigens are used. Comparable skin tests are performed with antigens from certain fungi and other pathogens that characteristically elicit a cell-mediated response. It is now possible to examine cultured cells for reactivity to specific microbial antigens, but these tests are demanding and expensive.

Significance of Antibodies

After known exposure to a pathogen, an individual may want to learn whether he or she has immunity, as with a man exposed to mumps or a pregnant woman exposed to rubella. Knowledge of prior immune status is sometimes helpful in deciding whether to administer vaccines that are in scarce supply or cause unpleasant or dangerous side effects. The question of immune status is easily answered if serum is examined immediately after exposure. Absence of antibody indicates susceptibility to disease, and presence of antibody indicates immunity. Because of the dangers of an intrauterine rubella infection, many states have adopted laws that require a rubella antibody titer (concentration of rubella antibodies) to be determined in a woman applying for a marriage license. If no antibodies are present or if the titer is low, it is recommended that the woman receive rubella vaccine before becoming pregnant.

The presence of antibodies may be significant if uncertainty exists about the time of exposure to a pathogen or whether a certain pathogen was present. When serum is examined well after exposure, absence of antibody still indicates susceptibility, but presence of antibody is more difficult to interpret. The antibody could have been present for years, indicating prior immunity, or it could have arisen as a prompt reaction to the recent immunizing event. Under these circumstances, it can be very useful to determine Ig class. Predominance of IgM suggests recent primary immunization, whereas antibodies that are wholly or predominantly IgG indicate previously established immunity.

Significance of Skin Tests

Skin tests for cell-mediated immunity are used for epidemiologic studies and to make therapeutic decisions. A healthy person who fails to react to tuberculin or other comparable antigens is considered free of present or previous infection. Some adults in the United States and most adults in many economically or hygienically deprived areas have a positive tuberculin test result. This indicates past experience with the organism, even if there is no history of present or past clinical illness. If an individual known to have had a negative test becomes positive on a subsequent test, this documents recent infective exposure and is an indication to institute treatment. When a person is found to have infective tuberculosis, it is customary to administer skin tests to the patient's close contacts. A positive skin test result in a child or young person is assumed to reflect recent infection from the original patient; even without signs of illness, antituberculosis therapy is given. Older contacts found to have a positive skin test may or may not be considered recently infected, depending on past circumstances and the results of previous tests, if known. Table 9–4 outlines some of the ways in which tuberculin testing affects clinical judgments.

Childhood Diseases

Many diseases with a distinctive clinical course confer long-lasting protection after a single episode of illness. If the organism is widely distributed, this immunity will be periodically reinforced by subsequent encounters. Infections with other organisms provoke less individualized clinical manifestations. For example, a number of respiratory and gastrointestinal organisms produce clinical syndromes that so closely resemble one another that it is impossible, without extensive microbiologic investigation, to assign a specific organism to each episode. In these circumstances, immunity against individual organisms has little practical importance, inasmuch as repeated episodes of very similar illness occur on successive encounters with different organisms.

The diseases sometimes called the **usual childhood diseases** are characterized by distinctive clinical syndromes, by a high level of interpersonal contagion, and by

TABLE 9–4. **Significance of the Tuberculin Test**

Test Result	Associated Circumstances	Interpretation
Negative test	1. In healthy child or adult 2. In serious illness suggestive of tuberculosis	1. No present or previous disease 2. Depression of cell-mediated immunity (anergy)
Positive test, no previous results known	1. In seemingly healthy young child 2. In seemingly healthy adult 3. In adult with illness suggestive of tuberculosis	1. Active infection; treatment indicated 2. Previous exposure to tuberculosis 3. Diagnosis of tuberculosis more probable, but not proven
Positive test, previous test(s) known to have been negative	1. In seemingly healthy adult or child 2. In adult or child with illness suggestive of tuberculosis	1. Recent infective exposure; treatment indicated 2. Strengthens likelihood of diagnosis, but proof by culture still desirable
Negative test, previous test(s) known to have been positive	1. In seemingly healthy adult 2. In adult with serious illness suggestive of tuberculosis 3. In adult with illness not suggestive of tuberculosis	1. May indicate either complete eradication of organism or unsuspected presence of illness that depressed cell-mediated immunity 2. May or may not indicate tuberculosis, but does indicate depressed cell-mediated immunity 3. Malignant or immune disease may be cause of depressed cell-mediated immunity

subsequent establishment of lifelong immunity. Before immunization for these conditions was widely prevalent, measles, mumps, chickenpox, whooping cough, diphtheria, and scarlet fever affected larger numbers of young children, a population in which close interpersonal contacts occurred among children with little established immunity. In such circumstances, children who contracted the pathogen and recovered from the characteristic illness did not again suffer from that disease. Widespread vaccination has made these diseases infrequent in economically developed countries, but in developing parts of the world, distinctive contagious diseases continue to afflict most children.

Age at Exposure

Pathogens highly prevalent in an environment are more likely to cause disease in children than in adults. After maternal antibodies wane, the child is vulnerable to every newly encountered microorganism. With each successive infection, the child expands the list of organisms to which he or she is immune and reduces the number of pathogens capable of causing illness. As long as the pool of pathogenic agents remains constant, symptomatic infections become less and less frequent as age and microbial exposure increase. A change in the pool of organisms or in the state of individual immunity restores susceptibility. Children exposed to the altered social environment of a new school, for example, commonly bring home organisms sufficiently different from those of the parents' previous exposures that the entire household experiences a surge in infections.

Some endemic organisms cause illness that is trivial in children, but far more significant when older persons are infected. Hepatitis A virus and the Epstein-Barr virus (EBV), which causes infectious mononucleosis, are examples. These viruses cause subclinical infection in infants and children, who thereafter possess permanent immunity. Persons who escape childhood exposure and acquire infection only as adolescents or adults often become significantly ill. In unimmunized populations in which poliovirus is common, most children acquire immunity through subclinical gastrointestinal infection early in life; however, if primary infection occurs in later childhood or adulthood, severe or fatal neurologic involvement may result.

Failure of Protection

So-called lifelong immunity is not absolute; levels of protection tend to diminish with time. The immunity that follows clinical illness tends to persist at higher levels than protection induced by artificial immunization. If an infecting dose is large and the level of immunity is low, disease may develop before the anamnestic response can become effective. At any level of immunity, a sufficiently large dose can overcome the protective effect; this is especially likely if other circumstances have compromised innate defense mechanisms. Even in persons with previously normal immune function, severe debility, malnutrition, the presence of burns or inflammatory disorders, and the effects of many medications all increase susceptibility to infection. However, the disease may be less severe than it would have been in a comparably impaired patient without prior immunity.

Some systemic conditions make infections more frequent and more severe, regardless of prior immune status. Notable in this regard are diabetes mellitus, alcoholism, and widespread malignant neoplasms. Adrenal corticosteroids, given as therapy for a wide range of conditions, suppress nonspecific inflammatory defense mechanisms, depress previous levels of immunity, and increase predisposition to infection. Many cytotoxic drugs have a comparable effect. Malignant conditions, diseases of autoimmune etiology, chronic infections, and malnutrition are other common events that make infections more numerous and more severe. Acquired immune defects are discussed in greater detail in Chapter 10.

Some examples of seemingly failed protection result from mistaken identity, in which several different organisms cause indistinguishable clinical illnesses. For example, otherwise healthy individuals rarely suffer twice from the distinctive illnesses of measles or whooping cough, but widespread skin rashes or epiglottitis can occur several times in the same person, caused by several antigenically distinct organisms.

IMMUNITY AT SURFACES

As long as it is intact, the skin with its multilayered epithelium is an effective barrier against microbial invasion. Mucosal surfaces are much thinner and hence much more vulnerable. Three forms of acquired immunity augment the defensive effect of intact epithelium in protecting surfaces. The most conspicuous is the **presence of antibodies,** largely IgA, in secretions. **Cell-mediated events** and the actions of **IgE** also help protect body surfaces from pathogenic microorganisms.

Antibodies in Secretions

The IgA present in secretions provides a protective surface and prevents adherence and entry of bacteria and viruses into the underlying epithelium. IgA originates in plasma cells of the mucosa-associated lymphoid tissue (MALT); plasma antibodies do not seep into secretions. Specialized epithelial cells called **M cells** cover Peyer's patches of the gut and regulate the passage of antigens across the mucosa. Inhaled or ingested antigens stimulate systemic responses as well as surface immune activity. Antigen presentation occurs either in MALT or in regional lymph nodes that drain the epithelium. Intramuscularly injected antigens rarely stimulate secretory antibodies. Most secreted IgA reflects antigens that stimulate the mucosa directly. However, antigen presented at a single mucosal site may induce antibody at additional surface locations.

IgA is the only antibody class significantly present in normal secretions. Persons with congenital IgA deficiency may have IgM in their secretions. Receptors on epithelial cells recognize the J chain associated with IgA or IgM and help transport the antibodies from the basal to the luminal epithelial surface. Epithelial receptors have a much greater affinity for dimeric or trimeric IgA than for IgM, but if IgA is absent, IgM pentamers engage the receptors and are transported across the epithelium.

Effects of IgA

Secretory IgA prevents antigenic or pathogenic material from penetrating the epithelium and entering the body. The antibody complexes with soluble antigens to reduce absorption of potentially immunizing material. Several antibodies neutralize intraluminal toxins and metabolites, thus preventing damage to epithelial cells.

Whatever toxins and antigens manage to enter the bloodstream are probably further inactivated by the monomeric IgA present in plasma, but this role for circulating IgA has not been proved.

IgA antibodies against bacteria and viruses prevent these pathogens from adhering to epithelial cells. Possible mechanisms for this effect include reducing motility of the potential invader, blocking receptor sites for epithelial attachment, altering the solubility and the surface electrical charge of the organisms, and enveloping the invaders in a macromolecular complex of antibody, mucus, and antigen. IgA antibodies do not agglutinate organisms but may attach to the surface and exert an opsonic effect, rendering potential pathogens attractive to phagocytic cells that possess receptors for the alpha chain. Inflammatory cells with alpha chain-Fc receptors are relatively rare in internal tissues but are more numerous in epithelium. Although IgA does not activate complement by the classical pathway, protein aggregates that contain IgA can initiate the alternative pathway and generate the chemotactic and opsonic effects that occur after C3 is cleaved.

IgE-Mediated Mechanisms

The skin and the epithelial surfaces of the gut and the respiratory tracts contain numerous tissue basophils, called **mast cells,** which bind IgE to their membrane through high-affinity receptors. Encounter with antigen stimulates mucosal T cells to elaborate lymphokines that enhance local production of IgE and increase the number of mast cells. After IgeE binds to mast cells and the membrane-bound IgE interacts with antigen, the mast cells release products that induce inflammation, promote smooth muscle contraction, and increase vascular and epithelial permeability. These mechanisms appear to provide a major defense against intestinal parasites, especially helminths, such as *Schistosoma* species and *Trichinella spiralis*. The inflammatory response allows proteins from the bloodstream to enter the tissue fluid, thus exposing the worms and their larvae to antibodies of all classes. Inflammatory mediators attract macrophages and granulocytes, especially eosinophils, into the antibody-rich area. IgG is opsonic for phagocytic effector cells and serves as the target for antibody-dependent cell-mediated cytotoxicity (ADCC; see Chapter 7). IgE is also produced in allergies and is the cause of type I hypersensitivity reactions (see Chapter 12).

Antihelminthic Effects

IgE molecules that are not bound to mast cells have special actions against helminths; antigen-specific IgE can bind to macrophages and stimulate them to attack specific target organisms. Mast cell degranulation releases eosinophil chemotactic factors that mobilize bone marrow eosinophils to enter the circulation. Therefore, parasite infestation is often associated with eosinophilia. Eosinophils have receptors for IgE and therefore recognize parasites that become coated with IgE. Eosinophils contain many enzymes capable of damaging parasites and also release activating factors that bring platelets and macrophages into the battle. Products released from mast cells promote smooth muscle contraction and secretion of mucus, and this assists in expulsion of parasites already damaged by the mechanisms described above. Humoral antiparasitic protection is far from totally effective; individuals with high levels of IgE antibodies against helminths may at the same time be heavily infested with the organisms. In addition, parasites have developed numerous methods of evading and suppressing the host immune response to establish long-term infection.

Cell-Mediated Immunity at Surfaces

Mucosal surfaces are abundantly supplied with T cells, B cells, macrophages, and other types of specialized antigen-presenting cells. M cells take up microbes and macromolecules from the intestinal lumen and transport them to lymphoid follicles localized in the intestinal wall. In the skin, dendritic cells called Langerhans' cells are capable of trapping antigen and presenting it to lymphocytes. Antigen-stimulated T cells elaborate lymphokines, which not only enhance antibody production and mucus secretion but also promote accumulation of macrophages, neutrophils, eosinophils, and mast cells.

EFFECTS OF ANTIBODIES

Antibodies are the major immune defense against bacterial infection, acting to prevent bacterial invasion, eliminate those organisms that manage to enter and multiply, and inactivate many bacterial products. Against viruses, antibodies serve more to prevent infection than to eradicate established intracellular organisms. Many fungal and parasitic infections provoke antibodies, but these antibodies may not effectively eliminate these pathogens. Organisms that have a significant extracellular phase characteristically elicit a humoral response, whereas a cell-mediated response follows intracellular multiplication of most viruses and many fungi, protozoa, and certain bacteria.

Specific Effects on Bacteria

Antibodies against cell-wall, flagella, or capsular components inhibit the movement and multiplication of bacteria and their attachment to target cells. During infection, bacteria synthesize an enormous range of structural, metabolic, and secreted materials that mediate motility, cellular adhesion, evasion of phagocytosis, and incorporation of nutrients. Antibodies against these materials reduce the efficiency with which the organisms cause infection. The organisms may not be directly killed, but if antibody-mediated actions reduce their numbers and viability, they are more vulnerable to nonspecific host defense mechanisms.

IgM antibodies produce many *in vitro* effects, but it is unclear how many are physiologically significant in the living host. It is doubtful whether agglutination occurs commonly, although it may serve to clear pathogens from the bloodstream. Complement-mediated lysis of bacteria and some viruses is known to occur, but this mechanism seems to have significant antimicrobial effects only against *Neisseria meningitidis* and *Haemophilus influenzae*.

IgM, Complement and Inflammation

Complement activation is crucially important in promoting opsonization and initiating the anaphylatoxic effects that magnify inflammation. Only a few IgM molecules need combine with antigen to initiate the classical pathway, which generates large amounts of C3a and C5a. These complement products attract inflammatory cells and promote localized accumulation of blood-borne proteins, such as antibodies, fibrinogen, complement proteins, fibronectin, and kinin precursors. Combination of antibody with surface antigen causes numerous C3b molecules to attach to the cell surface. Macrophages and neutrophils, which have C3b receptors, are attracted to the site by the anaphylatoxic effects of complement, and their phagocytic actions are enhanced by the opsonic effects of complement. Attachment of C3d to an antigen increases its immunogenicity and therefore enhances the immune response to this antigen.

IgG antibodies develop late in the primary response and predominate in anamnestic reactions to organisms previously encountered. Large numbers of IgG molecules must complex with an organism to activate complement. IgG coating by itself has significant opsonic effect, because numerous phagocytic cells have high-affinity receptors for the Fc portion of gamma chains. Microorganisms coated with both IgG and C3b are even more attractive to macrophages and granulocytes than those coated with either protein alone. Antibody-coated organisms are also susceptible to ADCC.

Antibodies to Metabolites

The metabolites of multiplying bacteria often exert independent pathogenic effects, such as inhibition of coagulation, lysis of tissue proteins, repulsion of inflammatory cells, or inhibition of essential physiologic interactions. Antibodies that neutralize these products reduce the competitive advantage that their unmodified action gives to the infecting bacteria. In some diseases, the major clinical effects result from the actions of bacterial toxins rather than from the multiplication of the organisms. Examples are enterotoxic diarrhea in cholera, the systemic events in staphylococcal toxic shock syndrome, neurotoxic effects in tetanus and botulism, and damage to cardiac and neurologic functions in diphtheria. Antibodies against these toxins are therapeutically more useful than those directed against bacterial cell-body antigens. Hence, the substance used in tetanus vaccinations is a chemically modified clostridial toxin **(toxoid).**

Some bacterial diseases should not, strictly speaking, even be called infections because no bacteria multiply in the host. Staphylococcal food poisoning is a relatively innocuous example, and botulism is a potentially fatal example of problems that follow ingestion of preformed bacterial toxins. Treatment for botulism is not antibiotic medication but administration of antibody to the type of toxin identified.

Bacteria produce and release proteins called **heat shock proteins (HSPs)** when subjected in the host to elevated temperatures due to fever or phagocytosis. HSPs are highly antigenic and therefore help stimulate an effective immune response against the invading bacteria.

Antiviral Antibodies

Viruses are obligate intracellular parasites; they replicate only within living cells in which it is difficult for immune mechanisms to penetrate. The virus must enter the body, arrive at the target organ, and then invade individual cells. Antiviral antibodies have several opportunities to interrupt this sequence, but once the virus is inside the cell, cell-mediated immunity (CMI) is the major defense. Antibodies are more effective in preventing than in curing viral diseases.

Antibodies may counteract the effects of viral proteins, block attachment of virus to a host cell, prevent penetration of the target cell, or directly lyse the intact virus. IgA antibodies in epithelial secretions protect susceptible cells against many respiratory or gastrointestinal viruses; antibodies in the bloodstream attack organisms traveling from their site of entry to distant target organs. The complement cascade may produce direct lysis or may interfere with mechanisms for attachment and penetration. Cells infected by virus often express virus-derived surface antigens, which can combine with complement-activating antibodies that initiate lysis of the infected cell. This is beneficial only if antibody in the surrounding tissue fluid destroys organisms released by lysis of the initially infected cell. When viruses spread directly from one cell to another, antibodies are not effective and therefore CMI provides the better defense.

Nonprotective Marker Antibodies

Most viruses have both surface and interior epitopes. Because protective antibodies are generally those that react with surface antigens, immunization procedures are intended to evoke these antibodies. Antigens inside the virus activate the immune system only if viral multiplication occurs within the host's cells. Antibodies to surface antigens can result from artificial immunization, but the presence of antibodies to interior viral antigens indicates ongoing or past infection. These antibodies provide useful diagnostic markers but provide little protection. Antibodies against enzymes of the viral coat or interior similarly indicate present or past viral multiplication. Fluid-borne antibodies to these enzymes do not protect against infection because the processes mediated by these enzymes occur inside the invaded cells.

Immunosuppressive Viruses

Some viruses acquire an unfair advantage by depressing immune mechanisms of the infected host. The most notorious example is HIV-1, the retrovirus that causes AIDS. It uses the CD4 antigen to invade T cells, destroying the infected helper T cells and profoundly diminishing immune reactivity. Other viruses, notably cytomegalovirus and EBV, exert significant but less dramatic and less permanent immunosuppressive effects on lymphocyte populations.

CELL-MEDIATED IMMUNE EVENTS

Complement-mediated membrane damage is a direct consequence of humoral immunity, but most other immune defenses involve cellular activity, either alone or in association with antibody actions. Antibodies augment cellular defenses through opsonization, ADCC, and enhancement of acute inflammatory events. The cell-mediated arm of immune defense comprises, as we have seen in Chapter 7, a variety of phagocytic and nonphagocytic events that may help protect against microbial invasion.

Effects of Lymphokines

In the form of CMI described as delayed-type hypersensitivity (DTH), a small number of antigenically specific T cells secrete lymphokines that activate nonspecifically lymphocytes, granulocytes, and macrophages. Immune reactivity of this type is effective against many organisms that resist antibody defenses either because their intracellular location prevents contact with antibody or because their surfaces fail to evoke protective antibodies. The classic examples of DTH are the etiologic agents for tuberculosis and leprosy, which remain infective and metabolically active inside macrophages. Comparable effects are seen with various fungi and with *Listeria*, another intracellular bacterium.

On Tissue

In DTH, antigen-activated T_H1 cells produce interleukin-2 (IL-2) and interferon-γ (IFN-γ) which promote the effector actions of macrophages. Macrophages are attracted to the site of microbial invasion and the antimicrobial effectiveness of the macrophages is enhanced. The actions of lymphokines include enhancing phagocytosis and intracellular bacterial killing, inducing increased surface receptors for complement and Ig, and increasing the generation of bactericidal oxygen metabolites. The secretion of many proteins is stimulated, including transport mechanisms, coagulation factors, and enzymes that cleave proteins, fats, and carbohydrates. Also enhanced is production of leukotrienes and prostaglandins, and of IL-1 with all its systemic effects (see Chapter 7).

The type of helper T-cell subpopulation that develops during an immune response can profoundly affect the course of disease. A good example of the influence of T_H1 or T_H2 cells is leprosy. Two distinct clinical forms of leprosy occur: tuberculoid and lepromatous. Tuberculoid leprosy which accounts for most cases, is the milder form of the disease. Affected patients show strong DTH reactions and therefore stimulation of T_H1 cells. Patients with the lepromatous form of leprosy do not show a strong cell-mediated response, but do make high levels of antibody to *Mycobacterium leprae*. In these patients, T_H2 cells are preferentially stimulated and large amounts of IL-4 and IL-10 are produced. IL-10 inhibits macrophage activation and the production of IFN-γ and TNF-α. Since *M. leprae* is an intracellular organism and has cell-wall components resistant to antibody-mediated killing, a T_H2 response is ineffective in controlling growth of this bacteria. The prognosis of patients with lepromatous leprosy is not as good as those with the tuberculoid form.

Immunity to Viruses

Cell-mediated immunity exerts significant effects on cellular antigens and intervenes in infectious events in two additional ways. Certain viruses—notably measles, cytomegalovirus, and some herpesviruses—acquire surface proteins from the cells in which they have multiplied. Viruses with these acquired antigens stimulate T lymphocytes to DTH actions that the unmodified virus might not otherwise elicit. Viruses also contribute antigens to the membrane of host cells. Infected cells characteristically acquire membrane antigens that arise from expression of viral genes in the host nucleus. Because cells expressing these viral antigens continue to make their own major histocompatibility complex (MHC-1) antigens, they become targets for cytotoxic CD8 cells that recognize foreign antigens in the context of autologous class I antigens. Infected host cells also become more attractive to natural killer (NK) cells, which do not recognize specific antigens but characteristically interact more effectively with infected cells than with normal cells of the same tissue type. These antiviral mechanisms are illustrated in Figure 9–3.

WAYS THAT VIRAL INFECTIONS
CREATE TARGETS FOR CMI

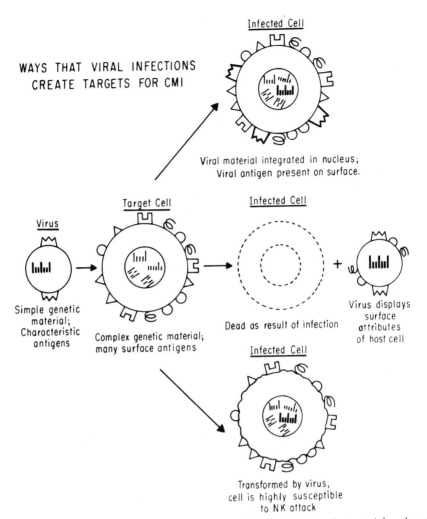

Infected Cell

Viral material integrated in nucleus;
Viral antigen present on surface.

Virus

Target Cell

Infected Cell

Simple genetic
material;
Characteristic
antigens

Complex genetic material;
many surface antigens

Dead as result of infection

Virus displays
surface
attributes
of host cell

+

Infected Cell

Transformed by virus,
cell is highly susceptible
to NK attack

FIGURE 9–3. (*Left*) The two figures show virus, with distinctive genetic material and surface antigens, infecting a host cell with many intrinsic genetic and surface attributes. Infection modifies the host cell in ways that elicit cell-mediated immunity. (*Top*) The figure shows that an infected cell may express on its membrane viral antigens that the immune system will perceive as foreign. (*Middle*) The figures show that virus, released into body fluids after infecting and rupturing a host cell, may manifest host-cell antigens that render the virus a target for major histocompatibility complex (MHC) restricted recognition. (*Bottom*) Viral infection has transformed the host cell so that it is more vulnerable to attack.

Interferons constitute another avenue of antimicrobial defense. Production of IFN-α and IFN-β does not require antigen-specific recognition. Secreted by macrophages, fibroblasts, and other cells, these products promote cellular resistance to viral invasion and enhance the actions of macrophages and antigen-specific lymphocytes. IFN-γ is an immune product secreted only by T cells that have recognized specific antigen; viral infection may constitute the immune stimulus, but many other antigens are also effective. Many complex cellular antigens elicit IFN-γ, but bacteria characteristically do not. IFN-γ intensifies nonspecific cellular defense events by enhancing the actions of macrophages and NK cells. In fact, NK cells are critical during early phases of viral infection, and patients deficient in NK cells may suffer severe infections.

SUMMARY

1. Passive immunity refers almost exclusively to the transfer of antibodies from one individual to another. This process occurs naturally across the placenta from mother to unborn child. Breast milk is also a vehicle for passive immunity and contains antibacterial and antiviral antibodies of the IgA class as well as other nonspecific protective materials such as complement proteins, interferons, lysozyme and lactoferrin. Antibodies or globulin may be directly injected to treat persons after exposure to certain pathogens or to protect those with immunodeficiencies or immunodysfunctional conditions. Passive immunization is short-lived and decreases as immunoglobulins (Igs) undergo normal protein degradation.

2. Active immunization generally provides better and longer-lasting immunity than passive immunization. Active immunity may be naturally acquired through clinical or inapparent infection or artificially acquired through vaccination procedures. Vaccines may be organisms that have been killed, attenuated, or fractionated, or they may be materials made through recombinant deoxyribonucleic acid (DNA) techniques or perhaps anti-idiotype antibodies. Problems associated with active immunity include cross-reactivity of antibodies with host tissues or proteins, strain variation of microbes, nonprotective antibody production, adverse side effects of vaccines and complications in immunodeficient individuals.

3. Intrauterine exposure to microbes is rare. Few microbes can cross the placenta. Exposure to microbes during the latter part of gestation will stimulate precocious development of the immune system with production of IgM. Because maternal IgM does not cross the placenta, fetal IgM is diagnostic of intrauterine infection. Intrauterine infections are more often viral than bacterial and may cause serious congenital anomalies.

4. Subclinical infection with no overt symptoms of disease may result in active immunity. Immune status can be determined by detection of antibodies in the individual or skin testing.

5. With loss of maternal antibody, a newborn child becomes susceptible to infection. Widespread vaccination procedures in economically developed countries have dramatically decreased many of the usual childhood diseases. Infection by other less virulent microbes expands the child's immune repertoire. Change in environment exposes the child to new microbes and thereby increases susceptibility to new infection. Some endemic pathogens may be trivial to small children, but devastating to adults.

6. Immunity following clinical disease generally persists at higher levels than protection induced by artificial immunization (hence, booster shots). Infecting dose and preexisting conditions such as malnutrition, burns, diabetes, and inflammatory conditions in the host affect level of immunity.

7. Three forms of acquired immunity augment the defensive effects of intact epithelium in protecting body surfaces: the presence of IgA, the presence of IgE, and cell-mediated events.

    a. IgA produced by mucosa-associated plasma cells prevents adhesion and invasion by pathogens. IgA neutralizes toxins and other metabolites and can serve as an opsonin, thereby enhancing phagocytosis and complement activation via the alternative pathway.

    b. IgE binds to mast cells, and, upon interaction with antigen, the mast cell releases products that induce inflammation. Inflammatory mechanisms aid in removal of intestinal parasites through stimulation of smooth muscle contraction and induction of chemotaxis and cell-mediated cytotoxicity by macrophages and eosinophils.

    c. Mucosal surfaces are abundantly supplied with T cells, B cells, macrophages, M cells, and Langerhans' cells, which interact in antigen presentation, lymphokine production, and cell-mediated immune processes.

8. Antibodies are very effective against bacteria; regarding viruses, antibodies are better for preventing infection than eradicating an established infection. Antibody to bacterial cell walls, flagella, and capsule help prevent adhesion and motility and enhance removal by phagocytosis. IgM agglutination may help clear bacteria from the bloodstream. Other antibody-mediated defense mechanism include complement-mediated lysis, opsonization, anaphylatoxic effects of C3a and C5a, and the presence of C3b and Fc receptors on phagocytes that bind bacteria coated with antibody and complement. Antibodies can also inactivate metabolites of bacteria (enzymes, toxins, heat shock proteins) and thereby reduce the competitive advantage and clinical effects of infection.

9. Antiviral antibodies are most useful when viruses first enter the body or are released from infected cells. After viruses are inside the host cell, cell-mediated immunity (CMI) is the major defense. Antibody may counteract effects of viral proteins, block attachment or cause lysis of intact virus. Virally infected cells that express viral antigen on their cell surfaces are susceptible to complement-activating antibody and lysis. Presence of viral antibodies are useful diagnostic markers of infection. The screening test for AIDS detects HIV antibody, not virus particles.

10. Antibodies augment cellular defenses through opsonization, antibody-dependent cell-mediated cytotoxicity (ADCC), and enhancement of inflammatory events. In delayed-type hypersensitivity (DTH) responses, antigen-activated T_H1 cells produce the lymphokines, interleukin-2 (IL-2) and interferon-γ (IFN-γ), which promote effector activities of macrophages such as phagocytosis, intracellular bacterial killing and increased production of receptors for antibody and complement. The type of helper T cell and their repertoire of secreted lymphokines help determine whether a humoral or cell-mediated response predominates. CMI with participation by CD8-positive cells and NK cells, and production of interferons is critical for clearance of viruses.

REVIEW QUESTIONS

1. An example(s) of passive immunity is/are _____.
   a. maternal antibodies in the newborn child
   b. anti–snake venom treatment
   c. immune serum globulin given after known exposure to hepatitis
   d. variolation
   e. a, b, and c

2. Maternal antibodies circulating in the fetus may cause _____.
   a. serum sickness
   b. food allergies in the newborn
   c. hemolytic disease of the newborn (HDN)
   d. congenital anomalies
   e. hypogammaglobulinemia

3. Which of the following are characteristics of passive immunization?
   a. Involves humoral and cell-mediated immunity
   b. Is short-lived
   c. In certain circumstances is a useful therapeutic approach
   d. a and b
   e. b and c

4. Important protective components of breast milk include _____.
   a. IgG
   b. IgA
   c. lactoferrin
   d. a and b
   e. b and c

5. Most states require a couple seeking a marriage license to have a blood test for detection of antibody to syphilis; in addition, the woman must be tested for antibodies to rubella because
   a. presence of antibodies implies previous infection
   b. demonstration of antibody implies previous vaccination
   c. rubella may cross the placenta and cause congenital disease in a fetus
   d. maternal antibodies to rubella will protect mother and child from measles infection
   e. all of the above

6. The presence of _____ in fetal or cord blood is indicative of intrauterine infection.
   a. IgG
   b. IgA
   c. IgM
   d. Ige
   e. IgD

7. A seemingly healthy adult displays a positive tuberculin skin test result; previous results are unknown. The most likely interpretation of this result is _____.
   a. active infection, treatment indicated
   b. prior exposure to tuberculosis
   c. depressed cell-mediated immunity
   d. a and b
   e. b and c

8. Which of the following statements are true concerning Epstein-Barr virus (EBV)?
   a. It is the cause of infectious mononucleosis.
   b. It causes subclinical infection in children.
   c. No permanent immunity follows EBV infection, and therefore a person may acquire the disease multiple times.
   d. a and b
   e. a, b, and c

9. Factors that can increase susceptibility to infection even with prior immuniza-tion include _____.
   a. malnutrition
   b. inflammatory conditions
   c. alcoholism
   d. corticosteroids
   e. all of the above

10. Macrophages in cell-mediated immunity are activated primarily by _____.
    a. interferon-α (IFN-α)
    b. interferon-γ (IFN-γ)
    c. interleukin-2 (IL-2)
    d. a and b
    e. b and c

11. IgE binds to _____ and aids in removal of _____.
    a. mast cells . . . parasites
    b. eosinophils . . . parasites
    c. mast cells . . . fungi
    d. eosinophils . . . fungi
    e. macrophages . . . bacteria

12. Cell-mediated responses are most effective against _____.
    a. *Staphyloccus aureus*
    b. *Herpes simplex*
    c. *Listeria monocytogenes*
    d. a and b
    e. b and c

13. _____ is the antibody class primarily present in normal secretions.
    a. IgG
    b. IgM
    c. IgA
    d. IgE
    e. Igd

14. _____ is/are associated with delayed-type hypersensitivity (DTH).
    a. T_H1 cells
    b. T_H2 cells
    c. macrophages
    d. a and c
    e. b and c

15. Virally infected cells can be killed if viral antigens are expressed on cell surfaces. What else is necessary?
    a. Major histocompatibility complex (MHC I)
    b. MHC II
    c. Natural killer (NK) cells
    d. a and c
    e. b and c

MATCHING QUESTIONS

Match the disease in Column I with the type of vaccine in Column 2.

Column 1	*Column 2*
16. Hepatitis B	a. Killed microorganism
17. Tetanus	b. Attenuated live virus
18. Measles	c. Toxoid
19. Pertussis	d. Fractionated microorganism
20. Pneumococcal infection	

ESSAY QUESTION

21. What types of materials can be used as vaccines and what are some of the potential problems associated with the use of each of these types of materials?

SUGGESTIONS FOR FURTHER READING

Beagley KW, Elson CO: Cells and cytokines in mucosal immunity and inflammation. Gastroenterol Clin North Am 1992;21:347–365

Dempsey PW, Allison M, Akkaraja S, et al: C3d of complement as a molecular adjuvant: Bridging innate and acquired immunity. Science 1996;211:348–350

Gounni AS, Lamkhioued B, Ochiai K, et al: High affinity IgE receptor on eosinophils is involved in defense against parasites. Nature 1994;367:183–186

Liew FY,Li Y, Millot S: Tumor necrosis factor-a synergies with IFN-g in mediating killing of Leishmania major through the induction of nitric oxide. J Immunol 1990;145:4306–4310

McGhee JR, Kiyono H: Effective mucosal immunity. Intl J Technol Assess Health Care 1994;10(1):93–106

Paul WE: Infectious disease and the immune system. Sci Am 1993;269:91–97

Sieling PA, Abrams JS, Yamamura M: Immunosuppressive roles for IL-10 and IL-4 in human infection. J Immunol 1993;150:5501–5510

REVIEW ANSWERS

1. e	6. c	11. a	16. d
2. c	7. b	12. e	17. c
3. e	8. d	13. c	18. b
4. e	9. e	14. d	19. a
5. e	10. e	15. d	20. d

10 Immunodeficiency Conditions

The complexity of the immune system provides innumerable opportunities for deficiency and malfunction. Defects can be classified into the following categories: B cells and immunoglobulin (Ig) levels, T cells and cell-mediated events, combined B-cell and T-cell relationships, complement factors and regulators, and functions of phagocytic cells. Defects in one area frequently affect other functions, but this overall classification is useful in organizing a complex subject. It is also useful to divide immunodeficiency conditions into inherited or congenital defects (primary immunodeficiencies) and immunodeficiencies resulting from environmental events (acquired or secondary immunodeficiencies). Table 10–1 outlines some of the ways in which different defects of cell types cause disease.

TABLE 10–1. **Sites of Defects in Acquired or Congenital Immunodeficiency States**

Element Affected	Pathologic Event
Marrow Stem Cells	Reticular dysgenesis Severe combined immunodeficiency syndrome Immunosuppressive drugs; x-ray exposure
T Lymphocytes Thymus Numbers of mature cells	DiGeorge syndrome Corticosteroids Malignant disorders Some viral infections Thermal burns
Function of mature cells	Chronic mucocutaneous candidiasis Acquired metabolic disorders (e.g., diabetes, alcoholism, uremia) Autoimmune disorders
B Lymphocytes Pre–B cells Numbers of mature cells Immunoglobulin (Ig) synthesis	Infantile hypogammaglobulinemia (X-linked) Corticosteroids; malignant disorders Selective Ig class deficiencies ? Common variable immunodeficiency Malignant disorders Malnutrition
Ig levels	Hypercatabolism Protein-losing diseases
Phagocytic Cells Marrow production	Autoimmune disorders Many drugs, viral infections
Motility and chemotactic recognition	Complement disorders Acquired metabolic disorders (e.g., diabetes, steroids, alcohol, aspirin)
Phagocytosis	Splenectomy Hyperhemolysis (e.g., sickle cell disease, malaria) Complement disorders
Enzyme release and intracellular bacterial killing	Chronic granulomatous disease Chédiak-Higashi syndrome Inborn enzyme deficiencies Thermal burns

MANIFESTATIONS OF IMMUNODEFICIENCY

Defective immunity predisposes to infection. In immunodeficient individuals, there is an increase in number, severity, range of etiologic organisms, and clinical complications of infectious conditions. With inherited or congenital immunodeficiencies, infections begin early in life, and untreated patients may not survive long enough to manifest later complications. However, therapeutic strategies in current use permit many individuals to survive years of immunodeficiency, only to experience autoimmune problems or malignant lymphoreticular neoplasms in later life.

Time Sequence

Infants born to an immunologically normal mother begin life with an impressive array of IgG antibodies, and bacterial infections are relatively rare in the newborn period. In normal infants, viral infections are more numerous than bacterial infections, especially those due to viruses that elicit antibodies with no protective effects. Maternal cells do not cross the placenta; therefore, the mother's cell-mediated immunity (CMI) does not pass to the infant. Intracellular bacteria, many fungi, and the more polymorphic viruses can and do cause infections in the normal newborn, but most infants manage to eliminate the majority of invaders.

Childhood Exposures

After maternal antibodies disappear and before active immunity develops, normal infants experience an interval of pronounced susceptibility to environmental agents. The infections that occur reflect the opportunities for exposure. An infant with intimate exposure to only a few adults in a few locations will have fewer infections than an infant who interacts with persons of varying ages in varying surroundings. With advancing age and an expanding social sphere, previously protected infants eventually encounter most of the common environmental pathogens. Regardless of previous social contacts, entering daycare or school nearly always increases the episodes of infection.

The immunodeficient child reacts abnormally to these normal environmental encounters. If CMI is defective, fungal or viral infections begin in the first few weeks and persist despite use of otherwise effective therapy. Defects of humoral immunity characteristically remain undetected until passive immunity dissipates at several months of age. Limited defects may not emerge until later in childhood, when infectious exposure is more extensive and subtle departures from the normal become more apparent. The age of onset for many primary immunodeficiencies is given in Table 10–2.

Range of Organisms

Patients with antibody deficiencies are considerably more susceptible to septicemia, infections of upper and lower respiratory tracts, and infections of the central nervous system. Commonly identified pathogens are the gram-positive and gram-negative cocci, enteroviruses, and agents that cause infectious diarrheas, notably *Rotavirus*, *Giardia*, and *Salmonella*.

TABLE 10–2. **Manifestations of Primary Immune Deficiency**

Most Common Age Period When Signs Occur	Immunologic Defect
Earliest infancy	Reticular dysgenesis
	Severe combined immunodeficiency syndrome
	DiGeorge syndrome
2–6 months	Infantile hypogammaglobulinemia
	Mucocutaneous candidiasis
6 months to 2 years	Transient hypogammaglobulinemia of infancy
	Chronic granulomatous disease
	Wiskott-Aldrich syndrome (bleeding may occur earlier)
Childhood	Ataxia-telangiectasia (ataxia may occur earlier)
	IgA deficiency (if symptomatic)
Adolescence or adulthood	Deficiency of C1 esterase inhibitor
	Deficiencies of C5–C8
	Common variable immunodeficiency

The pyogenic infections characteristic of antibody deficiency are more easily treated than are the infectious consequences of defective CMI in which lifelong vulnerability becomes apparent through persistent fungal infections and repeated viral infections of skin, mucosal surfaces, and respiratory tract. Other organisms common in patients with defective CMI include intracellular bacteria, such as *Mycobacterium* and *Listeria*; many viruses, especially those of the herpes, adenovirus and enterovirus groups; and opportunistic fungi and protozoa such as *Pneumocystis carinii*, *Cryptococcus neoformans*, and *Cryptosporidium* and *Toxoplasma* organisms.

Defects of Accessory Systems

Phagocytic defects become apparent either very early or somewhat later in childhood. Patients with defective phagocytosis have particular problems with staphylococci and gram-negative bacteria, which characteristically cause repeated and persistent infections rather than sudden or overwhelming sepsis. Fungal infections also frequently occur.

Patients deficient in the late components of complement have unexplained susceptibility to *Neisseria* infections. Disseminated gonococcal infection and meningococcal infections of the central nervous system or bloodstream are strikingly common. This may not become apparent until late childhood or adolescence when *Neisseria* exposure becomes more common. Other infections tend to be somewhat more frequent and more troublesome in these patients than in healthy individuals. Organisms that characteristically complicate immunodeficiency conditions are listed in Table 10–3.

ACQUIRED CONDITIONS OF DEPRESSED IMMUNITY

A small number of individuals have been identified with clearly defined immune defects that are genetically determined. Many insights about immune mechanisms have come from researchers investigating these patients and determining exactly how these defects are related to normal immune functions. However, the overwhelming majority of immune abnormalities result from age, environment, and acquired diseases. Secondary immune deficiencies are often associated with complex manifestations that defy single-cause explanations. Table 10–4 outlines some of the causes of acquired problems in immune function.

Systemic Conditions Affecting Immunity

Anything that impairs bodily economy can affect immune function. Vulnerable activities include cell division and multiplication, protein synthesis and secretion, metabolic interrelationships, and the ways in which cells and soluble molecules react with one another. Certain metabolic abnormalities and diseases are especially likely to depress immunity.

Generalized Changes

Overall nutritional state and the metabolism of oxygen, carbon dioxide, and simple nutrients significantly affect immune efficiency. States of malnutrition or protein deficiency depress cell multiplication and antibody production. When nutrition is poor, previously established protection diminishes and new exposures fail to evoke immunity. Any medical or surgical condition that impairs nutrition subjects the patient to the additional burden of depressed antimicrobial defense. In geographic areas where nutrition is poor because of severe economic deprivation, entire populations experience increased risk of infection.

Another cause of immune deterioration is advancing age, but individuals differ enormously in levels of deficiency. The physiology of aging is poorly understood, and immune changes are no exception. In general, antibody levels decline in and beyond the eighth decade. Cellular responsiveness, which is much more difficult to

TABLE 10–3. **Common Pathogens in Immunocompromised Conditions**

Defective Element	Common Microorganisms	
T-Cell Deficiencies	Bacteria:	Intracellular: *Mycobacterium tuberculosis, Listeria monocytogenes* Extracellular: *Salmonella, Legionella, Nocardia*
	Fungi:	*Candida, Histoplasma, Cryptococcus, Aspergillus, Pneumocystis*
	Viruses:	Cytomegalovirus, herpes simplex, herpes zoster
	Protozoa:	*Toxoplasma, Cryptosporidium*
B-Cell Dysfunction		
Hypogammaglobulinemia	Pyogenic extracellular bacteria	
IgA deficiency	Bacteria infecting sinuses, lungs: *Giardia lamblia*; hepatitis viruses	
Splenectomy	*Streptococcus pneumoniae, Salmonella*	
Phagocytic/Bactericidal Deficiency	Many staphylococci and streptococci, *Haemophilus influenzae, Candida*	
Complement Deficiencies		
C3	*S. pneumoniae*	
C5–C9	*Neisseria* species	

TABLE 10–4. **Conditions That Suppress Immune Function**

Cause	Induced Defects
Disease States*	
Diabetes mellitus	Depressed chemotaxis and phagocytosis
	Depressed T-cell functions
Alcoholism	Depressed delayed hypersensitivity (mild)
	Increased immunoglobulins, especially IgA
	Depressed neutrophil chemotaxis
Widespread tuberculosis	Anergy (severely depressed delayed hypersensitivity)
Uremia	Depressed macrophage functions
	Depressed T-cell functions
	Depressed neutrophil chemotaxis
Malnutrition	Depressed cellular multiplication and antibody production
	Depressed phagocytosis
	Depressed T-cell functions
Protein-losing gastrointestinal or renal conditions	Hypogammaglobulinemia
Thermal burns	Disruption of epithelial barrier
	Loss of serum proteins
	Accelerated degradation of serum proteins
	Depressed T-cell function
	Depressed phagocytosis and chemotaxis
Prolonged hemolysis (e.g., sickle cell disease, malaria)	Exhaustion of macrophage activity
External Events	
Splenectomy	Depressed antibodies to capsular polysaccharides
Adrenal corticosteroids	Depressed number and function of T cells and B cells
	Depressed neutrophil chemotaxis
	Depressed macrophage numbers, chemotaxis, phagocytosis
	Depressed synthesis of interferons
Cytotoxic drugs	Epithelial damage, leading to reduced barrier function
	Depressed numbers of all marrow-derived cells
	Depressed multiplication of T cells and B cells
	Activation of latent cytomegalovirus or Epstein-Barr virus infections (sometimes), leading to depressed T-cell functions
General anesthetics	Depressed T-cell functions
X-irradiation	Depressed number and function of lymphocytes, neutrophils
	Depressed macrophage function
	Damage to epithelial surfaces (sometimes)
Prolonged strenuous exercise	Decreased lymphocyte function
Bereavement, other traumatic emotional events	Decreased number and function of lymphocytes

*For effects of autoimmune and malignant diseases, see Chapters 11 and 12.

quantify, diminishes to an indeterminable degree. Older persons also exhibit increasing frequency of immune disfunction and autoimmune conditions.

Specific Conditions

Certain diseases exert an immunosuppressive effect disproportionate to measurable metabolic effects. **Diabetes mellitus,** both insulin-dependent and non–

insulin-dependent, impairs T-cell functions and also depresses activities of neu-trophils and macrophages. In severe **liver disease,** serum protein synthesis is de-pressed and complement levels fall. **Cirrhosis,** which alters hepatic circulation and distorts processing and presentation of many antigens, often provokes increased production of Igs that have no identifiable specificities, and the patient manifests decreased resistance to infection. **Alcohol abuse** impairs many cell functions, espe-cially the chemotactic and phagocytic aspects of inflammation and probably also T-cell activities. **Uremia** distorts many cellular activities, including those of T cells and possibly also of phagocytic cells.

Anesthetic agents depress T-cell activity for days or weeks after the acute ex-posure and may also affect B-cell responsiveness. The mechanism of depression is not known, but depressed immunity and increased susceptibility to infection almost invariably follow general anesthesia.

Other Conditions

Regular, moderate exercise appears to boost the immune system. However, strenuous exercise seems to suppress normal immune responses. Runners are most suscepti-ble to upper respiratory tract infections, and marathon participants show reduced lymphocyte function. Reduced function and number of lymphocytes may be corre-lated with increased corticosteroid levels and stress. Stress itself is a cause of im-mune disfunction, and increased corticosteroid levels can be traced to hypothalamic secretion of corticotropin-releasing hormone and subsequent secretion of adreno-corticotropic hormone (ACTH) by the pituitary. Lymphocytes have receptors for vari-ous neuroendocrine factors and glucocorticoids. Catecholamines and acetycholine can affect lymphocyte numbers, antibody production, natural killer (NK) cell activity, and cytokine production. The effects of stress and the manner in which mental states may affect the immune system have only recently been appreciated and have given rise to a new area of research called **psychoneuroimmunology (PNI).**

Protein Loss

If an increased loss or destruction of serum proteins occurs, antibody levels decline. The resulting **hypogammaglobulinemia,** if severe, may depress bacterial immunity. This is most conspicuous in **protein-losing enteropathies** (some of which probably have an immune cause) and in the renal and metabolic condition described as the **nephrotic syndrome.** Passive administration of immune serum globulin is ineffec-tive because the injected proteins are lost along with autologous Igs.

Thermal burns create special vulnerability to infection. Large-scale damage to skin removes the physical barrier to microbial entry and leaves an exposed surface that is excessively permeable to fluid and protein. Huge quantities of serum protein are lost across the warm, moist, weeping surfaces, which also provide excellent con-ditions for bacterial multiplication. Even though antibody synthesis may be unim-paired, further loss of plasma protein occurs because of accelerated degradation owing to the increased metabolism that follows extensive burns. Complicating the clinical picture is concomitant depression of cellular function, which affects both T cells and the chemotactic and phagocytic actions of inflammatory cells. Infection is the most common cause of death after severe burns.

Immunosuppressive Drugs

Many drugs depress immune functions. Drugs are often given specifically to diminish activity in dysfunctional immune states (see Chapter 12). In many other conditions, agents given for specific indications cause unwanted immunosuppression as an unavoidable consequence. Often lifelong immunosuppressive therapy is given after organ transplantations, and autoimmune or allergic diseases are often treated with immunosuppressive agents. Adrenal corticosteroids are probably the most commonly used agents. Used for a broad range of clinical problems, they inhibit proliferation and function of lymphocytes and interfere with many inflammatory interactions. Adrenal corticosteroid regimes are monitored to use the smallest effective dose in an attempt to reduce the immunosuppressive and other side effects of these potent agents.

Malignant diseases are treated with agents that suppress cellular multiplication at many different sites and phases. Cytotoxic drugs and radiation reduce proliferation of malignant cells but also suppress the normally multiplying cells of the immune system and bone marrow. Depressed immune and inflammatory functions and severe risk of infection are inevitable consequences of cytotoxic therapy.

Infections

HIV

Infectious organisms may cause immunosuppression in addition to local tissue damage. The most notorious example is human immunodeficiency virus (HIV-1), which causes AIDS. This retrovirus has envelope glycoproteins (gp120, gp41) which enable it to bind to CD4. Binding is followed by fusion with the host cell membrane, and thus this virus gains entry into CD4-positive (CD4+) cells. As a retrovirus, HIV contains the enzyme reverse transcriptase, which transcribes viral ribonucleic acid (RNA) into proviral deoxyribonucleic acid (DNA). The proviral DNA can then incorporate into the host cell DNA. CD4+ helper T cells are the major target for HIV; however, other cells such as macrophages are also susceptible. Direct infection and transfer of virus from infected cells to many other cell types is also possible. Once incorporated into the host cell DNA, replication is dependent on expression of viral regulatory genes.

HIV has three regulatory genes, *tat*, *ref*, and *rev*, and three structural genes, *gag*, *pol*, and *env*. The *gag* gene codes for glycoproteins that form viral capsids. The *pol* gene encodes the genetic information for viral enzymes, and the *env* gene contains the information for the envelope proteins gp120 and gp41. Interaction of viral regulatory genes with host intracellular proteins will lead to productive, latent, or abortive viral replication. Infection of CD4+ T lymphocytes and particularly activated lymphocytes leads to productive viral formation and cell death. HIV infection of macrophages does not result in cell death. Instead, viral particles accumulate, are slowly budded from the macrophage cell membrane and may be spread throughout the body. The macrophage and other antigen-presenting cells thus act as reservoirs of HIV throughout all stages of AIDS.

Over time, a profound loss of CD4+ cells occurs and patients become lymphopenic. Normal healthy individuals should have approximately twice as many CD4+ cells as CD8+ (CD4:CD8 ratio = 2:1). In patients with AIDS, the CD8+ cells eventually outnumber CD4+ cells and the ratio reverses to 1 : 2. Without helper T cells, CMI fails, and production and regulation of antibodies are severely distorted. Loss of CMI can be demonstrated by decreased *in vitro* responses to mitogen and antigen, decreased activity of cytoxic T cells and NK cells, and loss of delayed hypersensitivity. Patients with AIDS will not show positive skin tests to common bacterial antigens. They become **anergic.** Loss of immune activity leaves people with AIDS particularly susceptible to opportunistic diseases and malignant diseases that accompany acquired or inherited immune deficiencies.

Attempts to develop an effective vaccine are thwarted by the genetic variability of HIV. Nucleotide sequences of the *env* gene vary extensively, and new variants of HIV arise continuously. The envelope glycoproteins are the most vulnerable targets for antibodies; however, if new variants of HIV with antigenically different envelope proteins are produced, antibodies that neutralize one strain will not bind to another. The reason for this genetic variability is the inaccuracy of reverse transcriptase in its transcription of viral RNA into DNA. Small mistakes in the insertion of nucleotides result in HIV variants that differ not only in antigenicity, but also in pathogenicity.

Other Viruses and Bacteria

Other retroviruses that infect humans have been identified. HIV-2 has similarities to HIV-1, although it is more closely related to simian (monkey) immunodeficiency virus (SIV). HIV-2 is found more frequently in West Africa and seems to be less virulent than HIV-1. Patients show a longer time period before symptoms of AIDS occur.

Human T-lymphotrophic virus I (HTLV-1), HTLV-II, and HTLV-IV are associated with lymphocytic leukemias and lymphomas. Other viruses cause less permanent alteration of immune function. Cytomegalovirus multiplies in T cells and depresses cellular reactivity; Epstein-Barr virus infects B cells, but response to the B-cell infection causes an increase in the number and function of cytotoxic T cells. Rubella and rubeola (measles) viruses transiently depress T cells. Prolonged or repeated infection with many other common viruses may affect T-cell number or function.

Infections with mycobacteria (tuberculosis and leprosy) and many fungi characteristically activate cell-mediated specific and nonspecific defenses. Massive infection with these same agents may overwhelm cellular responses, leading to anergy.

The Lymphoreticular System

Neoplasms of lymphoreticular tissue inevitably depress or alter immune function. Neoplastic diseases frequently arise in the bone marrow, lymph nodes, and nonnodal reticuloendothelial tissues. Malignant disease originating in the bone marrow is called **leukemia.** Tumor formation in lymphoreticular tissue is called **lymphoma.** Special categories of lymphoreticular malignancies include multiple myeloma and macroglobulinemia. Besides depressing immune defenses, these diseases induce dysfunctional and autoimmune activity. Chapter 11 discusses conditions originating in the bone marrow in more detail.

Individuals with a dysfunctional spleen or whose spleen has been removed are more susceptible to blood-borne bacterial infections. Although *Streptococcus pneumoniae* (pneumococcus) is the most notorious agent, many other bacteria may produce sudden and overwhelming sepsis in asplenic individuals.

PRIMARY CONDITIONS AFFECTING BOTH T CELLS AND B CELLS

Common hematopoietic precursor cells generate multiple mature populations, so disorders of cellular development often affect several populations simultaneously. No inherited or congenital disorders globally suppress the marrow, because total hematopoietic failure would be incompatible with intrauterine survival.

Reticular Dysgenesis

The most severe form of the primary immunodeficiencies involves the multipotential hematopoietic stem cells. Defects in these stem cells result in lack of development of lymphocytes and granulocytes and a disease called **reticular dygenesis.** Growth occurs normally in the uterus, where inflammatory and immune capability are not needed but postuterine life is severely abbreviated. The typical form of this rare condition affects only lymphocytes and granulocytes, but variant forms with additional erythroid and megakaryocyte abnormalities have been reported. Affected patients exhibit severe lymphopenia and hypogammaglobulinemia, and the lymphoid organs are rudimentary. The thymus is severely maldeveloped, and lymph nodes, tonsils, and mucosa-associated lymphoid tissue are virtually absent. The clinical picture is one of early, intractable fungal infection of mucosal surfaces, followed by diarrhea, pneumonias, viral infections, and death in the first few months.

Severe Combined Immunodeficiency Syndrome

Severe combined immunodeficiency syndrome (SCIDS) is a term describing any of the immunodevelopmental failures that affect both T cells and B cells. Both autosomal and sex-linked forms exist; in some, specific enzymes or metabolites essential for cell multiplication can be identified as deficient, but most remain unexplained. Approximately 15 percent of cases of SCIDS involve enzymes associated with purine metabolism. All cells require these enzymes, but the resulting abnormalities produce more pronounced consequences in lymphocytes than in other cells. In enzyme-associated SCIDS, the defects in immune function may range in severity from total to relatively moderate; in other forms of SCIDS, immunodeficiency is uniform and profound.

Autosomal recessive SCIDS is sometimes called **Swiss-type agammaglobulinemia;** other forms have no distinctive name. The earliest manifestation of SCIDS is persistent candidal infection of mucosal surfaces, beginning in the first month of life. *Candida* cytomegalovirus, and *Pneumocystis* continue as particularly common pathogens. Patients may suffer widespread systemic infection if exposed to attenuated viruses used in many vaccines. Except for a subgroup of cases that exhibit increased numbers of B cells, the thymus and other lymphoid tissues are hypoplastic and lymphocytes and plasma cells are absent from blood and bone marrow. Repeated infections elicit no antibodies, and CMI is absent.

Bone marrow transplanted from an HLA-identical sibling can completely reconstitute the defect in SCIDS; if no suitable sibling exists, haploidentical marrow from a parent has sometimes been effective. These immunodeficient recipients are at severe risk, however, from **graft-versus-host disease (GVHD;** see Chapters 12 and 13), not only after bone marrow transplantation but even after blood transfusions that contain viable lymphocytes. Immunosuppression given after bone marrow transplantation in these patients is intended to prevent GVHD, not to prevent graft rejection. A new procedure using isolated hematopoietic stem cells from marrow or umbilical cords may bypass complications such as GVHD.

Gene Therapy

Gene therapy using genetically altered stem cells is a promising new treatment for some forms of SCIDS. Adenosine deaminase (ADA) is a specific enzyme associated with SCIDS, resulting in the toxic accumulation of purine metabolites and loss of T cells. The gene for ADA has been isolated and can be transferred to patient stem cells using a retrovirus. Incorporation of the normal ADA gene into stem cells restores purine metabolism, and subsequent transfusion of these altered stem cells back into the patient allows reestablishment of normal lymphocytes.

Wiskott-Aldrich Syndrome

Wiskott-Aldrich syndrome is characterized by X-linked transmission of immunodeficiency associated with thrombocytopenia and eczema. No single genetic defect has been identified to explain all the findings. Although the first few months of life may be free from immune abnormalities, early manifestations include bleeding due to thrombocytopenia and persistent and progressive eczematous rash. The most common infecting agent in Wiskott-Aldrich syndrome are bacteria (of the type associated with defective humoral immunity), but herpesviruses, cytomegaloviruses, and *Pneumocystis* infections frequently complicate the first years of life.

Patients with Wiskott-Aldrich syndrome show excessive degradation of Igs. They have low levels of IgM antibodies, including near absence of ABO blood group antibodies. IgG antibodies are quantitatively normal but seem to provide subnormal protective effects. Serum levels of IgA and IgE are increased. T lymphocytes are present and react normally on *in vitro* testing, but cell-mediated protection is clinically deficient.

Although survival is longer in patients with Wiskott-Aldrich syndrome than those with untreated SCIDS, patients with this poorly understood condition have a downhill course. Bleeding is a continuous threat, and repeated bacterial and viral infections take a progressive toll. Ig-producing cells are in a continuous hypermetabolic state; dysproteinemias are common and, as patients approach adolescence, lymphoreticular malignancies frequently develop. Bone marrow transplantation has shown some promise as definitive therapy.

Ataxia-Telangiectasia

Another inherited condition with no identifiable unifying defect is **ataxia-telangiectasia,** an autosomal recessive syndrome. This is a relatively common inherited immunologic defect; heterozygous possession of the gene is estimated at 1 percent. Although heterozygotes do not manifest the syndrome, they do experience increased liability to cancers of solid organs. Patients and family members have been shown to have an abnormality of the long arm of chromosome 14 and to have defects in repair of damaged DNA.

Ataxia is disturbance of gait and posture related to cerebellar dysfunction; this begins early and tends to progress. **Telangiectases** are superficial abnormalities of blood vessels, which, in this condition, become apparent after age 2 years. The most conspicuous immunologic abnormality is deficiency of secretory and serum IgA. Serum IgM tends to be high, and IgE tends to be low. Although IgG is quantitatively normal, antibody responses to specific immunogens are depressed, and chronic respiratory tract infections occur frequently. Most patients survive into adulthood, but the neurologic problems tend to worsen, and repeated infections cause pulmonary damage. Lymphoreticular malignancies are common in older patients.

PRIMARY DISORDERS OF T CELLS

DiGeorge Syndrome

Congenital **thymic hypoplasia,** also called DiGeorge syndrome or third/fourth pharyngeal pouch dysgenesis, is not genetically transmitted. It is a developmental defect that occurs sporadically in equal numbers of male and female infants. Structures in the anterior portion of the embryo develop abnormally, causing absence of the thymus and parathyroid glands, characteristic facial anomalies, and often malformations of the heart and blood vessels. The parathyroid deficiency causes symptomatic hypocalcemia. In the first few hours of life, the hypocalcemia along with facial deformities provokes diagnostic evaluation that uncovers absence of the thymus.

Defective immunity becomes apparent, such as superficial fungal infections, frequent diarrhea, susceptibility to pneumonia, and failure to thrive. T lymphocytes are severely reduced in number and function. B lymphocytes are present, and antibodies to T-independent antigens are normal, but because T-cell help is needed for most antibodies, there is increased susceptibility to a wide range of infections. Implantation of fetal thymus can restore T-cell activity, but the cardiovascular deformities and hypoparathyroidism remain independent problems.

Chronic Mucocutaneous Candidiasis

Chronic mucocutaneous candidiasis is a highly selective T-cell defect that affects both men and women. T cells respond inadequately to antigens of Candida albicans, leading to severe infection of skin and mucosal surfaces but not, ordinarily, of deeper tissues, T cells respond normally to antigens other than Candida, and B-cell function is unaffected. Abnormalities of IgA levels or of phagocytic activities have been noted in some patients, and other abnormalities occur frequently but unpredictably. The parathyroids, the adrenals, or the ovaries may be hypoactive; antigland autoantibodies may accompany or even precede the endocrine deficiency. Other sporadic problems include chronic hepatitis, diabetes mellitus, iron deficiency, and vitamin B_{12} deficiency. Neither the cause nor a cure for the immune defect has been found. Treatment is directed against the severe and often disfiguring skin infections and the glandular deficiencies.

PRIMARY DISORDERS OF B CELLS

B-cell abnormalities result in diminished production of Igs. Ig deficiencies may involve multiple classes or single-class deficiencies.

X-Linked Hypogammaglobulinemia

The first recognized immunodeficiency disease was **X-linked hypogammaglobulinemia,** described by Bruton in 1952. Patients demonstrate uniformly low levels of Igs and often a family history of infectious problems in male infants. These children appear normal as long as passively acquired maternal antibodies persist; after several months, *Pneumococcus, Streptococcus, Haemophilus,* and other pyogenic bacteria cause recurrent infections that affect especially the respiratory tract, the skin, and sometimes the central nervous system. Viral and fungal infections are uncommon except for hepatitis and enteroviruses. Frequent and persistent infections of lung or central nervous system often cause progressive tissue damage. Rheumatoid arthritis is common in those who survive past puberty. This deficiency of gammaglobulins has been traced to a genetic defect in a tyrosine kinase gene that is necessary for B-cell maturation.

Clinical Observations

The entire B-cell population in patients with X-linked hypogammaglobulinemia seems to be absent; blood and tissues lack cells with any of the B-lymphocyte markers. T cells are normal or increased in number and exhibit normal functions. Phagocytic cells are functionally normal, but absence of IgM and IgG antibodies reduces opsonic activity. The bactericidal actions of neutrophils are sharply reduced. Tissue sites normally rich in B lymphocytes are hypoplastic, but the thymus is normal.

Serum in X-linked hypogammaglobulinemia contains less than 250 mg/dL total Ig, most of which is IgG. Secretions contain virtually no IgA. Treatment is prophylactic administration of an Ig preparation (immune serum globulin), containing a wide range of antibody specificities (see Chapter 9). Episodes of infection are treated promptly with appropriate antimicrobials. Antibiotics are less effective in these patients than in persons with normal antibodies and opsonic activity. Passive immunotherapy cannot correct antibody levels in epithelial secretions; therefore, upper respiratory tract infections, dental caries, and diarrhea remain troublesome. Optimal treatment allows survival into adulthood, but life expectancy is reduced. Patients with X-linked hypogammaglobulinemia often suffer from allergic and autoimmune phenomena with leukemia and lymphomas as common late complications. Overwhelming infections with fungi, *Pneumocystis, Pseudomonas,* and *Proteus* may prove fatal despite seemingly optimal therapy.

Other Hypogammaglobulinemias

Some infants fail in the second half of their first year to develop normal Ig levels. Some come to medical attention because of repeated infections, but others are found only incidentally during studies of families with known immunodeficiencies.

Continued observation often demonstrates eventual but belated antibody production and normal responses to most bacterial challenges, although a few patients have persistently depressed IgA production. This condition has been called **transient hypogammaglobulinemia of infancy.** It appears to be self-limited. Passive administration of Igs is contraindicated because it may actually suppress antibody formation.

Patients with **X-linked hyperimmunoglobulin M syndrome** have very low IgG and IgA levels, but IgM levels are normal or elevated. These patients suffer repeated respiratory infections. The volume of lymphoid tissue is normal or increased, but B cells produce only IgM. This disease is a result of a defect in the patient's CD40 ligand (see Chapter 6). Malignant proliferation of IgM-producing cells may occur later in life. Red blood cells (RBCs) and neutrophils frequently exhibit autoimmune impairment; neutrophil defects probably contribute to the increased susceptibility to *Pseudomonas* and *Pneumocystis*, which persists despite passive immunotherapy.

Common Variable Immunodeficiency

Also known as acquired hypogammaglobulinemia or idiopathic late-onset immunodeficiency, **common variable immunodeficiency** becomes apparent only after one or several decades of normal immune activity. Normal numbers of B cells persist, but Ig concentration and antigen-specific responses decline. With experimental stimulation, cultured B cells fail to multiply or to differentiate. The defect is thought to be constitutional, even though normal immune activity occurs in the first years of life. Some patients who initially exhibit the X-linked hyperimmunoglobulin M (IgM) condition described in the preceding paragraph gradually lose all Ig-producing capacity. Infections tend to be less severe than in Bruton's agammaglobulinemia, but the frequency of autoimmune phenomena and malignant disease is even higher. Intestinal malabsorption syndromes and protein-losing enteropathy are common, as is chronic lung disease. Some patients eventually develop deficiencies of T-cell function as well, which expands the spectrum of infections to which they are susceptible. Family members have a high incidence of Ig abnormalities and autoimmune diseases.

Selective IgA Deficiency

The most common immunoglobulin deficiency in the general population is **selective absence of IgA.** Frequency estimates range from 1 in 320 to 1 in 800 in Caucasians populations surveyed. In patients with allergic or autoimmune disorders, prevalence is even higher. The diagnosis is made from depression of serum IgA concentration, which is usually below 5 mg/dL, but the pathologic manifestations result from deficiency of IgA in secretions. The cause of the defect is unknown. Many different abnormalities have been observed: increased suppressor activity directed against IgA-producing cells, inability of IgA-producing plasma cells to mature, abnormal distribution of isotypes on cells destined to produce IgA, and abnormal reactivity to chemical agents. Some family members may also have selective IgA deficiency, and others may have common variable immunodeficiency.

Selective IgA deficiency produces diverse clinical effects. Some patients experience respiratory infections or chronic diarrhea as a result of inadequate mucosal defenses. Allergies against environmental antigens, especially cow's milk, are unduly common in persons with deficient serum and secretory IgA. Another condition frequently associated with IgA deficiency is autoimmune disease of the collagen-vascular type (see Chapter 12). Some affected persons have no symptoms and are identified only through population surveys.

Antibodies Against IgA

IgA-deficient patients often have antibodies against all Igs of the IgA class. Severe anaphylactic reactions have occurred in a very few IgA-deficient persons transfused with IgA-containing blood components. Although circulating anti-IgA antibodies are found relatively frequently, anaphylactic transfusion reactions are very rare. Cell-bound IgE, not circulating antibody, mediates anaphylactic transfusion reactions, but the presence of anti-IgA in serum should prompt caution in undertaking transfusion.

In patients with selective IgA deficiency, infections are treated only as they occur, and allergic or autoimmune manifestations are treated as needed. Passive administration of IgA is contraindicated, because injections do not restore antibody levels in secretions and could possibly provoke class-specific antibodies.

Deficiencies of Other Isotypes

Aside from IgA, selective isotypic deficiencies are rare. Some patients who lack IgA also lack IgG2. When added to IgA deficiency, IgG2 deficiency seems to cause no incremental clinical consequences. Some patients with ataxia-telangiectasia have subclass-specific depression of IgG2.

Selective IgM deficiency has been very rarely observed. These patients have experienced meningococcal septicemia, pyogenic infections of the upper and lower respiratory tracts, staphylococcal skin infections, and tuberculosis. In the few cases studied, other Ig classes were normal.

An isolated disturbance of kappa-chain production has been reported; lambda-chain production was increased in compensation and Ig status was functionally normal.

DEFICIENCIES IN THE COMPLEMENT SYSTEM

Deficiency of virtually any of the components, factors, or regulators of complement can occur. C2 deficiency is the most common complement deficiency in the white population. The gene for absence of C2 has been estimated to occur in 1.2 percent of the white population, giving an expected homozygote frequency of 1 in 28,000. The HLA haplotype A10,B12 has strong linkage disequilibrium with the C2-null gene. Deficiencies of early components in the classical pathway have been reported only in whites. Blacks with complement deficiencies have lacked components 5 through 8, which are activated in both classical and alternative pathways. The site for properdin synthesis is on the X chromosome. Genes for C4, C2, and factor B are located within the MHC class II region. Chromosome 1 carries a cluster of genes important for regulation of complement activation. Genes for C4 bp, CD55, CR1, CR2, CD46, and factor H all are located on the long arm of chromosome 1.

Clinical Consequences

Given the importance of complement in inflammation and opsonization, it is not surprising that complement deficiencies cause increased susceptibility to bacterial infection. Less readily explained is the striking prevalence of autoimmune diseases in patients lacking the early components of the classical pathway. Late-sequence deficiencies cause susceptibility to neisserial infection, both *Neisseria meningitidis* (meningococcus) and *N. gonorrhaeae* (gonococcus). Nearly 25 percent of persons lacking C5 through C9 have no clinical abnormalities, and 16 percent of persons deficient in C1, C2, or C4 report no associated problems. Persons who lack C3, the pivotal protein in both the classical and the alternative pathways, are susceptible both to infections and to autoimmune diseases.

The autoimmune diseases seen most often in patients with complement deficiency are systemic lupus erythematosus, diskoid lupus, glomerulonephritis, and vasculitis. These affect 85 to 90 percent of patients with defects of C1, C2, or C4 and about 65 percent of C3-deficient patients. About one-third of patients with C3 deficiency have increased susceptibility to pneumococcal infection as their only problem. In patients with late-phase deficiencies, abnormalities other than neisserial susceptibility have been seen only with C5 defects, which show an association with glomerulonephritis.

Deficient Control Protein

Hereditary angioedema, which results from deficiency of the control protein **C1 esterase inhibitor** (C1 inhibitor, C1-INH), is an inherited deficiency that does not cause immune dysfunction. This α_2-globulin prevents generation of the C1qrs esterase by attaching to the C1q molecule in a fashion that causes C1r and C1s to dissociate (see Chapter 8). C1-INH is a normal constituent of plasma. It prevents ongoing activation not only of C1 but also of the plasminogen system, which cleaves fibrin and fibrinogen, and of the kinin system, which generates proteins that mediate increased vascular permeability.

All these proteins have interrelated roles in the coagulation and inflammatory systems, and normal physiologic function depends on precise adjustment of activation and inhibition. In persons who lack C1-IHN activity, uncontrolled activation of C1qrs leads to excessive cleavage of C4 and C2, generating powerful kinin-related proteins that cause increased vascular permeability. There are no signs of complement deficiency, presumably because the alternative pathway can generate sufficient C3 convertase to compensate for defective classical-pathway activation. Problems arise, however, from the inappropriate excess of vascular permeability. Patients suffer recurrent episodes of localized edema affecting the gastrointestinal tract, the upper respiratory tract, and the skin. Skin problems are the most visible but least dangerous. Gastrointestinal involvement causes episodic abdominal pain or diarrhea, and angioedema of the larynx may cause death by asphyxiation.

The C1-INH deficiency derives from an autosomal dominant gene, of which there are two varieties. The more common variety causes absence of the protein, whereas the less common (15%) form codes for a protein that has no physiologic activity. Diagnosis rests upon demonstrating absent or very low C1-INH and, during acute episodes, marked depletion of C4 and C2.

ABNORMALITIES OF PHAGOCYTOSIS

Antibody and complement deficiencies severely impair phagocytic defenses, but an additional category of defects specifically affects phagocytic cells. Defects in phagocytic cells result in problems primarily with bacterial defense. Very severe depression of phagocytosis predisposes to fungal infections, but these occur much less commonly than recurrent or persistent bacterial infections.

TABLE 10–5. **Major Inherited Defects of Immune Function**

Defective Element	Name of Syndrome	Inheritance Pattern
Precursor cell for lymphocytes, macrophages, granulocytes	Reticular dysgenesis	Autosomal recessive
B and T lymphocytes	SCIDS, common type	Autosomal recessive or X-linked
	SCIDS with enzyme defects	Autosomal recessive
	Wiskott-Aldrich syndrome	X-linked
	Ataxia-telangiectasia	Autosomal recessive
Primarily T lymphocytes	DiGeorge's syndrome	Developmental defect, probably not inherited
	Chronic mucocutaneous candidiasis	Autosomal recessive
Primarily B lymphocytes	Infantile hypogamma-globulinemia	
	Bruton's type,	X-lined
	Affecting females	Unknown
	Transient hypogamma-globulinemia of infancy	Familial; more common in families with SCIDS syndromes
	Common variable immunodeficiency*	Familial, but transmission pattern not understood
	Selective IgA deficiency	Various: both autosomal recessive and dominant patterns; sometimes familial association with common variable immunodeficiency
Complement proteins		
C1-INH	Hereditary angioedema	Autosomal dominant
C1 through 9	Complement deficiency	Probably autosomal recessive
Phagocytic functions	Chronic granulomatous disease	Most common form is X-linked
	Chédiak-Higashi syndrome	Autosomal recessive
	Glucose-6-phosphate dehydrogenase deficiency	X-linked
	Defective leukocyte chemotaxis	Various; some associated with carbohydrate storage diseases

SCIDS, severe combined immunodeficiency syndrome.
*Some element of T-cell dysfunction.

Chronic Granulomatous Disease

Patients with **chronic granulomatous disease (CGD)** have a neutrophil dysfunction and suffer frequent infections with organisms that have low virulence in normal persons, notably *Staphylococcus epidermidis* and species of *Serratia* and *Aspergillus*. Characteristic problems are chronically enlarged and draining lymph nodes, persistent mucosal infections, osteomyelitis, and chronic intestinal symptoms. Treatment requires high doses of powerful bactericidal agents.

CGD is a result of defects in the intracellular processes that kill ingested organisms. Phagocytosis occurs normally, but the cells fail to generate toxic oxygen metabolites that kill the phagocytized organisms. Nicotine adenine dinucleotide phosphate (NADPH) oxidase is a complex enzyme consisting of four peptide chains necessary for the production of oxygen and hydrogen peroxide. Genetic defects can occur in any of these peptides. In the X-linked form of CGD, the missing or defective protein is a component of the cytochrome B complex. Normal production of oxygen metabolites by neutrophils cause reduction and precipitation of the dye nitroblue tetrazolium (NBT) in the cytoplasm. If neutrophils from a patient suspected to have CGD are exposed to NBT, failure to form blue-black deposits confirms the diagnosis.

TABLE 10–6. **Evaluation of Immune Competence**

Screening
  History: frequent or unusual infections, eczema; growth retardation or developmental
    defects; affected family members
  Complete blood cell count with differential white cell count
  Test for antibody to HIV-1
  Skin tests for delayed hypersensitivity to commonly encountered antigens
  Serum protein evaluation: protein electrophoresis; levels of anti-A and anti-B; levels of
    IgM, IgG, IgA
  Nitroblue tetrazolium (NBT) test for neutrophil function
  Hemolytic complement evaluation (CH50)

T-Cell Evaluation
  Chest x-ray for thymus in infants, thymic tumors in adults
  Quantify peripheral lymphocytes with antibodies to CD3 (all T cells), CD4, and CD8
  Lymph node biopsy to identify number, distribution, and morphology of T cells
  In vitro tests of functional competence: blast transformation to mitogens; stimulation by
    allogeneic cells; lymphokine production after challenge

Evaluation of Humoral Immunity
  Immunoelectrophoresis
  Antibody titers before and after specific immunization
  Quantity and distribution of IgG subclasses
  Enumerate peripheral lymphocytes that express mIg or receptors for Fc and Epstein-Barr
    virus
  Bone marrow evaluation for pre–B cells, plasma cells
  Lymph node biopsy, for number, distribution of cells with B-related differentiation markers
  In vitro test of functional competence: blast transformation to mitogens

Phagocytes and Complement
  Quantify C3, C4; other components if necessary
  Tests for chemotaxis: skin window, *in vivo*; Boyden chamber, *in vitro*
  Specific intracellular enzymes
  Quantitative tests of bacterial killing, opsonic response

Other Enzyme Deficiencies and Dysfunctions

Deficiencies in many different enzyme systems can impair granulocyte and macrophage function. Depressed levels of **myeloperoxidase** and **alkaline phosphatase** affect cells throughout the body, but only cells of the granulocyte/macrophage lineage express significant functional deficiency. Patients with severe **glucose-6-phosphate dehydrogenase** deficiency may have depressed intracellular bactericidal function comparable to that of CGD. Two other conditions in which defective phagocytosis is part of a clinical constellation are **Chédiak-Higashi syndrome** and the condition known as **Job's syndrome;** both are multiorgan diseases with familial distribution but unknown molecular basis.

Neutrophils may also be defective in their chemotactic abilities. They fail to migrate and congregate at sites of microbial invasion. Defective chemotaxis can be due to defects in the production of chemotactic factors, such as C5a, or to an intrinsic defect of the neutrophils themselves. Lazy leukocyte syndrome is a disorder in which neutrophils show poor migration.

A related class of disorders affecting neutrophils is inherited deficiencies of intracellular adhesion molecules (ICAMs). Abnormalities of CD11b/CD18 result in deficient chemotaxis and inability to bind to endothelial cells. Neutrophils are then unable to enter the tissues and participate in phagocytic defense.

Table 10–5 (p. 213) summarizes the major forms of primary immune dysfunction. Table 10–6 (p. 214) lists some of the tests used to identify and diagnose both primary and secondary immunodeficiencies.

SUMMARY

1. Developmental defects, deficiencies, and malfunctions in the immune system result in immunodeficiency diseases. Defects can be inherited or congenital (primary) or acquired (secondary) and can involve B cells, T cells, combined B and T relationships, phagocytic cells, or complement deficiencies. In those with inherited or congenital immunodeficiencies, infections begin early in life. Those with antibody deficiencies are most susceptible to bacterial septicemias. If cell-mediated immunity (CMI) is defective, fungal and viral infections are more prevalent.

2. Acquired immunodeficiencies are much more common than primary immunodeficiencies. Systemic conditions affecting acquired immunodeficiencies include age, environment, nutritional status, metabolism disorders (diabetes, liver disease), anesthesia, strenuous exercise, stress, glucocorticoids, burns, immunosuppressive drugs, and neoplasia.

3. The most notorious of infectious organisms capable of causing immune deficiency is HIV. HIV binds to CD4+ cells and with its reverse transcriptase, is able to transcribe viral ribonucleic acid (RNA) into proviral deoxyribonucleic acid (DNA). Incorporation of proviral DNA into host cell DNA enables HIV to replicate. Over the course of several years, a profound loss of CD4+ lymphocytes occurs. Macrophages do not necessarily die because of HIV infection,

Continued on following page

but can become reservoirs of HIV. With loss of CMI, patients with AIDS become anergic and susceptible to opportunistic infections. Other retroviruses exist that are associated with leukemia and lymphoma. Viruses such as cytomegalovirus (CMV) and Epstein-Barr virus (EBV) infect T and B cells without causing immune deficiency. Massive infection with some bacteria and fungi can also lead to anergy.

4. Primary immune deficiencies that affect both B cells and T cells include reticular dysgenesis, severe combined immunodeficiency syndrome (SCIDS), Wiskott-Aldrich syndrome, and ataxia-telangiectasia.

    a. Reticular dysgenesis is a rare condition resulting from a defect in hematopoietic stem cell development, which usually affects lymphocytes and granulocytes. Patients exhibit severe lymphopenia, maldeveloped thymus, and lymph nodes. Intractable infections result in death within a few months after birth.

    b. SCIDS is caused by a developmental defect of B cells and T cells. Autosomal and sex-linked forms exist, with some forms identified with specific enzyme or metabolite deficiencies. Affected persons suffer severe opportunistic infections, but bone marrow transplantation or gene therapy is possible.

    c. Wiskott-Aldrich syndrome is an X-linked immunodeficiency associated with thrombocytopenia and bleeding, eczema, increased IgA and IgE, and lymphoreticular malignancies.

    d. Ataxia-telangiectasia is an autosomal recessive syndrome with an abnormality of the long arm of chromosome 14 and defective DNA repair mechanisms. A deficiency of IgA and resulting respiratory infections, neurologic problems, and lymphoreticular malignancies are characteristic of the disease.

5. Primary disorders affecting T cells include DiGeorge syndrome and chronic mucocutaneous candidiasis. Thymic hypoplasia occurs in DiGeorge syndrome along with absence of parathyroid glands, characteristic facial anomalies, and malformations of heart and blood vessels. Lack of thymic development results in lack of T cells and CMI. Chronic mucocutaneous candidiasis is a highly specific T-cell defect in response to *Candida albicans*.

6. Primary disorders of B cells result in diminished production of immunoglobulins (Igs) and may involve multiple classes of Igs or single isotypes. Individuals with X-linked hypogammaglobulinemia demonstrate uniformly low levels of Igs and are particularly susceptible to recurrent pyogenic bacterial infections. A defect in a tyrosine kinase gene necessary for B-cell maturation has been identified in affected patients. Treatment is possible with immune serum globulin and bone marrow transplantation. Other Ig deficiencies include transient hypogammaglobulinemia of infancy, which in most cases is self-limiting. X-linked hyperimmunoglobulin M syndrome is associated with a defect in CD40 and failure to switch isotypes from IgM to IgG, IgA, and so on. Less severe B-cell−related defects are common variable immunodeficiency and selective deficiency of IgA.

7. Complement deficiencies can involve any of the various factors, components, or regulators. C2 deficiencies are most common in whites, and strong association with HLA haplotype A10B12 exists. Deficiencies of C5 through C8

occur more frequently in blacks. Because of the importance of complement in opsonization and inflammation, complement deficiencies result in increased susceptibility to infection. An unexplained association also exists with autoimmune disease.

8. Hereditary angioedema is an autosomal dominant disorder, which results in deficiency of C1 esterase inhibition (C1-INH). Persons who lack C1-INH have uncontrolled activation of C1qrs, which leads to cleavage of C2 and C4 and generation of kinins regulating vascular permeability.

9. Genetic abnormalities can also occur in phagocytic cells. Patients with chronic granulomatous disease have genetic defects in their ability to generate toxic oxygen metabolites. Depressed levels of myeloperoxidase and alkaline phosphatase, defects of chemotaxis and abilities of phagocytes to adhere to endothelium also result in increased susceptibility to bacterial and fungal infection.

REVIEW QUESTIONS

1. Which statement is <u>untrue</u> concerning inherited or congenital immunodeficiencies?
    a. Recurrent infections begin early in life.
    b. Strong linkage disequilibrium exists with HLA haplotype A10B12.
    c. Survival is often associated with development of autoimmune disease.
    d. Malignant lymphoreticular neoplasms may occur later in life.
    e. The affected neonate is protected by maternal antibody.

2. Regardless of previous social contacts, a child entering kindergarten will experience _____ episodes of infection because of _____ exposure to pathogens.
    a. increased . . . increased
    b. decreased . . . decreased
    c. increased . . . decreased
    d. decreased . . . increased

3. If _____ is defective, the patient is more susceptible to _____.
    a. CMI . . . bacterial infections
    b. humoral immunity . . . fungal
    c. CMI . . . fungal and viral infection
    d. humoral immunity . . . intracellular pathogens

4. Factor(s) that can affect acquired immunodeficiencies include(s) _____.
    a. age
    b. nutrition level
    c. liver disease
    d. strenuous exercise
    e. all of the above

5. _____ function and number of lymphocytes may be correlated with _____ steroid level and stress.
    a. Increased . . . increased
    b. Decreased . . . increased
    c. Decreased . . . decreased
    d. Increased . . . decreased

6. Treatments that depress immune function include _____.
   a. radiation
   b. cancer drugs
   c. blood transfusions
   d. a and b
   e. a, b, and c

7. HIV-1 binds to _____ via _____.
   a. CD4 . . . gp150, gp21
   b. CD8 . . . gp120, gp41
   c. CD4 . . . gp120, gp41
   d. CD2 . . . gp150, gp21
   e. CD3 . . . gp120, gp41

8. HIV-1 infects _____ and does not necessarily kill these cells.
   a. Th cells
   b. B cells
   c. macrophages
   d. neutrophils
   e. eosinophils

9. Patients with chronic granulomatous disease _____.
   a. frequently show edema
   b. have a neutrophil dysfunction
   c. cannot form toxic O_2 metabolites
   d. a and b
   e. b and c

10. A young man is found to test negative for a tuberculin skin test as well as skin
    tests for *Staphylococcus aureus* and *Streptococcus pyogenes*. He has _____.
    a. thymic hypoplasia
    b. anergy
    c. hypogammaglobulinemia
    d. hypocalcemia
    e. hyperglobulinemia.

11. _____ is a specific enzyme defect associated with severe combined immuno-
    deficiency syndrome (SCIDS).
    a. AGA
    b. ADA
    c. PNI
    d. LAP
    e. SOD

12. Which of the following are X-linked immunodeficiencies?
    a. Wiskott-Aldrich syndrome
    b. Bruton's hypogammaglobulinemia
    c. Reticular dysgenesis
    d. a and b
    e. a, b, and c

MATCHING QUESTIONS

Match the disease in Column 1 to the affected cell type in Column 2.

Column 1	*Column 2*
13. Severe combined immunodeficiency syndrome (SCID)	a. T cells
	b. B cells
14. Chronic granulomatous disease (CGD)	c. T cells and B cells
15. Bruton's hypogammaglobulinemia	d. Neutrophils
16. Chronic mucocutaneous candidiasis	e. c and d
17. Reticular dysgenesis	

Match the defect in Column 1 with the disease in Column 2.

Column 1	*Column 2*
18. Lack of CD40 receptor	a. DiGeorge syndrome
19. Negative nitroblue tetrazolium (NBT) test	b. Ataxia-telangiectasia
	c. Chronic granulomatous disease (CGD)
20. Lack of C1-INH	
21. Defective NADPH oxidase	d. Hereditary angioedema
22. Defective DNA repair	e. Hyperimmunoglobulin M syndrome mechanism
23. Thymic hypoplasia	

ESSAY QUESTIONS

24. Discuss three primary immunodeficiency diseases due to developmental defects. How do these diseases differ? What cell types are involved and what happens to the affected person?

SUGGESTIONS FOR FURTHER READING

Callard RE, Armitage RJ Fanslow WC, et al: CD40 ligand and its role in X-linked hyperIgM syndrome. Immunol Today 1993;14(11):559–564

Davis AE III: C1 inhibitor and hereditary angioneurotic edema. Ann Rev Immunol 1988;6:595–628

Dunn AJ: Psychoneuroimmunology, stress and infection. In: Friedman H, Klein TW, Friedman AL, eds. Psychoneuroimmunology, Stress and Infection. Boca Raton, FL: CRC Press, 1996:25–46

Kinnon C, Levinsky RJ: Molecular genetics of inherited immunodeficiency diseases. In: Noel R. Rose, Everly Conway de Macario, John L. Fahey, Herman Friedman, Gerald M. Penn, eds. Manual of Clinical Laboratory Immunology, 4th ed. Washington, DC: ASM Press, 1992:894–900

Levy JA: HIV and the Pathogenesis of AIDS. Washington, DC: ASM Press, 1994

Root RK: The compromised host. In: Wyngaarden JB, Smith LH, Jr, eds: Cecil Textbook of Medicine, 18th ed. Philadelphia: WB Saunders, 1988:1529–1538

Schur PH: Inherited complement component abnormalities. Ann Rev Med 1986;37:333–346

REVIEW ANSWERS

1. b	8. c	15. b	22. b
2. a	9. e	16. a	23. a
3. c	10. b	17. e	
4. e	11. b	18. e	
5. b	12. d	19. c	
6. d	13. c	20. d	
7. c	14. d	21. c	

11 Neoplasms of the Immune System

Without cellular multiplication, immune responses could not occur. With this propensity to divide, however, it is not surprising that cells of the lymphoreticular system often exhibit neoplastic proliferation. Malignancies of the lymphoreticular system can be classified best by the nature and maturational state of the cell of origin.

CLASSIFICATION OF NEOPLASMS

A **neoplasm** is an accumulation of cells derived from a single progenitor, a clone that proliferates autonomously, unconstrained by physiologic stimuli or external events. Other conditions can lead to overaccumulation of cells, but usually involve cells of several different genetic compositions; these processes reflect normally constituted cells responding in an excessive or abnormal fashion to an external stimulus. An example is a **leukemoid reaction,** in which increased numbers of mature and immature neutrophils enter the circulation in response to a severe infection. Neoplastic cells form a clone of identical cells. This monoclonal proliferation reflects derangement of the internal events that regulate cell division and growth. Neoplastic cells usually have a single clonal origin but can differ in their appearance and function, depending on the level of maturation, exposure to mediators, adequacy of blood supply, and other variables.

Benign versus Malignant

Not all neoplasms are malignant. Benign neoplasms are more likely than their malignant counterparts to stop growing spontaneously, to remain separate from the surrounding tissues, and to maintain a high level of differentiated appearance and function. Malignant neoplasms characteristically infiltrate surrounding tissue, establish new sites of multiplication at distant locations **(metastases)**, express immature and undifferentiated cellular characteristics, and may recur after surgical removal or treatment with cytotoxic agents.

Leukemia versus Lymphoma

Cells of certain types can experience either benign or malignant neoplastic proliferation, but neoplasms of the lymphoreticular system are malignant, almost without exception. Malignant proliferation that involves primarily circulating cells of blood and the bone marrow are called **leukemias;** neoplasms that originate in the solid tissues of the immune system are called **lymphomas.** Malignant leukemic cells may infiltrate solid tissues, and lymphoma cells may be found in the bloodstream; however, the diagnostic distinction—admittedly imperfect—is useful both clinically and theoretically.

Cells of Origin

Malignant cell proliferations arise from defects in regulation of the genetic processes that control replication. Cells at any stage of the differentiation process may escape from normal control. These cells will express the same dysregulation and will be at the same stage of differentiation as the parent cell. In classifying malignancies of the lymphoreticular system, the techniques used to identify normal populations can be applied to neoplastic cells. Rearrangement of immunoglobulin (Ig) or T-cell receptor (TCR) genes, presence of Ig and cluster determinant (CD) markers can be used to identify the origin of the malignant lymphocytes. Unchecked multiplication, however, often distorts protein synthesis and intracellular organization, so the malignant population may bear little immediate morphologic resemblance to normal cells of the same lineage. Characterization of cells that have lost their normal appearance and function can best be done with monoclonal antibodies to surface molecules and by genetic analysis of deoxyribonucleic acid (DNA) sequences. Identification of origin and stage of development is important for establishing prognosis and treatment modes.

Lymphoreticular neoplasms may arise from B cells, T cells, or mononuclear phagocytes, and the proliferating clone may reflect any stage of differentiation. Different neoplasms exhibit different patterns of age distribution, clinical course, and response to treatment. Table 11–1 outlines the developmental origins of most lymphoreticular neoplasms.

Cytogenetics

Nuclear events control the fate of all cells—normal and abnormal. Cytogenetic techniques that have been especially useful in examining chromosomes and individ-

TABLE 11–1. **Malignancies of the Lymphoreticular System**

Cell of Origin	Usual Clinical Condition
Lymphoblast, no other distinguishing features	"Null cell" acute lymphoblastic leukemia (ALL)
pre–B cell	ALL positive for the common-ALL antigen (CALLA. CD10)
Prothymocyte	T-cell ALL
Thymocyte	T-cell lymphoblastic lymphoma
Mature or partially differentiated B cell	Chronic lymphocytic leukemia (CLL) Burkitt's lymphoma Various non-Hodgkin's lymphomas Hairy cell leukemia
Immunoglobulin-secreting B cell/plasma cell	Multiple myeloma Waldenström's macroglobulinemia Heavy-chain disease Mediterranean lymphoma
Mature T cell	Adult T-cell leukemia/lymphoma T-cell chronic lymphocytic leukemia (TCLL) Sezary syndrome Mycosis fungoides Various non-Hodgkin's lymphomas
Monocyte/macrophage lineage	Hodgkin's disease (probably) True histiocytic lymphoma Histiocytosis X Monocytic or monoblastic leukemia

ual gene sequences are **karyotype analysis,** DNA probing by **restriction fragment length polymorphisms (RFLP;** see Chapter 5) and **fluorescent *in situ* hybridization.** Karyotype analysis reveals the morphology of chromosomes captured during mitosis. Histochemical, immunologic, and photographic techniques are used to characterize the size and shape of individual chromosomes and to identify abnormalities of appearance, number, and location of chromosomal segments. Specific chromosomal abnormalities are associated with certain types of neoplasms; therefore, cytogenetic studies can help identify disease, can provide clues to disease progression, and monitor remission. With RFLP techniques, the DNA sequence of specific segments can be mapped and compared with segments of known characteristics.

DNA probes can be made for specific gene abnormalities, and it is then possible to "paint" chromosomes with these probes and visually identify and pinpoint the location of an abnormal gene. The DNA probe is designed to hybridize or bind to complementary nucleotide sequences on the host cell DNA. If the abnormal gene is present, probe DNA binds. The probe carries a fluorescent tag so that its location can be visualized by fluorescence microscopy. This technique is called **FISH** for fluorescent *in situ* hybridization.

In diagnosing lymphoreticular malignancies, identification of genetic rearrangements are used to assign cells to B or T classifications and to discriminate proliferating neoplastic clones from other cells with which they are admixed. If specific cytogenetic abnormalities are frequently associated with certain neoplasms, it suggests that individual gene sequences influence development of specific kinds of neoplastic multiplication. Mapping procedures have revealed the presence and location of DNA segments, called **proto-oncogenes,** which are present in normal cells but which, after activation by various known or unknown stimuli, become **oncogenes** that mediate unregulated cell multiplication.

MALIGNANCIES OF LYMPHOID PRECURSORS

Neoplastic proliferation of minimally differentiated lymphoid cells is called **acute lymphoblastic leukemia (ALL).** Morphology, immunophenotype, and cytogenetic changes are cellular characteristics used to classify types of ALL. Morphologic classification is usually performed according to the French-American-British (FAB) system. With this system, types of ALL are divided into morphologic classes based on size and cytoplasmic and nuclear features. Unique cytogenetic abnormalities and identification of CD numbers can assign these prefunctional cells to individual lineages. However, the untreated clinical course of all such neoplasms is relatively uniform.

Acute Leukemia

Acute leukemia reflects a blockage in early differentiation events. Extremely immature cells overrun sites at which lymphocytes normally multiply, especially the bone marrow, where they suppress the division and maturation of red blood cells (RBCs), platelets, and granulocytes. Problems arise not only from unchecked multiplication of neoplastic cells, but also from absence of normal lymphocyte-mediated activities. The clinical picture usually includes anemia, with consequent weakness and impaired tissue function; thrombocytopenia, with bleeding from mucosal surfaces and into the skin; and granulocytopenia, leading to problems with infection. Impaired humoral and cell-mediated immunity (CMI) exacerbates the susceptibility to infection.

Predisposition and Prognosis

Any cell of bone marrow origin can exhibit leukemic proliferation; lymphocytes and granulocytes are most commonly involved. In general, ALL affects children, whereas acute leukemia of granulocyte precursors (myeloblastic leukemia) begins after puberty. Sometimes children suffer from acute myeloblastic leukemia, and adults may have ALL. Occasionally patients with leukemia have had exposure to ionizing radiation or mutagenic chemicals, but for most cases, no predisposing event is apparent. Viral infection has been implicated as a causative agent in two lymphoid neoplasms: Burkitt's lymphoma and adult T-cell leukemia. Spontaneous or induced immunodeficiency conditions and certain congenital chromosomal abnormalities also impose an excess risk of developing leukemia.

Common Acute Lymphoblastic Leukemia

Acute leukemias are usually characterized by the presence of circulating blast cells. Identification of the type of blast cell is dependent on morphologic and cytochemical evaluation, immunophenotyping, cytogenetic, and molecular genetic analysis. ALL can be divided into subtypes by the presence of specific receptors or antigens on the cell membrane of leukemic blast cells. The most frequently identified antigen on leukemic cells of both adult and childhood ALL is called **common acute lymphoblastic leukemia antigen (CALLA).** This surface marker, also designated CD10, is not specific for leukemia; it is present on early lymphoid precursor cells and is a marker for cellular immaturity. In normal marrow at all ages, approximately 1 percent of cells express CALLA. Common ALL blast cells do not express markers such as cytoplasmic Igs or surface Igs characteristic of more mature B cells. Nonhematopoietic cells that are CD10-positive include renal epithelium in adults and fetuses, fetal intestinal cells, and myoepithelial cells of the adult breast. Occasionally, CALLA may be seen on malignant blasts present in the terminal stage of chronic granulocytic leukemia.

Other Markers

Leukemic cells that express CALLA are also frequently positive for CD19 and the enzyme, terminal deoxynucleotidyl transferase (TdT). Although sometimes considered a marker for immature T cells, TdT is also present in the nucleus of early B-lineage cells where it aids in the rearrangement and production of diversity in Ig genes. About 10 percent of lymphoblastic leukemias are CALLA-negative, lack B-cell, T-cell, and pre–B-cell markers, but express HLA-DR, CD19, and TdT and have undergone Ig gene rearrangement. These leukemias are termed early pre–B cell ALL, or progenitor B-cell ALL.

More Differentiated Precursors

Of patients with childhood ALL, 10 to 15 percent have cells of T-cell lineages. Blast cells in these cases express the T-cell antigens CD7, CD2 (the sheep-cell rosette receptor) or the cortical thymocyte antigen T6 (CD1). T-cell ALL carries a worse clinical prognosis than progenitor B-cell or CALLA-positive lymphoblastic leukemia. In all types of childhood ALL, predictors of an unfavorable clinical course include male sex, high white blood cell numbers at presentation, and older age at onset. Patients with T-cell ALL also tend to have malignant cells in solid organs, particularly those sites where normal T cells pass from the circulation into solid tissue.

Cells that have mu heavy chains in the cytoplasm are considered pre–B cells; 15 to 20 percent of ALL cases involve pre–B cells, which are also positive for CALLA and for TdT. They lack Ig monomers on the membrane, the hallmark of the mature B cell, but do have CD21, the receptor for Epstein-Barr virus (EBV) recognition (see Fig. 5–10). Rarely, ALL involves mature B cells, which express membrane Ig and Fc receptors and lack CALLA and TdT. Only 2 to 5 percent of ALL cases fall into this category; affected patients respond very poorly to therapy and rarely survive more than 4 to 6 months.

As the disease progresses, markers on the neoplastic cells may change. CALLA may disappear if initially present or develop if initially absent. Features that distinguish T from B cells do not change. T-cell forms do not acquire B-cell characteristics or vice versa, and null cells do not later assume distinguishing features.

NEOPLASMS OF MATURE B LYMPHOCYTES

The mature B cell displays surface immunoglobulin (sIg) and other markers described in Chapter 5, but has not differentiated into an Ig-producing plasma cell. Neoplasms of mature B lymphocytes include both solid-tissue malignancies (lymphomas) and primary bone marrow conditions (leukemias).

Chronic Lymphocytic Leukemia

In **chronic lymphocytic leukemia (CLL),** the bone marrow is heavily populated by partially mature B lymphocytes that do not secrete Ig and are essentially nonfunctional. Adequate production of other normal cells in the bone marrow does occur during early phases of the disease. The neoplastic cells of CLL multiply much less rapidly than those of lymphoblastic leukemia. The leukemic cells have an abnormally prolonged life span, and eventually enormous numbers of cells accumulate. The disease usually remains indolent until the late stages during which there is loss of normal marrow function and infiltration of lymph nodes, spleen, and other tissues by leukemic cells. During terminal stages of the disease, the previously mature neoplastic cells may undergo irreversible transformation to immature blast configuration. Even if blast crisis does not occur, cells that previously appeared normal become larger and more atypical as the disease progresses.

Serum Ig concentration may be quantitatively normal, but functional immunity is often impaired. With reduced normal immune responses, there is an increased likelihood of dysfunctional immune activity. Autoantibodies to RBCs occur fairly frequently, sometimes causing significant hemolysis. Autoantibodies to platelets occur less commonly, but may cause symptomatic thrombocytopenia. As in many other immunodeficiency and dysfunctional states, patients with CLL have an increased likelihood of developing other malignant neoplasms.

Hairy Cell Leukemia

The name **hairy cell leukemia** derives from the peculiar filamentous projections of cytoplasm characteristic of these neoplastic cells (Fig. 11–1). Features characteristic of B cells include rearrangement of heavy-chain and light-chain genes, the presence of sIg, and existence of receptors for gamma-chain Fc, but not usually for C3. Unlike normal B cells, hairy cells are capable of limited phagocytosis, and they exhibit some reactivity with antibody against one of the monocyte-macrophage antigens. Another distinctive feature is strong expression of CD25, the receptor for interleukin-2 (IL-2). An early name for this molecule was Tac, denoting a marker for T-cell activation. IL-2 is now known to stimulate B cells as well as T cells, so the presence of its receptor need not identify the underlying cell as a T cell. Hairy cells seem most plausibly to be B lymphocytes in the phase of activation that precedes evolution into Ig-secreting plasma cells.

The clinical course of hairy cell leukemia is less aggressive than that of ALL, but somewhat more aggressive than most chronic lymphocytic leukemias. Middle-aged men are most frequently affected; splenomegaly and leukopenia are characteristic findings on presentation. Splenectomy has long been the treatment of choice for hairy cell leukemia, but interferon-α and new chemotherapeutic drugs have recently been used with excellent results in this type of leukemia. The most common and severe complications result from infections, but many patients also manifest autoimmune problems of various kinds.

Lymphomas

Lymphomas are solid tumors of the lymphoreticular system. Because many clinical syndromes and morphologic entities exist, classification systems of the lymphomas are confusing and controversial. Most lymphomas involve cells in middle or late stages of differentiation. The small proportion of cases called **lymphoblastic lymphomas** involve early T-cell precursors and have a very poor prognosis despite aggressive therapy.

Different classification systems place varying emphasis on cellular appearance, on the putative origin of the cells, on the overall tissue patterns, and on the clinical course. A reasonable summary is that lymphomas in which small, fairly uniform-looking cells grow in a nondestructive pattern have a less aggressive clinical course

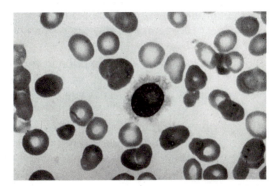

FIGURE 11–1. This "hairy cell" takes its name from the irregular cytoplasmic filaments seen in this Wright-stained preparation. On scanning electron microscopy, these cells have a densely ruffled contour.

and embody a later stage of maturation than conditions with large or pleomrpic cells and a growth pattern that disrupts normal architectural features.

Other than Burkitt's lymphoma (see following text), the occurrence of B-cell lymphomas increases with age. As lymphomas become more aggressive, normal B-cell activity diminishes and predisposition to autoimmune abnormalities increases. Bone marrow involvement occurs late or not at all, so abnormalities of RBCs, granulocytes, and platelets are less common than in leukemias. Anemia of chronic disease, weight loss, and other dysfunctions characteristic of systemic malignancies occur in advanced phases.

Burkitt's Lymphoma

Burkitt's lymphoma is a tumor of mature B lymphocytes first described in Africa, where it predominantly affects children. In affected tissues, diffusely proliferating lymphocytes are interspersed with large, pale macrophages and produce a "starry-sky" pattern when observed with low-power microscopy.

Untreated Burkitt's lymphoma is highly aggressive, growing and destroying the bone or other site of origin and spreading rapidly to other tissues. Prompt and intensive chemotherapy often induces a rapid, dramatic, and longlasting response. Although recurrence sometimes follows successful therapy, many patients experience lifelong remission. In certain areas of Africa, the tumor occurs so frequently that it is described as endemic. Sporadic cases of Burkitt's lymphoma occur in other parts of the world. Bones of the jaw are the most common primary site for tumors in Africans, followed by sites in the abdomen. Lymph nodes, the mucosa of the upper respiratory tract, and the bone marrow are seldom involved. In non-African cases, primary sites include the nervous system, kidneys, gonads, retroperitoneal tissue, liver, and spleen. In African but not sporadic cases, Epstein-Barr virus (EBV) is closely associated with the lymphoma. The chromatin of tumor cells contains genetic elements of EBV, and virus can be recovered from cultures.

Translocation and Oncogene

Burkitt's lymphoma provides an exciting illustration of consistent chromosomal abnormality and the association of an oncogene with neoplasia. The neoplastic cells of Burkitt's lymphoma characteristically express a translocation in which chromosomal material from the long arm of chromosome 8 is translocated to the long arm of chromosome 14, but sometimes the short arm of chromosome 2 or the long arm of 22 (Fig. 11–2). The break in chromosome 8 occurs at the location of the proto-oncogene called c-*myc*. The break in the other chromosomes occurs between the *v* and *c* genes that control production of the Ig heavy chain (chromosome 14) or the kappa and the lambda light chains on chromosome 2 and 22. c-*myc* is a proto-oncogene whose product is a transcription factor. Binding of transcription factors to promoter regions of genes turns on protein synthesis. Translocation of c-*myc* promotes conversion from a proto-oncogene to an oncogene. The resulting deregulation of normal function leads to uncontrolled cell proliferation. Chromosomal translocation is only one mechanism for oncogene activation. Other mechanisms include deletion, base pair mutation, and gene amplification. Oncogene activation and resulting deregulation of function is believed to play a role in the development of most if not all lymphomas.

Translocation (8;14) in Burkitt's Lymphoma

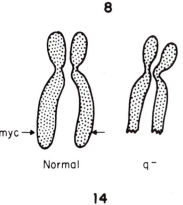

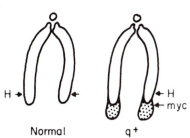

FIGURE 11–2. Normal examples of chromosome 8 (*top*) and 14 (*below*) are on the left. The proto-oncogene *myc* is located near the end of the long arm of chromosome 8. The site that directs production of immunoglobulin heavy chains (designated H) is near the end of chromosome 14. With an 8 : 14 translocation, shown in the two figures on the right, chromosome 8 loses a fragment that breaks at the *myc* site and chromosome 14 acquires the additional material, resulting in conversion of *myc* to an oncogene and the H-chain site in close proximity.

Significance of Epstein-Barr Virus

Burkitt's lymphoma is associated with EBV and primarily occurs in Africa. EBV is known to modify cell growth and multiplication. Insertion of DNA from EBV into the genome of cultured cells causes the recipient cells to become "transformed." They express growth and metabolic properties characteristic of cultured neoplastic cells, and they continue dividing indefinitely as long as culture conditions are favorable. In vivo, EBV infects B lymphocytes through the CD21 antigen, which serves as a virus receptor. EBV is the cause of infectious mononucleosis and as a result of infection of B cells, T-cell behavior is affected. Enhanced numbers and activity of cytotoxic/suppressor T cells is seen. These cells are referred to as "atypical" lymphocytes and demonstrate morphologic features characteristic of this disease.

EBV infection is widespread throughout Africa, but Burkitt's lymphoma is endemic only in certain areas, which are also characterized by intense prevalence of malaria. Malaria is known to distort T-cell function. It is plausible to assume that abnormal immune regulation might occur in children whose immune systems are challenged by repeated malarial infections. The normal response of cytotoxic/ suppressor T cells to EBV infection is to kill or suppress *in vivo* proliferation of infected B cells, but T-cell abnormalities induced by malaria could well interrupt this regulatory function. Because translocational events are more likely to occur during exuberant cell division, unchecked multiplication of EBV-infected cells could provoke damage to chromosome 8 and transposition of the oncogene. Adding plausibility to this hypothesis is the increased occurrence of Burkitt's lymphoma in patients with AIDS, who are known to have aberrant T-cell function and in whom EBV infection is extremely common. Possibly the numerous non-African cases of Burkitt's lymphoma reflect other types of prolonged or repeated immune dysregulation. Such a scenario does not explain why the crucial chromosomal sites are selectively involved, nor does it explain the unique sensitivity of the lymphoma to cytotoxic chemotherapy.

NEOPLASMS OF PLASMA CELLS

Plasma cells that are fully differentiated Ig-secreting cells may undergo malignant proliferation. Igs derived from the multiplying cells often can be found in the serum and usually cause serum protein abnormalities. Either a normal molecule is present in abnormal quantities or a protein accumulates that is not normally present in blood or body fluids. The presence of any serum protein abnormality is called a **dysproteinemia;** the term **paraproteinemia** usually refers to protein that is qualitatively abnormal. Most dysproteinemias reflect excess production of structurally normal Igs or their constituent chains, but in some proliferative disorders, structurally variant proteins accumulate in serum or tissues.

Monoclonal Gammopathy

Monoclonal gammopathy denotes accumulation of protein that originates from a single proliferating clone. The traditional way to demonstrate monoclonal origin has been electrophoretic analysis of the protein, but newer analytic techniques permit direct demonstration of uniform molecular properties in the proliferating protein-producing cells.

Migration of a protein in an electric field is determined by molecular size, shape, and charge, which reflect the amino acid sequence and associated side chains. Molecules of different structures express different migration patterns on an electrophoretic strip; densitometer analysis of the strip gives a tracing that depicts the migration rate and relative concentration of the separated proteins. When several different molecules migrate close to one another, the group of incompletely separated proteins appears as a diffuse, irregular-shaped elevation on the densitometer tracing. A single protein at high concentration produces intense staining at the sharply focused site where that molecule accumulates. On the densitometer tracing, this appears as a narrow, sharply defined peak with height proportional to the concentration of monoclonal protein (Fig. 11–3). Such a peak is called an **M spike;** M stands for monoclonal or myeloma (the most common cause of this diagnostic finding), not for mu chain or IgM class.

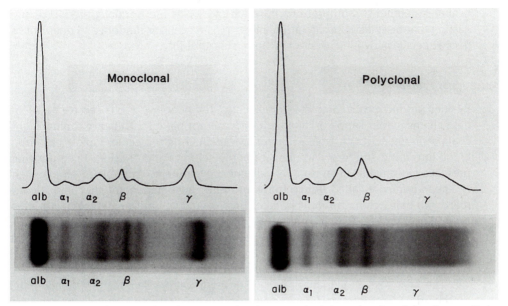

FIGURE 11–3. In the monoclonal gammopathy shown on the left, molecules of the abnormally increased globulin have migrated on the gel strip as a dense, homogeneous band in the gamma region. The densitometer tracing depicts a clearly defined peak. In the polyclonal increase shown at right, the entire gamma region is diffusely dark, and the densitometer tracing shows an irregular hump.

Multiple Myeloma

Multiple myeloma is a malignant neoplasm of plasma cells that largely affects older adults. It is characterized by masses of neoplastic cells in bone and marrow at various sites; "myelo" denotes marrow, and "-oma" means mass. Early in the process, the plasma cells have nearly normal appearance and function, but as neoplastic multiplication progresses, the cells lose differentiation of function and appearance.

Clinical Events

The bone is usually painful at the site of neoplastic cell accumulation and may be so weakened that fractures occur spontaneously. Although monoclonal protein is conspicuous in serum, overall levels of Ig decline, and susceptibility to infection increases. Anemia is common, reflecting depression of erythropoiesis rather than marrow infiltration by neoplastic plasma cells. Serum calcium is usually high and, along with abnormalities of urine protein levels, often impairs renal function. Therapy usually induces a favorable response, and survival is characteristically measured in years. Common causes of death are infection, hematologic complications, and renal failure.

The most striking diagnostic feature in multiple myeloma is accumulation of monoclonal protein, its nature determined by the phenotype of the proliferating plasma cell. The monoclonal protein is IgG in 50 percent of cases, IgA in 25 percent of cases, IgM in 15 to 20 percent, and IgD or IgE much less commonly. These percentages parallel the proportions in which Ig classes are normally produced, suggesting that neoplastic proliferation affects plasma cells at random and does not reflect a specific activating event or intrinsic susceptibility.

Bence Jones Protein

Besides production of complete Ig molecules, the neoplastic cells secrete excessive light chains, either kappa or lambda, which are not paired with heavy chains. Light-chain monomers, much smaller than the four-chain Ig molecule, rapidly pass from blood into urine and rarely accumulate in the serum. For more than a century, their presence in urine has been used as a diagnostic feature for multiple myeloma. Light chains in urine are called **Bence Jones protein.** These unpaired light chains do not react with many chemical indicators for protein and will not be detected with most urine dipsticks. The unique property of Bence Jones protein is that it precipitates when heated to about 55°C and then redissolves at temperatures near the boiling point. Most proteins are irreversibly denatured by heat, and the cloudy precipitate that forms on heating remains despite further heating or cooling (Fig. 11–4).

The heat test is a dramatic but insensitive way to demonstrate Bence Jones proteinuria. Electrophoresis of concentrated urinary proteins, a more sensitive technique, demonstrates Bence Jones protein in urine of 50 to 70 percent of patients with multiple myeloma. About 20 percent of myeloma patients have Bence Jones proteinuria as the only indication of dysproteinemia. Highly concentrated light chains in the urine damage renal epithelium; in patients with myeloma the development of renal failure parallels the magnitude and duration of Bence Jones proteinuria. Patients with isolated Bence Jones proteinuria without an M spike in serum more often suffer from amyloidosis (see later section) and generally have a poorer prognosis than those whose neoplasms secrete intact Ig molecules (Fig. 11–5).

BENCE-JONES PROTEIN vs. OTHER URINARY PROTEINS

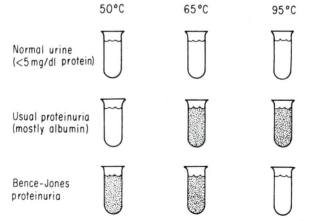

FIGURE 11–4. Heat precipitates most proteins. Heating normal urine (*top panel*) causes no precipitation because little or no protein is present. In most pathologic states, urine protein is largely albumin (*middle panel*) which precipitates irreversibly at about 65°C. Bence Jones protein, (*bottom panel*) precipitates at a lower temperature than does albumin, but redissolves when the temperature approaches the boiling point.

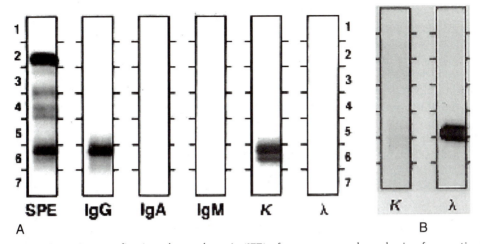

FIGURE 11–5. Immunofixation electrophoresis (IFE) of a serum sample and urine from patients with multiple myeloma. In order to identify the exact immunoglobulin produced in excess by the neoplastic lymphocyte/plasma cell, a serum or urine sample is placed in each lane of an agarose gel support medium. The agarose gel is subjected to electrophoresis and then each lane is overlaid with antibody specific for immunoglobulin heavy chains or light chains (anti-alpha, -mu, -gamma, -kappa, or -lambda). Precipitation will occur between immunoglobulin and anti-immunoglobulin antibody. The gel is washed and stained. Only immunoprecipitates remain in the gel. Identification of excess immunoglobulins is shown by darkly stained bands in specific lanes. In *Figure* A, this multiple myeloma case shows production of a monoclonal IgG with kappa light chains. The first lane to the left is the serum protein electrophoresis (SPE) stained with Coomassie blue. The next lane reveals the monoclonal IgG identified as a discrete homogeneous band. Kappa chains are bound to heavy chains as they migrate in the same position as the IgG. *Figure* B is a urine IFE from another multiple myeloma patient with Bence Jones proteins of lambda type. (Photographs kindly provided by Dr. G. Kukes, Veteran's Affairs Medical Center, Long Beach, CA.)

Other Problems

Clinical problems in multiple myeloma include hyperviscosity of blood and elevation of serum calcium. The hyperviscosity occurs because of the high levels of circulating Ig. Hypercalcemia is thought to result both from bone destruction by the proliferating malignant cells and from abnormalities of renal and bone metabolism.

WALDENSTRÖM'S MACROGLOBULINEMIA

Conceptually similar to multiple myeloma but clinically distinct is **Waldenström's macroglobulinemia,** in which the paraprotein is IgM, usually the pentamer but sometimes also in the monomeric form. This disease is caused by a clone of neoplastic cells that appear to be in an intermediate stage of development between the mature lymphocyte and the early plasma cell. The typical site of cellular proliferation is the solid tissue of the lymphoreticular system, rather than the bone marrow. Patients are generally somewhat older than those with multiple myeloma, and the clinical course ranges from relatively indolent to fairly aggressive. Common presenting complaints are anemia and symptoms caused by abnormal serum proteins.

Accumulating IgM exerts many harmful effects. It causes a bleeding tendency by interfering with platelet function and with the finely regulated interaction of coagulation proteins. Large numbers of individual and aggregated IgM molecules make the blood flow sluggishly, especially in the peripheral portions of the circulation where RBCs may stick to each other and interact abnormally with the cells that line blood vessels. The resulting defects of flow often cause clinical symptoms in the brain, the eyes, and the fingers and toes. Kidney damage is common in Waldenström's macroglobulinemia; contributing factors include deposition of protein, accumulation of aggregated cells in vessels and interstitium, and immune activity against soluble or structural proteins.

Antibodies to Red Blood Cells

Occasionally monoclonal IgMs express specificity for antigens on the patient's RBCs. If the antibody reacts at physiologic temperatures, the result may be the syndrome called **cold agglutinin disease.** Circulating blood achieves somewhat lower temperatures in peripheral areas like the fingers, toes, and tips of the ears than in more central locations. IgM autoantibodies, which react better at cooler temperatures than at 37°C, may agglutinate RBCs and obstruct small vessels in cooler peripheral sites, or they may activate the complement cascade. The affected cells may either lyse within the vessels because of membrane attack by activated complement, termed **intravascular hemolysis,** or they may return to the central circulation and may be damaged by splenic macrophages that express C3 receptors, a phenomenon called **extravascular hemolysis.**

Heavy-Chain Dysproteinemias

Unpaired overproduction occurs less commonly for heavy chains than for light chains. In heavy-chain dysproteinemias, abnormally rearranged genetic material often causes production of structurally abnormal chains. Patients characteristically experience depressed levels of normal Ig, predisposition to infection, and generalized marrow depression. Any heavy-chain isotype except epsilon may be involved, but only alpha-chain disease occurs with any frequency.

Clinical Syndromes

In **alpha heavy-chain disease,** also called **Mediterranean lymphoma,** the lymphoid tissue of the gut is massively infiltrated by lymphocytes and plasma cells of appearance ranging from relatively normal to highly bizarre. Diarrhea, malabsorption, and abnormal muscular activity accompany the mucosal changes. This condition occurs in geographic areas in which the population suffers frequent and recurrent intestinal infections with numerous bacteria, viruses, and parasites. A similar mucosal abnormality affecting only the respiratory tract occurs sporadically in Europe and the United States. In some patients with intestinal manifestations, antimicrobial therapy has induced complete remission. Antilymphoma therapy has been successful in other patients, but many patients have a progressively fatal course despite all therapy.

Amyloidosis

Amyloid is a fibrillar protein that accumulates in many different tissues under various clinical circumstances. Tissues with amyloid deposits stain dark blue with iodine; hence the term amyloid (starchlike). When amyloidosis occurs in patients with the chronic immune stimulation of persistent infection or with disorders of plasma cells, the condition is called **secondary amyloidosis.** Other forms are **primary,** in which there is no other associated abnormality; **familial,** and **degenerative,** in which increasing age is associated with increasing deposition of protein in heart and brain.

Similarities to Ig Chains

Amyloid, which looks featureless and homogeneous on light microscopy, actually includes several different kinds of fibrillar material. Table 11−2 lists the main types of amyloid. The protein seen in patients with primary amyloidosis and in those with plasma cell disorders shares structural characteristics with the Ig light chain, more

TABLE 11−2. **Proteins Associated with B-Cell Neoplasms**

Protein	Disease	Structure	Clinical Features
Monoclonal Ig	Multiple myeloma	Normal four-chain immunoglobulin	Hyperviscosity may occur Frequency of involved isotypes parallels normal Ig proportions
Bence Jones	Multiple myeloma	Normal kappa or lambda light chain	Present in urine but not serum Precipitates at 55°C, redisolves at 95°C
Macroglobulin	Waldenström's macroglobulinemia	Normal IgM, sometimes as monomer	Hyperviscosity is common Autoantibody to red cells may cause hemolysis or vascular occlusion
Alpha heavy chain	Mediterranean lymphoma	Alpha heavy chain, often of abnormal structure	Masses of cells infiltrate gut, cause gastrointestinal tract symptoms
Amyloid AL form	Primary amyloidosis, Myeloma or macroglobulinemia-associated	Antibody fragments	Present in muscle, skin, liver, spleen, kidneys, and so on
AA form	Chronic infections	Unique configuration	May accumulate anywhere
AB form	Alzheimer's disease Down's syndrome	B-protein precursor	Present in heart, brain

Ig; immunoglobulin.
Adapted from the 1990 guidelines for the nomenclature and classification of amyloid and amyloidosis.

TABLE 11–3. **Selected Neoplasms of B Lymphocytes**

Disease	Presumed Cell of Origin	Predominant Population Affected	Significant Clinical Events	Prognosis (With Appropriate Treatment)
Acute lymphoblastic leukemia (ALL)	Pre–pre B or pre-B	Prepubertal children	Normal marrow replaced by leukemic cells Infections, bleeding common	Up to 70% long-term survival when onset between ages 2 and 10
Chronic lymphocytic leukemia (CLL)	Partially to fully mature B cell	Older adults	Peripheral blood lymphocytosis Autoimmune problems Second tumors common	Prolonged course (3–20 years) but no cures
Hairy cell leukemia	B cells, possibly in activated state	Middle-aged men	Splenomegaly Pronounced marrow infiltration Neutropenia and infections	Usual course 3–5 years
Burkitt's lymphoma	Mature B cells	Children and adolescents (M:F ratio = 2:1)	Rapidly enlarging extranodal tumors Translocation of chromosome 8 Association with Epstein-Barr virus in African type	Up to 50% long-term survival after prompt, intensive treatment
Non-Hodgkin's lymphomas (approx. 65%)	Various phases	Older adults	Painless lymphadenopathy Extranodal tumors	Moderate to poor
Multiple myeloma	Plasma cells	Middle-aged and elderly	Monoclonal gammopathy Bence Jones protein Bone lesions and hypercalcemia	Survival 3–6 years
Waldenström's macroglobulinemia	Ig-secreting lymphocytes	Elderly	Hyperviscosity Cold-agglutinin syndrome	Plasma exchange ameliorates symptoms Survival approx. 3 years
Mediterranean lymphoma	IgA-secreting plasma cells	Young adults	Mucosal tumors of small intestine	Variable; some cures, some rapid progression

often lambda than kappa. Amyloid with similarities to Ig light chains includes the V portion of the light chain; some examples also express part or all of the C domain. Molecular weight varies between 5 and 25 kD. It is not clear why amyloid accumulates or whether the deposited material reflects degradation of previously intact chains.

Other Forms

Some forms of amyloidosis are protein abnormalities associated with immune system dysfunction, but many are not. The structure of the amyloid that accompanies chronic infections and other chronic illnesses has a unique structure unrelated to any other known protein. The form that accumulates in senile heart and brain is chemically related to prealbumin. No specific therapy exists for any of these conditions. For amyloidosis of chronic infection or plasma-cell disorders, treating the primary disease prevents further progression, but the material already deposited does not regress.

Benign Monoclonal Gammopathy

Electrophoresis of serum proteins from some seemingly normal older individuals reveals an M spike. Of otherwise normal persons older than 70 years, 5 to 8 percent have this abnormality, but its significance is inconclusive. Some patients subsequently develop malignant monoclonal proliferative conditions; in others, the monoclonal protein remains stable for many years and lymphoreticular abnormalities never develop. The term **benign monoclonal gammopathy** or **monoclonal gammopathy of undetermined significance (MGUS)** is used when an M spike is found as the only abnormality in an otherwise healthy person. If cellular proliferation develops, the diagnosis becomes that of the evolving disorder. If the serum protein abnormality remains stable and asymptomatic, the diagnosis of benign monoclonal gammopathy stands. Because this condition affects older people and because plasma cell disorders take many years to become apparent, it is probable that many "benign" monoclonal conditions never reveal their malignant aspect because the patient dies of unrelated causes.

Table 11–3 summarizes significant neoplasms of B-cell origin.

MALIGNANCIES OF MATURE T LYMPHOCYTES

Despite the fact that T cells constitute about 70 percent of peripheral blood lymphocytes, proliferative disorders of T cells involve solid tissues more often than bone marrow or circulating blood. Of the chronic lymphocytic leukemias, only 2 to 5 percent involve T cells. Although morphologically indistinguishable from cells in B-cell chronic lymphocytic leukemia, the leukemic cells show genetic rearrangement of the T-receptor sites and express the pan–T antigen CD2, the sheep-cell rosette receptor. In most T-cell chronic leukemias, the cells have cytoplasmic granules and high enzyme levels, suggesting possible kinship with large granular lymphocytes or with T cells at the prolymphocyte stage of maturation.

TABLE 11–4. Selected Neoplasms of T Lymphocytes

Disease	Presumed Cell of Origin	Predominant Group Affected	Predominant Clinical Events	Post-Treatment Prognosis
Acute lymphoblastic leukemia (ALL)	Immature T cell	Children > 5 years; M > F	Normal marrow replaced by leukemic cells Infections, bleeding common	Less favorable than B-cell types
Lymphoblastic lymphoma	Partially differentiated thymocyte	Older children and young adults; elderly	Mediastinal mass Dissemination to meninges, marrow	Generally poor
Adult T-cell leukemia/lymphoma	Mature T cell expressing CD4	Adults, especially blacks	Association with HTLV-1 Bone lesions and hypercalcemia; solid-tissue infiltration	Very poor
Cutaneous lymphomas	CD4+ T cells	Adults	Localized skin lesions; blood, other organs involved later	Local therapy helps skin lesions; survival worsens when disease disseminates

Adult T-Cell Leukemia/Lymphoma

Adult T-cell leukemia/lymphoma is most commonly found in southwestern Japan and the Caribbean basin. This aggressive process involves the skin in addition to blood and the solid lymphoreticular tissues. The leukemic cells display markers of mature T cells, including CD4 and the IL-2 receptor. Functionally active, they exert a suppressor effect on other lymphocytes, and they secrete a lymphokine that leads to bone damage and hypercalcemia. Uniquely significant is the association of this disease with infection by the retrovirus called human T-lymphotropic virus type I (HTLV-I) or human T-cell leukemia virus. Viruses have long been implicated in animal and avian leukemias, but this is the first virus proven to cause human leukemia.

Cutaneous T-Cell Lymphoma

CD4+ lymphocytes infiltrate the skin in a group of conditions known as **mycosis fungoides** and **Sézary syndrome.** In Sézary syndrome, neoplastic cells of uniform appearance are present both in skin and in circulating blood. In mycosis fungoides, there is greater diversity of cells in the skin, but circulatory involvement is rare. Both pursue an indolent course, but, in longstanding cases, the neoplastic cells eventually infiltrate lymph nodes, spleen, and liver. Hypergammaglobulinemia and elevation of serum IgE and IgA are common, but CMI remains active until the advanced phases; liability to infection is rarely a problem.

Systemic Lymphomas

Relatively few lymphomas have T-cell phenotypes, but, as a group, they are marked by an aggressive course and comparatively poor prognosis. The neoplastic cells vary in size and shape and have a diffuse growth pattern that obliterates preexisting architectural features. Inflammatory cells frequently accompany the neoplastic cells, possibly in response to chemotactic lymphokines. These diffuse mixed-cell lymphomas express CD4 more often than CD8. A category of large-celled, highly aggressive lymphomas called **immunoblastic sarcoma** usually derives from B cells, but 5 to 15 percent are of T-cell origin. These tumors, which respond poorly to therapy, often occur in patients with preexisting immune dysfunction.

Mature T cells and their lymphokines are implicated in a condition variously called **angiocentric immunoproliferative lesion,** atypical lymphocytic vasculitis, and polymorphic reticulosis. Lymphocytes and inflammatory cells infiltrate and progressively destroy blood or lymphatic vessels. The lymphokine-stimulated cells display conspicuous phagocytosis of blood cells, especially erythrocytes.

Table 11–4 summarizes significant neoplasms of T-cell origin.

HODGKIN'S DISEASE

Lymphomas are a very heterogeneous group of diseases that arise from lymphoid tissue (lymphocytes, macrophages, and reticulum cells). The lymphomas are often broadly divided into two major categories: Hodgkin's disease or Hodgkin's lymphoma and non-Hodgkin's lymphoma. The characteristic cell type associated with

Hodgkin's disease is the **Reed-Sternberg cell,** a large cell with abundant cytoplasm and, classically, two or more nuclei with prominent nucleoli. With identification of CD markers, cell culture, and with the polymerase chain reaction (PCR) techniques to amplify genes expressed by Reed-Sternberg cells, these cells seem to be neoplastic cells capable of expressing phenotypes of multiple cell lineages. Other cell types that form the bulk of Hodgkin's disease tumors are lymphocytes, plasma cells, granulocytes, and fibroblasts. These cells may be precursors to Reed-Sternberg cells, host inflammatory cells, and cells recruited to the site in response to cytokines produced by the Reed-Sternberg cells. Although Hodgkin's disease does not appear to be a primary T-cell neoplasm, depressed T-cell activity occurs even in early phases.

Classification

Different cases of HD present different histologic appearances and clinical syndromes. These have been systematized into several classifications used to predict prognosis and, to a certain extent, to plan therapy (Table 11–5). Age distribution is bimodal. One peak occurs in young adults, and then few cases occur until gradually increasing numbers of cases develop after age 50. The forms that occur in young adults respond much better to therapy than those of older patients. Many young

TABLE 11–5. **Features of Hodgkin's Disease**

Cells Involved
  Reed-Sternberg cell: ? monocytoid, ? interdigitating cell
  Reactive cells: lymphocytes, plasma cells, granulocytes, fibroblasts

Patterns of Lymph Node Change (Rye Classification)
  Lymphocyte predominance: 5–15% of cases: often asymptomatic, excellent prognosis
  Nodular sclerosis: 40–75% of cases, multiple nodes involved, often in young women, good
    prognosis
  Mixed cellularity: 20–40% of cases, usually asymptomatic; patients are middle-aged; fair
    prognosis
  Lymphocyte depletion: 5–15% of cases, presents at advanced stage; poor prognosis

Clinical Staging (Ann Arbor Classification)
  (A) denotes absence, (B) denotes presence of fever, night sweats, weight loss of >10% of
    body weight
    I: Single node region or localized, single extralymphatic site
    II: Two or more node regions or one node region and one localized extralymphatic site
        on same side of diaphragm
    III: Node regions on both sides of diaphragm, with or without involvement of spleen or
        localized involvement of extralymphatic site
    IV: Multiple or disseminated extralymphatic sites, with or without lymph nodes

Therapeutic Approaches, With 5-year Disease-free Survival Rates
  Localized radiation therapy, for stages I and II, A or B: 70–90%
  Total irradiation, with or without chemotherapy, for some stage IIIA: 70–80%
  Combined chemotherapy, with or without irradiation, for some stage IIIA: 65–75%
  Combination chemotherapy, for stage IIIB: 60%
  Combination chemotherapy, for stage IV, A or B: 50%

Adapted from Glick JH: Hodgkin's disease. In: Wyngaarden JB, Smith LH, Jr. eds: Cecil Textbook of Medicine, 18th ed. Philadelphia: WB Saunders, 1988:1014–1022

adults have been aggressively treated and are alive and healthy many years later, but older patients rarely have an outcome as favorable.

In the most favorable form, called **lymphocyte predominance,** Reed-Sternberg cells are few, small lymphocytes are numerous and uniform, and there is little inflammatory cell admixture. Another pattern with an excellent prognosis, **nodular sclerosis,** occurs primarily in young women. It is characterized by abundant fibrous tissue that encircles nodules of reactive and neoplastic cells in varying proportions. The form called **mixed cellularity** is common in older patients; it has numerous and sometimes atypical Reed-Sternberg cells and a reactive cell population that includes variable proportions of lymphocytes, plasma cells, neutrophils, eosinophils, histiocytes, and fibroblasts. The form of nodular sclerosis with the worst prognosis is called **lymphocyte depletion;** it has numerous, often strikingly pleomorphic, neoplastic cells and very few reactive cells.

Clinical Findings

Hodgkin's disease, although a primary neoplasm of lymph nodes, may involve any part of the lymphoreticular system and virtually any organ of the body. The primary complaint is usually enlarged lymph nodes, but sometimes investigation is precipitated by fever, anemia, or unexplained laboratory findings. Some cases come to medical attention only because enlarged lymph nodes are found on chest or abdominal x-rays taken for some other reason.

It is important to know how far the disease has progressed before beginning and subsequently evaluating therapy. Disease at presentation is classified into stages I through IV, according to the number and location of involved lymph nodes and the presence of disease in spleen or nonlymphoid organs. These are described in Table 11–5. Within each stage of extent, the letters A and B are used to connote the absence or presence of such symptoms as weight loss, fever, night sweats, and bone pain.

NEOPLASMS OF MONOCYTE/MACROPHAGES

Before solid tumors could be accurately phenotyped, many non-Hodgkin's lymphomas were described as histiocytic or reticulum cell tumors. With better diagnostic techniques, the neoplastic cells in most of these can now be identified as lymphocytes at varying stages of differentiation and maturation. Only a few lymphomas—possibly 5 to 10 percent—derive from monocyte/macrophage lines. In these lymphomas, the malignant cells possess receptors for Fc and complement and frequently manifest phagocytic capability. This group of non-Hodgkin's lymphomas is called **true histiocytic lymphoma** and carries a poor prognosis.

Monocytic Leukemia

Pure monocytic or monoblastic leukemia is malignant proliferation of bone marrow cells derived from myelocyte/monocyte precursors. It is a relatively uncommon subcategory of leukemia and is more a hematologic than a lymphoreticular neoplasm.

Histiocytosis X

Histiocytosis X includes several diverse clinical syndromes of unknown etiology. The most prominent conditions are **eosinophilic granuloma, Hand-Schüller-Christian disease,** and **Letterer-Siwe disease.** In all, there is systemic immunodeficiency and proliferation of nonphagocytic mononuclear cells that are probably related to the Langerhans' cell normally found in the skin. Bone and lung are the most common sites of the localized conditions, but destructive changes may affect almost any organ when the involvement is systemic. These conditions usually occur in early childhood.

SUMMARY

1. Neoplasms of the immune system may arise from B cells, T cells, or mononuclear phagocytes, and the proliferative clones may reflect any stage of differentiation. Most neoplasms of the lymphoreticular system are malignant and capable of metastases. Leukemias involve primarily circulating cells of the blood and bone marrow. Lymphomas originate in solid tissues of the immune system.

2. Neoplastic cells of the immune system often fail to differentiate beyond certain stages; therefore, characteristic surface markers or proteins are not expressed. Neoplastic cells may or may not undergo rearrangement of immunoglobulin (Ig) or T-cell receptor genes. Characteristic oncogenes may also be present. Identification of neoplastic cells may be accomplished by monoclonal antibodies to surface molecules, characterization of secreted proteins, and cytogenetic techniques such as karyotype analysis, restriction fragment length polymorphism (RFLP), and use of deoxyribonucleic acid (DNA) probes in fluorescent *in situ* hybridization (FISH).

3. Acute lymphoblastic leukemia (ALL) refers to neoplastic proliferation of minimally differentiated lymphoid cells. Further identification of cell type is based on distinctive cellular morphology, cytogenetic abnormalities, and the presence of cluster determinant (CD) markers. Clinical problems of acute leukemia arise from unchecked proliferation and loss of cell function. Anemia, thrombocytopenia, and granulocytopenia are commonly associated conditions.

4. Common acute lymphoblastic leukemia antigen (CALLA) is the most frequently identified antigen on leukemic cells of both adult and childhood ALL. It is also designated CD10 and is present on normal early lymphoid precursor cells. However, in normal marrow only 1 percent of cells express CALLA. Other markers associated with ALL are CD19 and terminal deoxynucleotidyl transferase (TdT). Depending on the presence of various markers, ALL may be classified as common ALL, early pre–B or progenitor–B-cell ALL, pre–B-cell, or T-cell ALL.

5. Neoplasms of mature B lymphocytes include chronic lymphocytic leukemia (CLL) and lymphomas. CLL consists of mature B cells that accumulate in the bone marrow and circulating blood because of prolonged cellular

life spans. Neoplastic B cells show reduced function and dysfunction in the form of autoantibodies and increased susceptibility to infections. Affected persons also have an increased likelihood of developing other malignant neoplasms.

6. Lymphomas are neoplasms of B cells or T cells usually in the middle or late stages of differentiation; they originate most frequently in lymph nodes, but can originate in any tissue of the body. Burkitt's lymphoma was first described in African children in whom it affects bones of the jaw. It occurs in other parts of the world and in other sites of the body. Burkitt's lymphoma is associated with Epstein-Barr virus (EBV) and characteristic chromosomal abnormalities (translocations and activation of the proto-oncogene c-*myc*.)

7. Plasma cells can also undergo malignant proliferation with continual production of Ig. Monoclonal gammopathies are characterized by accumulation of a single protein that originates from a single proliferating clone of plasma cells. By electrophoresis and densitometer tracing, an M spike can be identified. In multiple myeloma, malignant plasma cells accumulate in the bone, causing hypercalcemia and pathologic fractures. An M spike usually of IgG or IgA is present as well as excessive light chains, which, in the urine, is referred to as Bence Jones protein.

8. Other plasma cell neoplasms are also associated with dysproteinemia and paraproteins. Waldenström's macroglobulinemia is characterized by an IgM paraprotein that causes hyperviscosity of the blood and bleeding because of interference with platelets. In some cases, it may result in cold agglutinin disease. Heavy-chain dysproteinemia is characterized by unpaired heavy chains frequently of alpha type. Amyloid is associated with various diseases, and Igs accumulating in plasma cell disorders show some structural similarities.

9. Malignancies of mature T cells involve lymphomas more often than leukemias. Only 2 to 5 percent of chronic lymphocytic leukemias are T cell in origin. Adult T-cell leukemia is most commonly found in southwestern Japan and the Caribbean and is associated with HTLV-I. Cutaneous T-cell lymphoma, known as mycosis fungoides and Sézary syndrome, is characterized by infiltration of skin with CD4+ lymphocytes. Hypergammaglobulinemia and elevation of IgE and IgA are common clinical signs of the disease. T-cell lymphomas are infrequent, but generally aggressive with poor prognoses.

10. Hodgkin's disease is a lymphoma characterized by a distinctive neoplastic cell called a Reed-Sternberg cell. These cells are capable of expressing phenotypes of multiple cell lineages. Several forms of Hodgkin's disease occur with differing histologic appearance, clinical presentation, and response to therapy.

11. A small number of lymphomas derive from the monocyte/macrophage cell lines and are characterized by cells with Fc and complement receptors and capabilities of phagocytosis. These lymphomas are referred to as histiocytic lymphomas and carry a poor prognosis. Monocytic leukemias occur infrequently, and diseases involving probably neoplastic Langerhans' cells are categorized as histiocytosis X syndromes.

REVIEW QUESTIONS

1. A patient with severe gram-positive bacterial infection is found to have a white blood cell count of 50×10^9/L (normal range 5 to 10×10^9/L). Most of these cells were mature neutrophils. This patient most likely has _____.
   a. chronic myelocytic leukemia
   b. leukemoid reaction
   c. metastases
   d. Hodgkin's disease
   e. Wiskott-Aldrich syndrome

2. Characteristics of malignant neoplasm include _____.
   a. metastases
   b. immature, undifferentiated membrane markers
   c. encapsulation
   d. a and b
   e. a, b, and c

3. Technique useful for identifying neoplastic cells include _____.
   a. detection of surface immunoglobulin or cluster determinant (CD) markers with monoclonal antibodies
   b. karyotype analysis
   c. Fluorescent *in situ* hybridization (FISH)
   d. a and b
   e. a, b, and c

4. Which of the following statements concerning acute lymphoblastic leukemia (ALL) are *true*?
   a. ALL more frequently affects children.
   b. ALL is usually accompanied by anemia and thrombocytopenia.
   c. Exposure to ionizing radiation or mutagenic chemicals are common causes of ALL.
   d. a and b
   e. a, b, and c

5. The most frequently identified antigen on leukemic cells of both adult and childhood ALL is _____.
   a. CD8
   b. CD10
   c. CD12
   d. CD14
   e. CD19

6. In all types of childhood ALL, predictors of an unfavorable clinical course include _____.
   a. high number of white blood cells at presentation
   b. older age at onset
   c. female sex
   d. a and b
   e. a, b, and c

7. Characteristics of the cells associated with chronic lymphocytic leukemia include _____.
   a. nonfunctional B cells
   b. prolonged life span

    c. mu heavy chains in the cytoplasm
    d. a and b
    e. a, b, and c

8. Which of the following statements is *untrue* concerning B-cell lymphomas?
    a. Incidence of B-cell lymphoma increases with age.
    b. Predisposition to autoimmune disease exists.
    c. There is a poor prognosis despite aggressive therapy.
    d. Bone marrow involvement occurs late or not at all.
    e. Anemia of chronic disease and weight loss are seen in advanced phases.

9. African, but not sporadic cases of Burkitt's lymphoma are associated with _____.
    a. Epstein-Barr virus (EBV)
    b. Cytomegalovirus (CMV)
    c. HTLV-1
    d. HIV-2
    e. ERB

10. A translocation of chromosome 8 to chromosome 14 frequently occurs in _____.
    a. Hairy cell leukemia
    b. Burkitt's lymphoma
    c. T-cell ALL
    d. Waldenström's macroglobulinemia
    e. Sézary syndrome

11. An M spike is characteristically observed in _____.
    a. multiple myeloma
    b. monoclonal gammopathy of undetermined significance (MGUS)
    c. Sézary syndrome
    d. a and b
    e. a, b, and c

12. Which of the following concerning cold agglutinin disease is *untrue*?
    a. It is caused by IgG autoantibodies.
    b. It agglutinates red blood cells at 30°C.
    c. It is associated with Waldenström's macroglobulinemia.
    d. It causes increased intravascular hemolysis.
    e. It causes increased extravascular hemolysis.

MATCHING QUESTIONS

Match the distinguishing characteristic in Column 1 with the disease in Column 2.

Column 1

13. c-*myc* oncogene
14. Reed-Sternberg cell
15. EBV
16. CALLA
17. Bence Jones proteins
18. Treatment with interferon-α
19. Mature plasma cells

Column 2

a. Multiple myeloma
b. Hodgkin's lymphoma
c. ALL
d. Burkitt's lymphoma
e. Hairy cell leukemia

ESSAY QUESTIONS

20. What is the difference between a lymphocytic leukemia and lymphoma? How do the accompanying disease manifestations differ? Refer to specific examples in your discussion.

SUGGESTIONS FOR FURTHER READING

Juliasson G, Oscier DG, Fitchett M, et al: Prognostic subgroups in B-cell chronic lymphocytic leukemia defined by specific chromosomal abnormalities. N Engl J Med 1990;323:720–724

Kamat D, Daszewski MJ, Kemp JD, et al: The diagnostic utility of immunophenotyping and immunogenotyping in the pathologic evaluation of lymphoid proliferation. Mod Pathol 1990;3:105–112

Korsmeyer SJ: chromosomal translocations in lymphoid malignancies reveal proto-oncogenes. Am Rev Immunol 1993;10:785–807

Kyle RA: "Benign" monoclonal gammopathy—after 20 to 35 years of follow-up. Mayo Clin Proc 1993;68: 26–36

Rabbits TH: Chromosomal translocations in human cancer. Nature 1994;327:143–149

Sandhaus LM, Voelkerding KV, Dougherty J, et al: Combined utility of gene rearrangement analysis and flow cytometry in the diagnosis of lymphoproliferative disease in the bone marrow. Hematol Pathol 1990;4:135–148

Solomon E, Borrow J, Goddard AD: Chromosome aberrational cancer. Science 1991;254:1153–1159

Stone MJ: Amyloidosis: A final common pathway for protein deposition in tissues. Blood 1990;75:531–545

Waldman T: Immune receptors: targets for therapy of leukemia/lymphoma, autoimmune diseases, and for prevention of allograft rejection. Ann Rev Immunol 1993;10:675–704

REVIEW ANSWERS

1. b	8. c	15. d
2. d	9. a	16. c
3. e	10. b	17. a
4. d	11. d	18. e
5. b	12. a	19. a
6. d	13. d	
7. d	14. b	

12 Inflammation and Immune-Mediated Diseases

INFLAMMATION

Inflammation is the response of tissues to irritation or injury and is necessary for normal repair and healing. Inflammation is a protective mechanism that works hand in hand with the immune system. It is the means by which immunoglobulins (Igs), complement, and phagocytic and lymphocytic cells gain access to sites of microbial invasion and tissue damage. Immune events that trigger inflammatory responses include binding of antibody to antigen with subsequent activation of complement or activation of T cells. Nonimmune events include simply the presence of bacteria and release of bacterial products or components of dying tissue cells.

The immune system performs vital protective functions, as described in Chapter 9, and dire consequences follow absence of immune activity, as described in Chapter 10. Besides protecting against disease, immune events can *cause* disease. Unregulated or misdirected immune processes provoke or exacerbate many pathologic conditions. The study of immune-mediated diseases and how they cause tissue damage is known as **immunopathology.** However, before considering immunopathologic conditions, a better understanding of the process of inflammation is needed.

Acute Inflammation

Inflammation may take two forms: acute or chronic. Acute inflammation occurs very rapidly after injury and is of short duration. Neutrophils migrate to the site of injury, and their presence is characteristic of acute inflammation. Neutrophils are also known as polymorphonuclear neutrophils (PMNs) because of their nuclear configuration. Chronic inflammation lasts much longer, takes longer to develop, and is characterized by the presence of lymphocytes and macrophages. The ancient Greeks recognized four cardinal signs of inflammation: heat, redness, swelling, and pain. These signs are a direct result of changes in blood vessels at the site of injury. The first response in acute inflammation is a temporary constriction of local arterioles followed within seconds by dilation and increased blood flow (heat and redness). Vasodilation also results in increased permeability of the blood vessels. Endothelial cells become thinly stretched, thus allowing plasma to leak into the tissue resulting in edema (swelling). Pain is experienced as a result of edema and pressure of fluid against tissues and production of pain mediators.

Leukocyte Migration

The increased permeability of blood vessels allows infiltration of tissues by leukocytes. To migrate into the tissues, leukocytes must first bind to endothelial cells at the inflammatory site. Binding is a result of increased adhesiveness of the endothelial cells and expression of cell adhesion molecules. The endothelial cells express P-selectin (CD62P), which initially binds to CD15s on the neutrophil (PMN) cell surface. Initial binding via P-selectin and CD15s slows the flow of PMNs and stimulates further expression and increased binding via integrins on the neutrophil surface. Leukocyte function-associated antigen-1 (LFA-1 or CD11a) binds to intercellular adhesion molecule-2 (ICAM-2) on the endothelial cells. Local production of cytokines such as interleukin-1 (IL-1) stimulates expression of cell adhesion molecules and promotes vasodilation and migration of leukocytes into the tissue. Once bound to the endothelium, PMNs extend pseudopods between endothelial cells and migrate through the vessel wall and the underlying basement membrane to reach the damaged tissue. PMNs are more mobile than monocytes and thus arrive first in an inflammatory response. Once within the tissue, PMNs proceed to kill and phagocytose any foreign material. Monocytes migrate from the bloodstream to tissues in a similar fashion as do neutrophils, and together with macrophages they can also phagocytose dead and dying tissue cells.

Chemotaxis

Leukocytes are attracted to a site by **chemotactic factors.** These factors may be exogenous or endogenous. Exogenous factors include bacteria and their products such as formyl methionyl peptides, toxins, and so on. Endogenous factors include the complement components, C3a, C5a, collagen, and chemotactic factors produced by lymphocytes, platelets, and the neutrophils themselves. **Leukotriene B$_4$** is a potent chemotactic factor produced by neutrophils. **Chemokines** are a family of chemotactic factors characterized by the presence of closely spaced cysteine residues. Chemokines include macrophage inflammatory protein 1, monocyte chemoattractant protein, and RANTES protein, which are chemotactic for monocytes and macrophages. RANTES protein is produced by circulating T-cells and is an acronym for **R**egulated upon **A**ctivation, **N**ormal **T** cell **E**xpressed and **S**ecreted. This protein is chemotactic not only for monocytes but also for eosinophils and some T-cell subsets. RANTES also stimulates histamine release from basophils. IL-8 is a member of the chemokines and is chemotactic for neutrophils, basophils, and some T cells.

Chemokines can be made by a variety of cell types including the inflammatory cells themselves in response to infection or injury. The chemokines thus play a key role in mobilizing white blood cells (WBCs) to sites of inflammation. Overzealous activity of chemokines and other chemotactic factors can contribute to tissue damage in a wide range of inflammatory disease, including short-term conditions such as septic shock and persistent disorders such as rheumatoid arthritis. Methods to enhance or, in other situations, to specifically suppress the activity of chemokines is an area of intense interest to biotechnology and pharmaceutical companies.

Neutrophils enter the inflammatory site through gaps in the local capillary endothelium. Surrounding tissue may be damaged by release of proteolytic enzymes from lysozomes as neutrophils phagocytose invading microorganisms. Neutrophilic infiltration is followed by mononuclear cells (lymphocytes and macrophages). Activated macrophages are very effective phagocytic cells and will digest not only the microorganisms, but also necrotic tissue, inflammatory products, and dead neutrophils that have become damaged in the inflammatory process. If bacteria or the initiating inflammatory signal are eliminated, macrophages will clear the inflamed site, enzyme inhibition and oxygen scavengers will neutralize inflammatory products, and healing will commence. If tissue damage is extensive or the inflammatory signals persist, chronic inflammation occurs. Figure 12–1 summarizes the processes of leukocyte migration and chemotaxis.

LEUKOCYTE MIGRATION

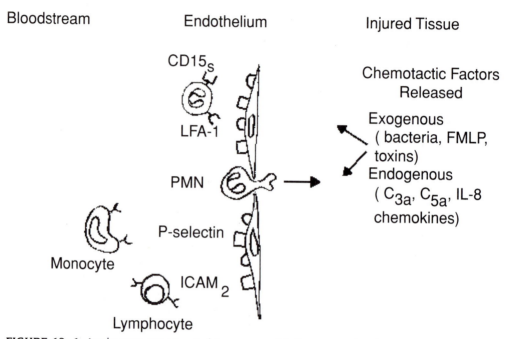

FIGURE 12–1. Leukocytes are attracted to an area of inflammation by the release of exogenous and endogenous chemotactic factors. The leukocytes attach to local endothelium via adhesion molecules and migrate between thinly stretched endothelial cells to reach the site of injury.

Chemical Mediators

The cells involved in the process of acute inflammation include mast cells, neutrophils, platelets, and eosinophils. These cells and others produce chemical mediators that initiate, maintain, and regulate the inflammatory response. The chemical mediators are signaling molecules that act on smooth muscle cells, endothelial cells, and WBCs. These agents first affect smooth muscle cells to produce dilation and increased blood flow. This early phase of inflammation is mediated by histamine and serotonin. Continued vasodilation and permeability involve other mediators derived from a variety of sources (Table 12–1).

Histamine

Mast cells are found in all tissues and are frequently located near small arterioles. When activated, they release their granules, which contain large concentrations of histamine. Histamine is formed from the amino acid L-histidine by the action of the enzyme L-histidine decarboxylase, which is found in the cytoplasm of mast cells and basophils. Exposure of mast cells to factors released by tissue damage induces degranulation. The released histamine then binds to receptors on various target cells.

TABLE 12–1. **Some Mediators Involved in Inflammation and Immediate Hypersensitivity**

Name	Functions
*Histamine	
Through H_1 receptors	Increases vascular permeability
	Stimulates smooth muscle of bronchioles, gastrointestinal tract
	Stimulates mucus production in upper respiratory tract
	Attracts eosinophils
	Promotes synthesis of prostaglandins
Through H_2 receptors	Stimulates secretion of gastric acid
	Increases vascular permeability
	Stimulates mucus production in lower respiratory tract
*Eosinophil chemotactic factor of anaphylaxis (ECF-A)	Attracts eosinophils and neutrophils
	Increases expression of complement receptors on eosinophils
	Deactivates eosinophils and neutrophils
*Heparin	Prevents coagulation
	Inhibits complement
	Binds to histamine
*Activators for prekallikrein, Hageman factor	Activates coagulation and contact cascades
*Kallikrein	Generates kinins
†Platelet activating factor	Aggregates platelets, also neutrophils and monocytes
	Promotes release of platelet factors affecting vasculature, coagulation, inflammation
	Promotes bronchoconstriction
†Lipoxygenase pathway products (leukotrienes)	Attract neutrophils, eosinophils
	Induce sustained smooth-muscle constriction
	Increase vascular permeability and dilation
†Cyclooxygenase pathway products (prostaglandins and thromboxanes)	Induce sustained increase in vascular permeability
	Induce smooth-muscle constriction and bronchoconstriction

*Preformed, released from granules after antigen-antibody reaction.
†Generated as secondary part of response.

Three types of histamine receptors, H_1, H_2, and H_3, have been identified. Binding of histamine to H_1 receptors induces contraction of intestinal and bronchial smooth muscles, increased permeability of venules, and increased mucus secretion by goblet cells. Interaction of histamine with H_2 receptors increases vasodilation and permeability and stimulates exocrine gland secretions. P-selectin expression is enhanced in venules and thus neutrophil binding to endothelium is increased.

Factors Derived From Arachidonic Acid

Other major mediators of inflammation are the **leukotrienes** and **prostaglandins,** which are derived from the membrane phospholipid **arachidonic acid.** Metabolism of arachidonic acid occurs not only in mast cells but also in macrophages, neutrophils, platelets, and most, if not all cells participating in the inflammatory response. Arachidonic acid is metabolized by two alternative pathways. The **cyclooxygenase pathway** gives rise to prostaglandins. The **lipoxygenase pathway** results in production of the leukotrienes. Leukotriene B_4 is a powerful chemoattractant for neutrophils and eosinophils. Leukotrienes C_4, D_4, and E_4 are powerful stimulants for vasodilation, smooth muscle spasms, and increased vascular permeability. The cyclooxygenase pathway generates prostaglandins, prostacyclins, and thromboxane, which also affect smooth muscle, vascular functions, and platelet activities. These cyclooxygenase metabolites variously promote or suppress inflammation and coagulation, depending on changing microenvironmental conditions that regulate their concentrations.

Inflammatory Peptides

Peptides that play a role in inflammation include the **kinins** and **anaphylatoxins.** Kinins are formed from precursors in the plasma and tissue fluids by the activity of proteolytic enzymes called **kallekreins.** Kallekreins are found in mast cells, basophils and platelets and may also be produced from plasma components by the action of the Hageman clotting factor (factor XII). Kinins promote the release of leukotrienes and prostaglandins, increase vascular permeability, and stimulate smooth muscle contraction. Kinins are also capable of stimulating pain receptors.

The anaphylotoxins are products derived from activation of the complement components C3 and C5. C3a and C5a promote histamine release form mast cells and thus participate in inflammation. C5a is a potent chemoattractant for neutrophils.

Cytokines in Inflammation

Local inflammatory responses are often accompanied by symptoms such as fever, fatigue, loss of appetite, and neutrophilia. These effects are primarily caused by IL-1, IL-6, and tumor necrosis factor-α (TNF-α). These cytokines are able to interact with brain cells regulating body temperature, the need for sleep, and appetite. Liver cells are also affected by these cytokines and produce **acute-phase proteins.** Important acute-phase proteins include **C-reactive protein (CRP), serum amyloid P and A (SAP, SAA),** and protease inhibitors such as α_1-**antitrypsin,** α_1-**chymotrypsin,** and α_2-**macroglobulin.** CRP promotes phagocytosis, can activate the complement system and also can inhibit neutrophil superoxide production and degranulation. SAA and the protease inhibitors also inhibit neutrophil function and therefore may help prevent excessive tissue damage in inflammation.

Chronic Inflammation

Macrophages usually infiltrate an inflammatory site several hours after the neutrophils and are attracted by many of the same chemotactic factors as well as by breakdown products of elastin, collagen, and fibronectin. The main function of the macrophage is to phagocytose damaged tissue components, microorganisms, and other cells. Potent secretory enzymes such as collagenase and elastases break down local connective tissue and aid in clearance of debris so that healing can commence. Secretion of the cytokines TNF and **platelet-derived growth factor (PDGF)** attract fibroblasts and promote proliferation and synthesis of new collagen in the inflammatory site. **Angiogenic factors** that promote growth of new capillaries are also produced by macrophages.

Chronic inflammation can cause tissue damage, loss of weight, and the wasting phenomenon associated with such diseases as AIDS and cancer. If the cause of inflammation is removed by the acute inflammatory process, then healing occurs rapidly. Chronic inflammation develops if the agent or antigen cannot be destroyed or removed. Microorganisms with cell-wall components that resist phagocytosis and degradation or inorganic material such as asbestos can cause chronic inflammation and significant tissue damage. Persistence of an antigen results in continual arrival of new macrophages and lymphocytes. Excessive deposition of collagen with accumulation of macrophages around the antigen can also occur and is characteristic of **granuloma formation.** Macrophages may fuse to form giant cells and with the accompanying collagen attempt to wall off the persistent antigen. Mycobacterium tuberculosis, the bacteria causing tuberculosis, often causes granuloma formation in the lungs, which is detectable by x-ray.

IMMUNE-MEDIATED INFLAMMATION

Binding of antibody and reactivity of specific lymphocytes to antigen with subsequent inflammation aids in removal of invading foreign microorganisms. However, inappropriate immune responses to antigen can cause tissue damage and even death (Table 12–2). Immunopathologic responses are called **hypersensitivities.** Hy-

TABLE 12–2. **Terms Used to Describe Immune Events**

Beneficial to the Host	
Immunity	Protection against specific environmental agents; from Latin for "exempt"
Immunization	Acquisition of protection by contract with antigenic material
Harmful or Unpleasant to the Host	
Hypersensitivity	Any pathologic effect of immune reactivity; from Greek for "above, higher" and Latin denoting "perception" or "response"
Allergy	Detrimental effects of immunity: connotes especially local events mediated by cell-bound antibodies: from Greek term that means "other"
Anaphylaxis	Systemic effects of mediators released after cell-bound antibodies react with antigen: from Greek, meaning "the reverse of protection"
Atopy	Predisposition to allergies against common agents in the environment; from Greek for "out of place"
Experimentally Induced Phenomena	
Arthus phenomenon	Immune complex reaction at injection site where antigen combines with circulating antibodies
Prausnitz-Küstner reaction	Transfer of immediate-type hypersensitivity by introducing antibody into an intact skin site, where it binds to basophils
Schultz-Dale reaction	Transfer of immediate-type hypersensitivity by introducing antibody into an isolated tissue preparation that contains basophils
Schwartzman phenomenon	Inflammatory and vascular response occurring locally or systemically after a second injection of bacterial endotoxin

TABLE 12–3. **An Outline of Immune-Mediated Disease**

Gell and Coombs Classification	Descriptive Term	Immune Mechanism	Mechanism of Injury	Antigens Often Involved
I	Immediate hypersensitivity	Reaction between antigen and cell-bound antibody stimulates cell to release mediators	Vascular and cellular changes provoked by mediators released from granulocytes	Hetero: Inhaled, ingested, or injected plant or animal proteins Allo: Very rare Auto: Extremely rare
II	Antibody-mediated	Attachment of antibody to antigen-bearing surface exerts direct effects	Inflammatory or lytic effects of complement, if activated Actions on inflammatory or immune cells with Fc receptors Inactivation of cell or molecule expressing antigen	Hetero: Rare; some drugs that attach to cell surfaces Allo: Surface antigens on transfused or transplanted cells Auto: Surface antigens of blood, endocrine, epithelial cells; basement membranes; receptor molecules on cell membranes
III	Immune complex	Combination of complement-activating antibody with soluble antigen	Inflammatory effects of complement	Hetero: Drugs, microbial antigens, inhaled plant or animal proteins Allo: Rare, to transfused proteins Auto: Nuclear and cytoplasmic cell constituents; serum globulins
IV	Cell-mediated	Mediators produced by activated T cells Direct cytotoxic action of T cells	Inflammatory actions of macrophages, lymphocytes Enzymes, other proteins secreted by activated macrophages Enhanced natural killer cell actions	Hetero: Microbial antigens, plant oils, organic or inorganic haptens, drugs Allo: MHC products on transplanted cells; graft-versus-host disease Auto: Functional cells of nearly any organ, especially liver, pancreas, central nervous system

Allo—Antigens from human individuals genetically different from host; Auto—Antigens native to host, but usually not unique to host; Hetero: Antigens from any source other than humans

persensitivities may involve either humoral or cell-mediated responses. Those immune-mediated diseases involving humoral responses and formation of antibody-antigen complexes are called **immediate hypersensitivity reactions** because symptoms occur within minutes or hours after encounter of a sensitized individual with antigen. Exposure of a sensitized individual to antigen that stimulates a cell-mediated response is called a **delayed-type hypersensitivity** because symptoms may not appear for several days. Hypersensitivity reactions can be classified into four basic types according to the **Gell and Coombs classification** system (Table 12–3).

Gell and Coombs Classification

Gell and Coombs attributed immune-mediated damage to four different mechanisms, categorized according to type. **Type I** immediate hypersensitivity occurs when IgE and some subclasses of IgG attach to mast cells and basophils through Fc receptors. Subsequent binding of antigen to cell-bound antibody triggers release of inflammatory mediators. In **type II** reactions, free antibody molecules react directly with antigen on a cell surface or tissue membrane. Reaction of antibody with cell-surface antigen damages or destroys cells because complement is often activated. **Type III** reactions occur when antibody reacts with free or fluid-borne antigen to generate complexes that precipitate in tissue and induce inflammation. Gell and Coombs originally gave only two examples—serum sickness and the Arthus phenomenon (discussed later in this chapter)—but many pathologic conditions can result from immune-complex deposition. **Type IV** reactions include delayed or "tuberculin-type" hypersensitivities. Delayed reactions are not dependent on antibody, but are dependent on reaction of antigen with specifically sensitized lymphocytes, **T-delayed-type hypersensitivity lymphocytes (T-DTH).** Activation of T-DTH cells leads to production and release of lymphokines, which attract macrophages. Tissue damage occurs as a result of phagocytosis and the release of macrophage cytokines. Table 12–3 summarizes these categories, which are discussed in detail later in the chapter.

TYPE I IMMUNOPATHOLOGY

Type I conditions are called **immediate hypersensitivity reactions** because manifestations can begin seconds or minutes after contact with the antigen. The mediators that induce these events are already present in the cells and need only to be released to begin immediate activity (Fig. 12–2). The reaction may continue for prolonged periods, however, while new mediators are produced and cause further chemical and cellular events.

Type I hypersensitivites, or **allergies,** are mediated by antibodies of the IgE class. It is not clear why some antigens provoke IgE antibodies and why some people exposed to such antigens develop these antibodies. It is known that clones of helper T cells promote production of specific Ig classes, but why some antigens stimulate IgE production more effectively than others is not known. Certainly heredity and the inheritance of a predisposition to develop allergies are major factors. Affected persons usually have elevated total serum IgE. Sometimes reactivity of IgE to specific antigens can be demonstrated, but serum IgE circulates in nanogram concentrations, rendering this kind of investigation difficult to perform.

TYPE I: IMMEDIATE HYPERSENSITIVITY

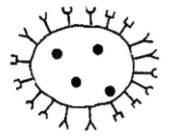

Basophil binds IgE
antibodies to membrane

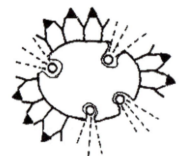

Specific antigen/allergen crosslinks
antibody, stimulates release
of granule contents

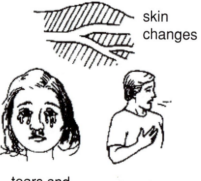

skin
changes

Mediators cause vascular changes,
smooth muscle contraction,
secretions from epithelium

tears and
runny nose   wheezing

FIGURE 12–2. Immediate hypersensitivity requires that specific IgE antibodies bind to the membrane of a mast cell or basophilic granulocyte (*top*). The immunologic reaction consists of crosslinking by the corresponding antigen (*middle*). This stimulates the cell to release previously synthesized materials stored in the granules. These materials cause the physiologic events perceived as hypersensitivity symptoms (*bottom*).

Cellular Events

IgE binds to mast cells via Fc receptors on the cell membrane. Once bound, IgE has a half-life of 11 to 12 days. Crosslinking of the Fab portions of IgE by antigen signals migration of mast cell granules to the cell surface and release of their contents into the surrounding area. A complex, highly modulated series of intracellular events involving tyrosine kinases, increased calcium levels, and cyclic adenosine monophosphate (cAMP) occur to mobilize actin and myosin microfilaments, which cause granules to move to the cell surface. Phospholipase A is also activated, which then acts on membrane phospholipid to produce arachidonic acid and subsequent metabolites.

Mediators of Immediate Hypersensitivity

Type I reactions occur predominantly in the skin, respiratory tract, and gastrointestinal tract. The first mediator discovered to cause type I reactions was **histamine,** and it is the first mediator released after cell-bound IgE binds to antigen. Cells that possess histamine receptors undergo changes that begin within seconds of exposure and end in 10 to 30 minutes. Cells with H_1 receptors are more significant in hypersensitivity reactions. Binding of histamine to H_1 receptors causes smooth muscle contraction in bronchioles and the upper respiratory tract, increased permeability of venules in mucosal surfaces, constriction of pulmonary blood vessels, and increased epithelial secretion in the upper respiratory tract. Activation of H_2 receptors causes widespread permeability of venules and capillaries, increased mucus production, and secretion of acid by cells that line the stomach. Histamine attracts eosinophils, which release materials that promote bronchoconstriction and elaborate proteolytic substances that may damage many parasitic worms. Eosinophil-derived materials also neutralize histamine actions. Tissues undergoing a type I reaction characteristically contain many eosinophils.

Other Secreted Materials

Several other substances released from basophil granules prolong and modify events initiated by histamine. The **eosinophil chemotactic factor of anaphylaxis (ECF-A)** attracts eosinophils to the area, and a closely related substance has a comparable effect for neutrophils. Eosinophil chemotactic factor of anaphylaxis stimulates eosinophils to release material harmful to helminths; it stimulates the antihistamine and anti–immune-complex actions of eosinophils but also exerts effects on eosinophils that neutralize their activity. Kallikrein released from mast cell granules cleaves a serum precursor to activate **bradykinin.** Bradykinin induces moderately prolonged smooth muscle contraction, increased vascular permeability, and increased secretory activity and is thought to be involved in stimulation or perception of pain and itching. **Heparin** and **serotonin** are also released from basophil granules and are known to be involved in anaphylaxis of animal models, but their functions in immediate-type hypersensitivity in humans are not clear.

Late-Developing Mediators

The prolonged consequences of type I reactions result from mediators generated in response to the initial events. Some are synthesized by granulocytes, some by endothelial cells in the involved blood vessels, and some by macrophages. **Platelet activating factor (PAF)** is generated by basophils and macrophages. As its name implies, it causes platelets to aggregate and to release materials that promote coagulation and inflammation. It also acts directly on tissues, causing pronounced bronchoconstriction and alterations of vascular function that cause skin reactions locally and, if introduced systemically, cause hypotension and cardiovascular collapse. Additional late effects arise from the cumulative actions of metabolites generated from the arachidonic acid pathway. The resulting leukotrienes, prostaglandins, prostacyclins, and thromboxanes affect smooth muscle, vascular function, and platelet activities.

Other Effects

A poorly understood aspect of immediate hypersensitivity, called **late-phase reactions,** includes cutaneous and respiratory events that occur hours after initial stimulation. Eosinophils and mononuclear cells that accumulate during earlier events are thought to be responsible, but specific mediators have not been characterized.

Table 12–1 lists the major mediators involved in immediate-type hypersensitivity.

Clinical Events

Most of the clinical events in type I reactions can be attributed to the mediators described in the previous text. Skin reactions begin with localized pallor followed by flushing, itching, and accumulation of fluid in swellings called **wheals** or **hives.** Vasoactive mediators promote the increased blood flow that causes flushing and the increased permeability that causes edema. The itching has been variously attributed to bradykinin, to direct effects of histamine, or to unknown interactions.

The most conspicuous upper respiratory change is **increased secretion** by mucous and tear glands, leading to the weeping eyes and runny nose all too familiar to allergy sufferers. The consequences of **edema** are nasal stuffiness, swelling around the eyes, and, most dangerous of all when it occurs, laryngeal edema. In the lower respiratory tract, increased production of mucus and constriction of smooth muscle cause narrowing of small bronchi and bronchioles. This leads to **wheezing** that is more noticeable on expiration than inspiration. Smooth muscle contraction in the gastrointestinal tract causes **diarrhea** or **vomiting.** Gastric hyperacidity and profuse watery secretions in small and large intestines occur when epithelial secretion is stimulated.

Atopy

Hay fever, some food sensitivities, many cases of asthma, and some skin rashes are type I reactions against antigens commonly encountered in the environment. The descriptive term for this group of conditions is **atopy** or, sometimes, the unmodified term "allergy." Predisposition to the atopic form of type I reactions is familial. Atopic conditions occur in an estimated 10 percent of the population. The child of two atopic parents has a 75 percent chance of being affected; if one parent is atopic, the chance is 50 percent.

Entry of Antigens

The heritable abnormality that causes the atopic state has not been characterized. The offending antigens or allergens are usually of moderate size (10 to 70 kD) and characteristically enter the body through the respiratory or gastrointestinal tract. Atopic manifestations in the skin usually reflect antigens that have been inhaled or ingested. Skin problems arising from materials that directly penetrate the skin are called **contact dermatitis** and are usually cell-mediated (see later section). Pollens, feathers, dust mites, animal danders, and airborne fungal spores are common inhaled allergens; proteins from fish, milk, eggs, nuts, and legumes are the foodstuffs most often incriminated. Affected patients seem more likely than normal persons to absorb these substances in antigenically active form.

The constitutional defect has been attributed to some or all of the following: reduced barrier function of mucosal surfaces, increased production of IgE, alteration in antigen processing or presentation, and some peculiarity of a poorly defined aspect of the major histocompatibility complex (MHC) called "immune response genes." Persons congenitally deficient in IgA are especially prone to atopic conditions. This suggests that secretions on mucosal surfaces normally exert protective action against exogenous materials.

Local Symptoms

Hay fever, asthma, atopic dermatitis, and allergic gastroenteritis are site-specific manifestations of local mediator release. Basophils in individual tissue locations bind antibodies against environmental antigens. Wherever antigen reaches the tissue in significant quantity, mediators are released at levels proportional to the degree of immune reactivity. As the atopic patient grows older, the intensity of reactions and the number of eliciting allergens that affect them often decline. Allergic asthma occurs more often and more severely in small children than in adults, partly because of age-related differences in sensitivity and partly because the child's small bronchi suffer proportionately greater narrowing from smooth-muscle constriction than the larger bronchi of adults. Atopic manifestations often change with age. The child who suffered from rashes or asthma may develop hay fever as an adult, or a person with gastrointestinal intolerance to eggs may later exhibit a rash after eating fish.

Anaphylaxis

In contrast to localized, often unpleasant but rarely dangerous atopic reactions, **anaphylaxis** is a generalized condition, which, if inadequately treated, can be fatal within a short period of time. Atopic individuals are not excessively subject to anaphylactic hypersensitivity. For those few who do experience anaphylaxis, antigenic material that enters the circulation (sometimes in minute quantities) causes system-wide release of mediator substances. The most familiar triggering agents are **venoms** of stinging insects (the Hymenoptera family), **penicillin,** and local **anesthetic agents** such as procaine. Many protein and nonprotein drugs have been incriminated with varying frequency, and in a few individuals such foods as seafood, legumes, or egg albumin cause anaphylaxis.

Laryngeal edema, intractable shock, and cardiac dysrhythmias are the most dangerous manifestations and can be life-threatening. Unpleasant but not life-threatening are severe wheezing, edema of the face or extremities, cramping pain of the intestines or uterus, diarrhea or vomiting, and urinary or fecal incontinence. Some anaphylactic reactions strike with full force in just a few minutes, but more often, symptoms increase over time, with superficial edema, respiratory distress, cramping, or hypotension as characteristic events indicating the need for prompt therapy. Table 12–4 summarizes clinical considerations in atopy and anaphylaxis.

Diagnosis

Diagnosing type I hypersensitivity reactions requires two steps: (1) establishing that IgE-mediated immune reactivity is in fact the cause of the clinical problems and (2) detecting which antigens are responsible. A careful clinical and family history is crucial for the first determination, because these conditions produce virtually no specific test findings. Eosinophilia in the blood or mucosal secretions may confirm a suspicion, but negative results do not rule out the diagnosis.

Skin Testing

Skin testing remains the most effective way to identify specific allergens. Even if manifestations are most prominent in the gastrointestinal or respiratory tract, introducing the responsible antigen into the skin reliably elicits local signs. Antigen-antibody combination induces acutely increased vascular dilatation and permeability within 15 to 20 minutes, generating the skin changes described as **wheal and flare.** The problem is to decide which potential allergens to test and to obtain pure, potent preparations suitable for skin challenge. Suitable controls are important to rule out hyperreactivity of the skin to every form of stimulation.

TABLE 12–4. **Atopy versus Anaphylaxis**

	Atopic Conditions	**Anaphylactic Reactions**
Immune mechanism	Type I hypersensitivity	Type I hypersensitivity
Nature of reaction	Localized	Systemic
Sites frequently involved	Upper respiratory tract	Soft tissue of face and neck
	Lower respiratory tract	Larynx
	Gastrointestinal tract	Small vessels of systemic circulation
	Skin	Respiratory bronchioles
		GI tract
Familial tendency	Pronounced	Minimal
Nature of antigen	Ubiquitous environmental proteins, often multiple	Specific agent, often insect venom or drug
Usual treatment	Antihistamines: sometimes subcutaneous adrenal steroids, bronchodilators	Epinephrine: sometimes massive adrenal steroids, bronchodilators, agents to elevate blood pressure

In Vitro *Testing*

A laboratory test to detect elevation of IgE with antigenic specificity is intellectually appealing but, in most cases, offers no greater sensitivity or specificity than skin testing. The procedure is called **radioallergosorbent testing (RAST)** (Fig. 12–3). The suspected allergen is adsorbed to a solid phase such as a disk, well, or microtiter plate. When serum is incubated with the solid-phase antigen, all antibody molecules that recognize that antigen attach to the solid phase. This includes antibodies of the IgG class, which are likely to be present in much higher concentration than IgE. The presence and quantity of bound IgE is determined by adding radiolabeled antiglobulin serum specific for IgE. (An enzyme label, as described in Chapter 18, can be used instead.)

Radioallergosorbent testing procedures present both technical and clinical problems. The test is only as good as the antigen used. Preparing pure and potent antigen is just as demanding for RAST as for skin testing, and selecting antigens for trial requires the same diagnostic decisions. Even when massively elevated, serum levels of IgE are several orders of magnitude lower than those of IgG, so the

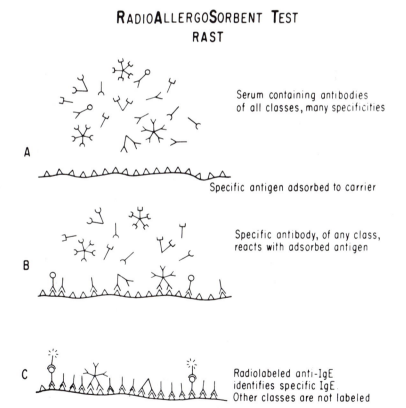

RADIOALLERGOSORBENT TEST
RAST

A

Serum containing antibodies
of all classes, many specificities

Specific antigen adsorbed to carrier

B

Specific antibody, of any class,
reacts with adsorbed antigen

C

Radiolabeled anti-IgE
identifies specific IgE.
Other classes are not labeled

FIGURE 12–3. The purpose of the radioimmunosorbent test (RAST) is to identify in serum IgE antibody of a single specificity. The selected antigen is adsorbed to a solid phase (panel A), and allowed to interact with serum. Antibodies of any class that are specific for that antigen will bind to the surface (panel B). Many antigen sites attract antibodies of IgG and other classes (panel C). The relatively few IgE molecules that bind are detected and quantified by a radiolabeled antiglobulin serum specific for the epilson chain of IgE.

antiglobulin reagent must be rigorously specific for IgE. There is no satisfactory way to obtain absolute nanogram concentration from the level of radioactivity generated. Results are expressed relative to a known positive control serum, but it can be difficult to extrapolate this relative reactivity to the clinical events seen in a specific patient. Many allergists believe that *in vitro* testing is more advantageous than skin testing only when there are widespread skin lesions that make such testing impossible, when the patient is on medications that will suppress reactivity, or when the patient's skin is so hyperreactive that needle prick alone can elicit a wheal and flare.

Treatment

Blocking Antibodies

Antigens that elicit IgE antibodies often elicit IgG antibodies as well. When soluble IgG antibody and cell-bound IgE of a single specificity compete for a limited amount of antigen, IgG usually prevails. This preferential reaction with IgG is exploited in the immunologic treatment of atopic and anaphylactic conditions. Very small doses of the incriminated antigen can be introduced in a repetitive schedule that elicits maximum anamnestic production of IgG. The presence in tissue fluid of so-called blocking IgG antibodies often prevents antigen from reaching and reacting with cell-bound IgE (Fig. 12–4). For many hay fever victims and those sensitive to Hymenoptera venoms, desensitization immunotherapy of this kind can provide satisfactory relief. For most drug and food allergens, the best treatment is avoidance.

Antihistamines

Antihistamines are therapeutically effective only after histamine has been released from granules. Antihistamines interact with histamine receptors, either H_1 or H_2. Most symptoms of atopic disease involve cells with H_1 receptors, so allergies are best treated with this class of antihistamines. Antagonists to H_2 receptors suppress gastric acid production and are useful in peptic ulcer disease but have relatively little immunologic application. Antihistamines affect only the clinical events mediated by histamine. They do not affect other life-threatening immune manifestations and do not modify the effects of other mediators.

Hormones

Pronounced and long-lasting changes in vascular permeability, smooth muscle constriction, and disturbances in cardiac rhythm initiate compensatory physiologic responses mediated through the autonomic nervous system. **Epinephrine,** the hormone of the adrenal medulla, causes vasoconstriction and smooth-muscle relaxation, thus directly reversing many of the effects we have been discussing. Epinephrine, or pharmacologic agents with selected effects of epinephrine, are used to treat systemic events mediated by IgE.

Another group of drugs useful in immune-mediated conditions are the **steroid hormones** of the adrenal cortex. Corticosteroids exert physiologic actions in many systems; in this context, they are useful as anti-inflammatory agents. They can be incorporated into bronchodilators and inhaled. Inhaled corticosteroids help reduce mucosal swelling without serious side effects.

BLOCKING ANTIBODIES

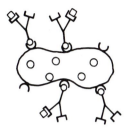

Cell-bound IgE has modest
avidity for antigen.

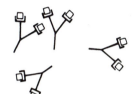

Soluble IgG has high
avidity for antigen.

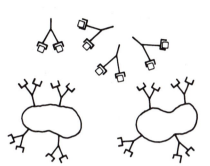

Antigen enters tissue, is rapidly
bound by IgG, does not reach IgE.

A   B

FIGURE 12–4. When the same antigenic specificity resides in antibodies of different classes, soluble IgG characteristically reacts with much greater avidity than cell-bound IgE (*panel* A). Panel B depicts tissue that contains both soluble IgG and cell-bound IgE specific for a single atopic allergen. As allergen enters the tissue, it is promptly bound by IgG and has no opportunity to elicit symptoms by crosslinking the cell-bound IgE.

Other Agents

Although their mechanisms of action are not fully understood, several other agents are useful in treating individual type I conditions. **Theophylline,** a substance related to caffeine, is a bronchodilator useful in treating asthma. **Disodium cromoglycate (cromolyn)** interferes in an unknown fashion with release of mediators from mast cells but does not counteract their tissue effects. Because cromolyn is not absorbed across membranes, its major use is topical application to the eyes, nose, or respiratory tract when exposure to inhaled allergens is likely.

TYPE II IMMUNOPATHOLOGY

Type II immunopathologies or hypersensitivities include tissue or cell damage resulting directly from antibody attachment.

Mechanisms of Damage

Effects of Complement

Antibodies that react with surface antigens may initiate several forms of tissue damage. Gell and Coombs originally emphasized the lytic effects of classical-pathway complement activation, and this remains the most dramatic and easily identified form of type II damage. The immune event involves a minimum of one IgM molecule or two closely adjacent IgG molecules. C1 then binds to the Fc portions of the bound Ig and can activate subsequent complement components. The released cleavage products C3a, C4a, and C5a are potent chemotactic agents that promote inflammation. Activation of later complement components results in cell lysis (Fig. 12–5).

Antibody on Cell Membranes

In addition to lysis and anaphylatoxic actions, C3 causes the antigen-bearing cell to become susceptible to prompt and efficient phagocytosis by cells with receptors for C3b. Opsonization can be a type II effect even without activation of complement. Surface-bound antibody enhances phagocytosis because cells with C3b receptors also have receptors for the Fc portion of IgG. In addition, antibody on a cell membrane exposes the coated cell to direct cytotoxic attack. Large granular lymphocytes and macrophages are the effectors of antibody-dependent cell-mediated cytotoxicity and quickly destroy antibody-coated cells (Fig. 12–6).

Antireceptor Actions

Antibodies against receptor molecules on cell membranes cause damage of a different kind. In most cases, antibodies that react with receptor molecules inactivate or impair the receptor and depress activity of the underlying cell. Characteristically, the receptor-antibody complexes are endocytosed, leaving the cell surface unable to interact with stimulatory agents (Fig. 12–7). A dramatic exception is the effect of antibody to the receptor for thyroid-stimulating hormone; when this antibody combines

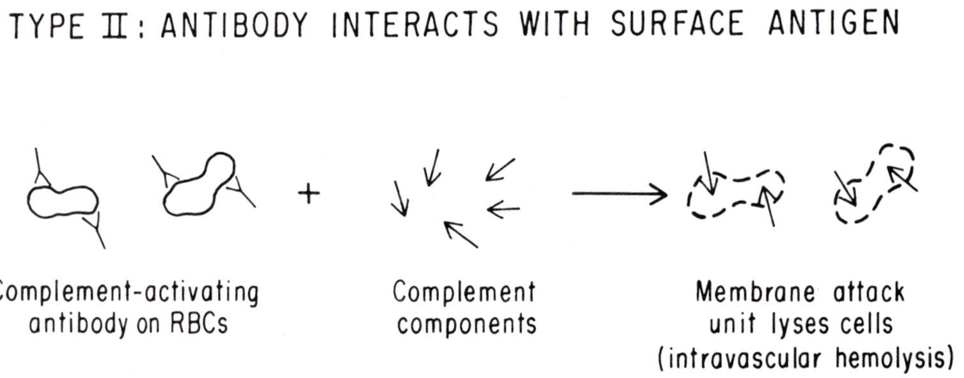

TYPE II: ANTIBODY INTERACTS WITH SURFACE ANTIGEN

Complement-activating antibody on RBCs

Complement components

Membrane attack unit lyses cells (intravascular hemolysis)

FIGURE 12–5. Complement-binding antibody specific for a red blood cell antigen attaches to the cell surface and initiates the complement cascade. At completion, the membrane attack unit lethally damages the membrane, and the circulating cell is hemolyzed. Intravascular hemolysis is almost always caused by IgM antibody.

TYPE II: ANTIBODY INTERACTS WITH SURFACE ANTIGEN

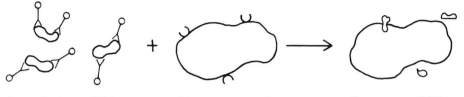

IgG antibody on RBCs   Macrophages with   Damage to RBCs
                          Fc-gamma receptors   (extravascular hemolysis)

FIGURE 12–6. IgG antibody specific for a red blood cell (RBC) antigen may remain attached to the cell as it travels through the spleen or other reticuloendothelial site. Macrophages with receptors for Fc-γ populate these sites. Macrophages bind and phagocytose IgG-coated RBCs. These RBCs are thereby removed from the circulation and destroyed.

with receptor, it crosslinks the receptor and stimulates the underlying thyroid cell to increase secretion of hormone. Anti-idiotype antibodies may stimulate immunoregulatory cells in a comparable fashion, leading to immune enhancement through a feedback mechanism. Table 12–5 summarizes the mechanisms of type II diseases.

Cytotoxic Antibodies to Blood Cells

Blood Transfusions

Blood transfusion introduces the recipient to numerous allogeneic antigens of red blood cells (RBCs), platelets, or WBCs. Depending on the blood type of the recipient, preexisting antibodies to RBC antigens are normally present in the circulation of A, B, or O individuals. Some recipients can develop antibodies against other RBC antigens in addition to A or B antigens. Such antibodies characteristically cause

TYPE II: ANTIBODY INTERACTS WITH SURFACE ANTIGEN

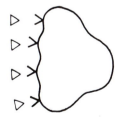 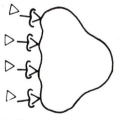 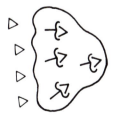

Receptors allow mediator   Antibody to receptor   Antibody–receptor
to stimulate target cell   prevents stimulation   complex is interiorized.
                                                    Membrane lacks receptors.

FIGURE 12–7. Stimulation by mediators requires accessible receptors on the target cell. Antibody against the receptor molecules not only blocks the steric interaction between mediator and receptor but often causes the mediators to disappear from the cell membrane.

TABLE 12-5. **Mechanisms of Tissue Injury in Type II Reactions**

Associated With Complement Activation
  Cell lysis, through membrane attack unit
  Opsonization, through surface-bound C3b
  Acute inflammation, through anaphylatoxic cleavage fragments

Independent of Complement Activity
  Opsonization, through surface-bound IgG
  Antibody-dependent cell-mediated cytotoxicity, through surface-bound IgG
  Depression of cell activity, through inactivation of receptor molecules
  Stimulation of cell activity, through crosslinking of receptor molecules

harm only if the individual later receives another transfusion of cells that express the same antigen. Pretransfusion compatibility testing detects most potentially harmful antibodies against RBCs, allowing transfusion of selected cells that lack the implicated antigens. If incompatible cells are transfused, the antibody causes cell damage either from complement-mediated intravascular lysis (see Fig. 12–5) or from phagocytosis by sinusoidal lining cells with Fc receptors (see Fig. 12–6). Antibodies can also be formed against platelets and WBC antigens, although these antibodies are more difficult to identify than RBC antibodies. Alloantibodies frequently cause reactions after transfusion of platelets or granulocytes.

Transplantation of solid organs exposes the recipient to foreign antigens that remain immunologically active as long as the graft remains in place. Both humoral and cell-mediated reactions occur against these allogeneic antigens. This is discussed in more detail in Chapter 13.

Hemolytic Disease of the Newborn

Hemolytic disease of the newborn (HDN) can develop if fetal RBCs enter the mother's circulation and provoke antibody formation against antigens that the fetus acquired from paternal genes. The antibodies do not harm the mother, because her cells lack the antigen. However, if the fetus of a later pregnancy is positive for the same antigen, IgG antibodies can cross the placenta, bind with antigen on the fetal cells, and cause the cells to undergo accelerated destruction. By far the most common antibody that causes severe HDN is anti-D, which develops in Rh-negative women who have successive Rh-positive infants. Injection of anti-D serum into the mother within 72 hours after birth prevents her from developing anti-D antibodies. Injection of anti-D serum (produced in male volunteers) was introduced in the late 1960s and has markedly reduced the frequency of symptomatic HDN. In rare cases, alloantibodies to granulocyte or platelet antigens may damage fetal neutrophils or platelets in a comparable manner. Another alloimmune event that can develop after natural exposure to sperm, is the formation of antisperm antibodies, which may impair fertility.

Drug-Associated Reactions

Damaging type II reactions against exogenous antigens are relatively rare. When they occur, the target antigen is often a drug. On entering the body, most drugs are dissolved or suspended in body fluids; however, reactions with anti-drug antibodies can lead to insoluble immune complexes that induce type III reactions. If the drug is fixed to a cell membrane, antibody that reacts with the drug may damage the underlying cell. If present at very high plasma concentrations, penicillin may adsorb to RBCs. Antibodies to penicillin are usually of IgG class and can react with the surface-bound drug. The cell thereby becomes coated with antibody. Through their Fc-gamma receptors, phagocytic cells in spleen, bone marrow, and liver may damage the membrane of the antibody-coated cell, even though the antibody is not directed against cell antigens.

TYPE III IMMUNOPATHOLOGY

Type III hypersensitivities occur when soluble antibody binds with soluble antigen and the macromolecular complexes precipitate out of solution. Damage results not from the union of antigen and antibody but from the associated activation of complement. Deposition of immune complexes promotes local accumulation of anaphylatoxic cleavage fragments and tissue damage because of immune-mediated inflammation. Most of the damage results from the anaphylatoxic effects of C3a and C5a. The membrane attack unit (C8 and C9) can lyse circulating RBCs coated with immune complexes, but tissue seldom undergoes lytic damage as in type II reactions (Fig. 12–8).

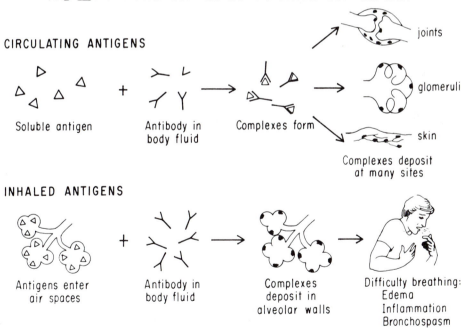

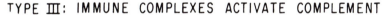

FIGURE 12–8. The consequences of type III hypersensitivity depend on the site of immune-complex deposition. Complexes containing soluble antigen and antibodies from the bloodstream may be deposited on membranes of blood vessels, joints, or kidney. At these sites, the anaphylatoxic effects of activated complement cause acute inflammation. When antigens are inhaled and react with circulating antibodies, complement-activating complexes rapidly deposit in the alveolar walls and cause prompt appearance of symptoms.

Mechanisms

Soluble molecules of antigen and antibody form complexes whose size depends largely on the relative concentration of each constituent. If excess antigen is present, saturation of combining sites on the antibody molecules occurs before an effective lattice can accumulate. With antibody excess, free antigen sites may be so sparse that multivalent antibody molecules cannot find multiple attachments to form a lattice. (See discussion of precipitation, Chapter 16.) In blood or body fluids, very small complexes either pass directly into the urine or remain suspended; they do not deposit in tissue. Very large complexes are removed and degraded by the reticuloendothelial system before they cause tissue damage. Immune complexes that form in conditions of mild antigen excess are just the right size to deposit in glomerular basement membranes, vascular endothelium, joint linings, and pulmonary alveolar membranes, where such complexes cause inflammatory disease.

Complement and Other Mediators

Precipitated complexes activate complement through the classical pathway. The anaphylatoxic effects of C3a and C5a attract neutrophils and promote degranulation of mast cells and subsequent inflammation. The damaged tissue then releases products that can perpetuate the inflammatory process. These events enhance the increased vascular permeability initiated by complement action and promote additional accumulation of proteins, including coagulation proteins that evolve into fibrin. As described in the section on type I reactions, materials released from mast cells promote platelet activation and further enhance vascular permeability. Generation of leukotrienes and prostaglandins further modulates the inflammatory events. Table 12–6 summarizes the sequence of tissue events.

Subsequent Events

If degradation of antigen or depletion of antibody interrupts the formation of immune complexes, these inflammatory processes may cease spontaneously. If complement activation is intense and explosive, depletion of complement may halt the process. However, if immune complexes continue to form and deposit, inflammation persists and produces permanent tissue loss and scarring. Table 12–7 lists some of the clinical events seen with these types of reactions, and Figure 12–8 illustrates the mechanisms.

Exogenous Antigens

Serum sickness and the Arthus reaction were the first forms of immune-complex disease to be recognized (Fig. 12–9). Spontaneous **Arthus reactions** occur infrequently. Classic **serum sickness** was common in the era before antibiotics, when passive immunization with animal serum was important in treating infections. The resulting syndrome caused malaise, fever, and generalized symptoms 1 to 2 weeks after injection of the animal serum. Antibodies to the foreign protein developed with sufficient speed that substantial amounts of the injected material remained in the system to combine with the evolving antibody. Injection of animal serum sometimes provoked more rapid and intense symptoms causing systemic cardiovascular

TABLE 12−6. **Sequence of Tissue-Damaging Mechanisms in Type III Reactions**

Initiating Events
Immune complex forms and deposits in tissue
Antibody in complex activates complement through classical pathway
Anaphylatoxic cleavage fragments are generated

Complement-Mediated Effects
Attraction of neutrophils and macrophages
Activation of macrophages and mast cells
Increase in vascular permeability
Contraction of smooth muscle

Second Events

Neutrophils	Damage to cells and extracellular proteins
Macrophages	Production of IL-1, other locally and systemically active proteins
Mast cells	Increased vascular permeability; platelet activation; smooth muscle constriction
Platelets	Promotion of coagulation events; release of platelet-derived growth factor; stimulation of vascular endothelium
Vascular changes	Accumulation of immunologically active proteins; formation of fibrin; generation of prostaglandins and leukotrienes

Long-Term Changes
Loss of tissue elements that cannot regenerate
Accumulation of scar tissue
Initiation of autoimmunity against damaged tissue constituents

IL-1 = interleukin-1.

catastrophe in patients with previous experience with the foreign protein and presence of already formed antibodies.

Drug Reactions

The term "serum sickness" is sometimes used for any systemic ill effects arising from immune-complex deposition after exposure to foreign material. Animal serums are so immunogenic that they have little current therapeutic use, but many widely used drugs provoke systemic immune-complex syndromes. Sulfonamides, penicillins and other antibiotics, thiazides, thiouracils, and hydantoins all have been implicated in immune-complex reactions characterized by fever and widespread inflammatory or hemorrhagic manifestations in skin, joints, or kidneys.

A rare but dramatic form of **RBC destruction** occurs with immune complexes involving drugs. Quinine derivatives, some analgesics that are no longer marketed, and several other drug classes may provoke antibodies that unite with circulating drug to form complexes that precipitate on blood cells. The complexes activate the complement cascade, which swiftly generates the membrane attack unit causing intravascular lysis of the underlying cells, which may be RBCs or platelets. This kind of cell damage is sometimes called "innocent bystander" hemolysis.

Organisms and Inhaled Antigens

Infections may cause immune complex-mediated disease if **antigens of microorganisms** remain present long enough to react with antibodies elicited by the infection.

TABLE 12–7. **Some Diseases Caused by Type III Reactions**

Organ Involved	Initiating Event	Clinical Consequences
Kidney		
Poststreptococcal glomerulonephritis	Infection with "nephritogenic" strain of organism	Usually resolves spontaneously as antigens are eliminated
Glomerulonephritis of systemic lupus erythematosus (SLE)	Immune dysfunction allows formation of anti-DNA	Acute episodes remit with depletion of antibody and complement; recurrence and progressive damage common
Lungs		
Acute allergic alveolitis	Inhaled antigens combine with circulating antibodies	Acute episode resolves if exposure ceases; repeated episodes may cause scarring
Joint Lining		
Postinfectious arthritis	Infection, often viral, induces circulating antibody	Systemic malaise, other symptoms common; usually resolves with no permanent damage
Drug-sensitivity arthritis	Circulating drug combines with antibody induced by previous exposure	Usually resolves promptly when drug is discontinued; systemic symptoms often present
Rheumatoid arthritis (RA)	Immune dysfunction allows formation of autoantibodies to IgG	Progressive damage follows recurrent episodes; not all patients with RA have demonstrable antibody to IgG
Blood Cells	Immune complexes settle on circulating cells; inciting antigen is usually a drug	Sudden, dramatic destruction of red blood cells or platelets follows exposure to very small amounts of antigen; complete recovery follows removal of antigen
Blood Vessels		
Serum sickness	Reexposure to animal proteins	Cardiovascular collapse, multiple organ involvement if severe; usually resolves
Henoch-Schönlein purpura	Unknown; may be drug or microbial antigens	Hemorrhage into skin, joint pain, glomerulonephritis; gastrointestinal problems; usually remits in 7–10 days
Drug-induced vasculitis	Reexposure to immunizing drugs	Skin, kidneys usual sites of involvement; usually resolves if drug is identified and withdrawn
Polyarteritis nodosa	Usually autoimmune; may occur after hepatitis	Progressive necrotizing inflammation of medium-size arteries
Wegener's granulomatosis	Unknown; possibly hypersensitivity to inhaled antigens, possibly autoimmune	Necrotizing inflammation of small arteries and veins; nearly always involves lungs, upper respiratory tract; T cells and macrophages are also involved

THE ARTHUS PHENOMENON

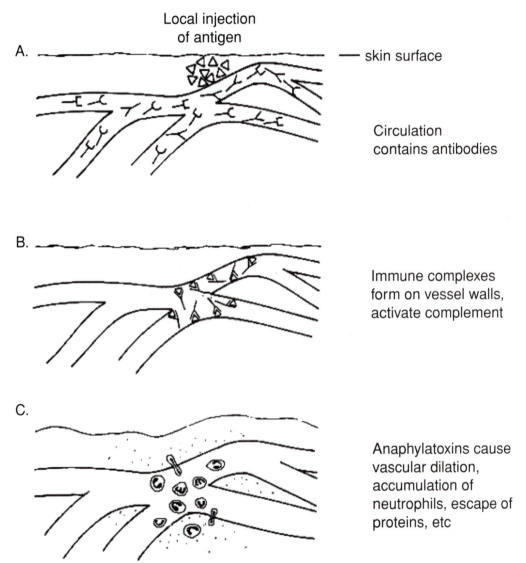

FIGURE 12-9. Panel A shows antigen injected into the skin of an individual with circulating antibody specific to the antigen. Immune complexes form and deposit on the walls of blood vessels (*panel* B). Complement is activated. Anaphylatoxic cleavage fragments cause dilatation and increased permeability of blood vessels, edema and swelling of the skin, and accumulation of neutrophils (*panel* C).

The classic example is **immune-complex glomerulonephritis,** which occurs 10 days to 2 weeks after infection with certain strains of *Streptococcus*. Skin and joint symptoms associated with viral hepatitis are also thought to result from immune-complex hypersensitivity. Less frequently, other viruses may also cause type III reactions.

Several kinds of **hypersensitivity pneumonitis** are due to inhaled antigens, but not all are type III conditions. **Extrinsic allergic alveolitis** is a type III inflammation of the lung alveoli that develops when a person with circulating antibodies inhales antigens. Alveolitis of this sort is usually due to moldy or contaminated hay, but other airborne plant or animal proteins can induce the syndrome in susceptible persons. Symptoms develop within a few hours of exposure and disappear when the inhaled antigen is removed. Pulmonary hypersensitivity conditions that develop more slowly and continue more persistently are usually cell-mediated and are described in a later section.

TYPE IV DELAYED HYPERSENSITIVITY DISORDERS

Type IV tissue damage results solely from cellular events. Antibody activity is not a factor, although there may be simultaneous formation of antibodies to the same antigens. In type IV conditions, antigen stimulates idiotype-specific T lymphocytes to perform direct cytotoxic actions or to secrete factors that activate macrophages and other cells to destructive activities. When the body defends against microorganisms, it is difficult to separate the beneficial and the harmful results of cellular events because cell-mediated attack on intracellular pathogens almost inevitably does some damage to the host tissues. Reactions to environmental antigens, on the other hand, have obvious harmful effects and few detectable benefits. Cell-mediated autoimmune reactions are clearly destructive, but they often represent physiologically useful activities gone wrong in target or intensity. Table 12–8 lists some of the diseases in which cell-mediated immunity damages tissue.

Tissue Changes

T-delayed-type hypersensitivity (T-DTH) lymphocytes, cytotoxic lymphocytes, and macrophages are prominent in tissue undergoing cell-mediated damage. Con-

TABLE 12–8. **Examples of Type IV Immune Conditions**

Exogenous Antigens
   Contact dermatitis
   Adult-type tuberculosis
   Infections with many intracellular bacteria and fungi
   Lepromatous leprosy
   Tertiary manifestations of syphilis
   Chronic hypersensitivity pneumonitis
   ? Sarcoidosis

Allogeneic Antigens
   Allograft rejection
   Graft-versus-host disease

Autologous Antigens
   Insulin-dependent diabetes mellitus
   Chronic active hepatitis
   Allergic encephalomyelitis
   Multiple sclerosis
   ? Sarcoidosis
   ? Granulomatous colitis
   ? Idiopathic myocarditis

tact with specific antigens provokes clonal expansion of effector T cells. Effector T cells secrete lymphokines that induce tissue effects, and other T cells may become T-DTH memory cells. If the antigen causing primary immunization is one that remains present for long periods, immune reactivity may become apparent days to weeks after initial exposure. For antigens that disappear or are degraded, type IV reactions can occur on reexposure to the same antigen because of the presence of the T-DTH memory cells. Lymphokines secreted by antigen-stimulated T cells promote accumulation of macrophages. The accumulating macrophages and lymphocytes express increased secretory capacities and augmented cytotoxic capabilities.

Tuberculin Reaction

The classic example of type IV cell-mediated immune response is the **tuberculin reaction** in which tissue effects are seen 12 to 48 hours after introduction of a previously encountered antigen. The involved tissue seldom experiences permanent damage because the vascular and cellular events degrade the small amount of injected material. As the antigen disappears, the reaction dissipates. However, individuals with very strong tuberculin reactivity may respond to the small amount of injected antigen with an inflammatory reaction, which results in tissue necrosis. Type IV reactions are consistently destructive if the eliciting antigen persists or renews itself and stimulates continuing cytotoxic, vasoactive, and proteolytic activity. The granulomatous skin lesions of leprosy or the granuloma formation in the lung associated with tuberculosis are examples of tissue damage due to chronic T-DTH reactions (Fig. 12–10).

Contact Sensitivity

The poison ivy reaction is undoubtedly the type IV condition with which the largest number of people are familiar. It belongs to the large category of **contact dermatitis**

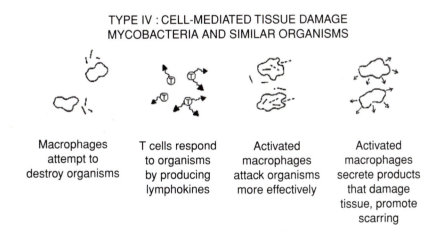

TYPE IV : CELL-MEDIATED TISSUE DAMAGE
MYCOBACTERIA AND SIMILAR ORGANISMS

| Macrophages attempt to destroy organisms | T cells respond to organisms by producing lymphokines | Activated macrophages attack organisms more effectively | Activated macrophages secrete products that damage tissue, promote scarring |

FIGURE 12–10. The destructive consequences of cell-mediated attack on microorganisms arise from events intended as protective. Antigen-specific T cells respond to microorganisms by secreting lymphokines, which enhance inflammatory mechanisms, especially by macrophages. This increases antimicrobial activity but also generates cellular and enzymatic events that destroy tissue and promote fibrosis.

reactions, in which antigen penetrates the skin to elicit a local cell-mediated immune response. Contact dermatitis illuminates the roles of **hapten** and **carrier** in the induction and expression of immunity. Characteristically, the allergen is very small (molecular weight less than 1 kD) and incapable of inducing primary immunization by itself. After penetrating the epidermal barrier, the allergen combines with the host's own proteins, which act as carriers to create a fully immunogenic complex. Langerhans' cells in the dermis serve as antigen-presenting cells. They can transport the complex to nearby lymph nodes and, on subsequent exposure to antigen, serve as foci for activated lymphocytes and macrophage cell-mediated responses (Fig. 12–11).

Poison Ivy Reactions

Poison ivy, poison oak, and poison sumac, which belong to the **Rhus** genus of plants, elaborate oils capable of penetrating intact skin. The skin reactions occur only after direct contact with the plant oil; contact with fluid from evolving blisters does not spread the rash. Sometimes new areas of rash and blisters appear well after an episode of known exposure or at a skin site that had no contact with the plant. These new lesions do not represent secondary spread from originally involved tissue. The late-reacting area has usually experienced unnoticed contact with a small amount of oil-bearing material; since the provoking dose is so small, the reaction takes longer to develop. The oily allergen can persist for many days on unwashed surfaces, so a person can experience type IV hypersensitivity long after contact with the plant. The oil can also spread by aerosol. Highly sensitive individuals standing downwind of burning foliage may experience severe skin or respiratory effects.

Reactions to Chemicals

Besides the *Rhus* allergens, common causes of contact dermatitis include nickel compounds, rubber compounds, dichromates, and paraphenylenediamine. Cross-reactivity is common; after a person develops a sensitivity, contact with related substances also elicits symptoms. Nickel is found in alloys used for jewelry and fasten-

TYPE IV : CELL-MEDIATED TISSUE DAMAGE
CONTACT SENSITIVITY

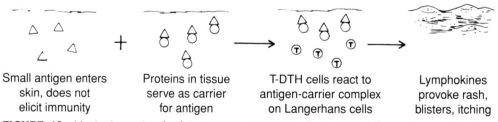

| Small antigen enters skin, does not elicit immunity | Proteins in tissue serve as carrier for antigen | T-DTH cells react to antigen-carrier complex on Langerhans cells | Lymphokines provoke rash, blisters, itching |

FIGURE 12–11. Antigens involved in contact sensitivity characteristically require combination with host proteins to elicit primary immunization. After sensitivity is established, exposure to very small quantities of antigen can provoke pronounced cell mediated symptoms.

ers on clothing; rashes develop where earrings, zippers, watch buckles, and other appliances touch the skin. Persons sensitive to rubber observe lesions on the hands after wearing rubber gloves. Dichromates are used in processing animal skin; this sensitivity affects tannery workers and those who wear or handle leather articles. Paraphenylenediamine sensitivity often becomes apparent as a reaction to para-aminobenzoic acid (PABA), a common ingredient in sunscreens. Related compounds like sulfonamides, azo dyes, sulfonylureas, or topical anesthetics of the benzocaine type are likely to cause skin problems in persons sensitive to PABA.

Photoallergic Events

A related form of contact dermatitis is **photoallergic dermatitis,** which requires the additional presence of ultraviolet (UV) radiation to modify or to activate the sensitizing events. Subsequent contact with the allergen produces a reaction only if UV is present at the same time. The lesions of photoallergic dermatitis can occur wherever skin is exposed to the sun. Chemicals in germicidal soaps and some ingredients of deodorants and cosmetics are common sensitizers.

Microbial Antigens

Cell-mediated immunity is important in protection against such invaders as Listeria, Salmonella, Cryptococcus, and Candida. Cell-mediated attack on the infecting organism can also damage the surrounding tissue. This is most conspicuous in infections with Mycobacterium tuberculosis and with the fungus Histoplasma capsulatum. In persons who lack immunity to these organisms, primary infection is often characterized by rapid multiplication and dissemination of the organisms, which may overrun the liver, bone marrow, spleen, and other reticuloendothelial sites. Disseminated M. tuberculosis infection occurs most often in young children, whose immune systems are immature, or in debilitated persons with depressed cellular immunity.

Tissue Destruction

Cellular immunity to these microbial organisms provokes an inflammatory reaction consisting of lymphocytes and large numbers of highly activated macrophages. Enzymes from the activated macrophages damage the infected tissue, often by slow but progressive necrosis. Fibrous tissue is abundant, partly from the scarring that follows tissue damage and partly in response to growth-promoting factors derived from the inflammatory cells. After extensive tissue loss, scarring and fibrosis distort the remaining functioning tissue. Although initiated by the infection, these tissue changes are largely the consequence of the immune response (Fig. 12–10). Therapy should be directed at halting the destructive process by containing and eliminating the organisms, not at suppressing immune activity. If other illness, malnutrition, drugs, or radiation depress the normal level of immune reactivity, microbes previously confined and inactivated by effective immunity may begin to multiply. In individuals with destructive but localized infection, anything that depresses cellular immunity may permit rapid multiplication and dissemination of the organisms. For example, patients with AIDS who had previously inactive tuberculosis granulomas may experience reactivation of their lesions.

Other Exogenous Antigens

Inhaled antigens may provoke cell-mediated pulmonary disease. Allergic alveolitis resulting from immune complexes (type III damage) is a brief, intense inflammation of the air spaces, with cough, dyspnea, and fever developing shortly after exposure to known allergens. In the cell-mediated forms of **hypersensitivity pneumonitis** (type IV disease), lymphocytes and macrophages cause problems that develop slowly and persist for long periods after exposure occurs. Cellular immunity to molds, dusts, or animal proteins cause many of the episodic or progressive lung conditions related to environmental or occupational events.

Allogeneic Antigens

Cell-mediated immunity is a major cause for **rejection of tissue grafts.** The purpose of the immune system is to attack non-self constituents to prevent disease, but with organ or tissue transplantation, immune destruction is considered harmful because the foreign tissue was intentionally introduced. Overall body health would be better served by allowing the non-self cells or tissue to remain, but the host's immune system has no way of knowing this. (Chapter 13 discusses transplantation at greater length.)

Graft-versus-host disease (GVHD) is a remarkable cell-mediated condition that occurs when transfused or transplanted T lymphocytes react against antigens of the recipient's tissue. Most recipients of foreign cells or tissue effectively eliminate T cells introduced with the blood or graft. If the recipient is severely immunodeficient, however, the donor's T cells can multiply unopposed and respond to their unfamiliar environment by attacking antigens of the host's tissues.

AUTOIMMUNE DISORDERS

The immune system provides for defense of the body by recognizing and responding to *foreign* antigens. It must not respond to *self* antigens. The lack of an immune response to self antigen is called **tolerance.** Tolerance is initially established in the thymus during fetal development. Thymocytes in the process of gene segment recombination, inversion, nucleotide addition, and so on, most likely form self-reactive T-cell receptors. However, many of these cells are selectively eliminated before they reach maturity and are allowed to enter the circulation. This would explain the high rate of observed thymocyte cell death. Other mechanisms by which self-reactive lymphocytes are eliminated or suppressed include insufficient costimulatory signals, very high doses of antigen resulting in immune paralysis, and cytotoxic or suppressor T-cell activity.

With breakdown of immune tolerance, all the destructive activities of the immune system are unleashed against self antigen, and **autoimmune disorders** are the result. Autoantibodies are produced, cytotoxic T cells and macrophages are mobilized for cell-mediated activity, complement is activated, and normal cells and tissues are destroyed. Fortunately, autoimmune diseases are fairly rare. Approximately 5 to 7 percent of adults in Europe and North America are affected, two-thirds of whom are women. Examples of important autoimmune diseases include diabetes, rheumatoid arthritis, multiple sclerosis, and systemic lupus erythematosus (Table 12–9).

TABLE 12-9. **Autoantibodies Associated With Specific Cells or Tissues**

Disease	Antigens	Mechanism
Autoimmune hemolytic anemia (AIHA)	On red-cell membranes	Cells damaged by macrophages with receptors for Fc
Immune thrombocytopenic purpura (ITP)	On platelet membranes	Same as for AIHA
Autoimmune neutropenia	Neutrophil antigens	Probably same as for AIHA
Pernicious anemia	Gastric parietal cells Intrinsic factor	Genetic predisposition Atrophic changes in epithelium; blockage of intrinsic factor activity
Lymphocytic thyroiditis	Thyroglobulin Microsomal antigens	Genetic predisposition ? Interaction of macrophages with colloid ? ADCC against epithelial cells
Graves' disease (toxic goiter)	Receptor for thyroid-stimulating hormone	Crosslinking of receptor stimulates hormone production
Addison's disease (adrenal insufficiency)	Microsomal antigens Adrenal epithelial cells	Genetic predisposition ? ADCC against epithelial cells
Pemphigus vulgaris	Desmosomes (protein structures that hold skin cells together)	Complement-mediated blister formation Detachment of skin cells from one another Possible secondary response to damaged tissue
Goodpasture's syndrome (glomerulonephritis or pulmonary hemorrhage)	Basement membrane	Acute inflammation mediated by complement activation
Myasthenia gravis	Acetylcholine receptor	Inactivation of receptor function
Insulin-resistant diabetic states	Insulin receptor	Inactivation of receptor function
Insulin-dependent diabetes mellitus (type I)	Islet cells	Inflammatory damage to insulin-producing cells (cell-mediated immunity also significant)

ADCC: Antibody-dependent cell-mediated cytotoxicity.

Autoantibodies as Garbage Collectors and Immune Regulators

Autoimmune diseases are rare, but autoantibodies are not. Autoantibodies can be found in normal individuals and increase with age. It has been hypothesized that autoantibodies may be useful for the disposal and clearance of defective or denatured molecules from the body. By binding to these molecules, immune complexes are formed, which can be phagocytosed and eliminated by the reticuloendothelial system. Thus, autoantibodies may serve as "garbage collectors." An example of how autoantibodies function as garbage collectors is the occurrence of autoantibodies to the anion transporter protein (band 3) on RBC membranes. As RBCs age, this glycoprotein is cleaved and a new epitope is exposed. Naturally occurring autoantibody to band 3 epitope has been identified and has a high affinity for C3. Binding of antibody and complement to old RBCs promotes phagocytosis by macrophages in the spleen. Band 3 glycoprotein is also found on lymphocytes, neutrophils, platelets, hepatocytes, and kidney cells. The widespread distribution of band 3 and the presence of autoantibodies may aid in the elimination of old cells of many different types.

Autoantibodies may also be important in regulating the immune response. The antigen-binding site (idiotype) on an Ig can function as a new epitope and cause the production of another antibody specific for the idiotype. This antibody is called an **anti-idiotype antibody** and will specifically bind to its matching idiotype forming an immune complex. Immune-complex formation promotes elimination of excess antibody. It is possible for antibodies to be produced against the anti-idiotype antibody, and theoretically this process can continue indefinitely. However, each anti-idiotypic response will reduce the previous response with the eventual termination of antibody production. Thus, idiotype-anti-idiotype networks of autoantibody may be important in regulating immune responses (Fig. 12–12).

Mechanisms of Autoimmune Disease

The exact mechanisms for loss of tolerance in autoimmune disease is not known. It *is* known that the regulatory and recognition mechanisms of the immune response are involved, as well as genetic and environmental factors. Many autoimmune diseases are chronic, with spontaneous and recurring acute episodes. No doubt many factors interact in determining susceptibility and severity of autoimmune disease.

Exposure to Altered or Hidden Antigen

Brain tissue and the testes are part of the body that normally are not exposed to circulating lymphocytes. The brain is protected by a blood-brain barrier that selectively prevents certain cells, drugs, and other products from entering. Likewise, sperm-forming tissue of the testes does not normally come in contact with immune cells and is therefore "hidden" or "sequestered" from the immune system. If the brain or testes is injured, antigens from damaged cells are exposed and an immune response may be generated. Virus infection of the brain can cause an immune-mediated encephalomyelitis. This can occasionally occur as a rare complication of chickenpox, measles, or even vaccination with attenuated virus. Infection of adult men by the virus that causes mumps can sometimes result in immune-mediated damage to the testes and subsequent sterility. This is a condition called **orchitis.** Another example of autoimmune disease resulting from exposure to altered or hidden antigen is the presence of autoantibodies to heart muscle components after a heart attack.

Cross-reactivity

Microbes are implicated in another mechanism by which autoimmune disease may occur. Antigens on microorganisms may mimic normal cell antigens in the host. As the patient (host) responds to invasion by the microorganism, antibodies are made that react not only with the microbe, but also with normal body cells. Subsequently, the microbe may be eliminated, but cross-reactive autoantibodies persist, resulting in autoimmune disease. **Antigenic** or **molecular mimicry** is the term applied to this

IDIOTYPES AND ANTI-IDIOTYPIC ANTIBODIES

A. Anti-idiotypic antibody production

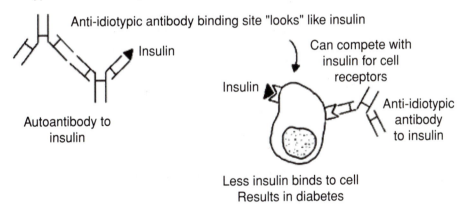

B. Regulation of autoantibodies by anti-idiotypic Ab

C. Anti-idiotypic antibodies may cause disease

FIGURE 12–12. Unique antigen binding sites are generated as new antibodies are produced. Panel A indicates the idiotype of antibody 1 and the anti-idiotypic antibody 2, which is made in response and demonstrates specific binding to idiotype 1. Panel B shows anti-idiotypic antibodies, which are produced and are specific for autoantibodies. Panel C shows that anti-idiotypic antibodies may reflect the structure of the original antigen and in this case "looks" like insulin and may interfere with the normal activities of insulin.

mechanism of autoimmune disease. An example of antigenic mimicry is seen in Chagas' disease, caused by a protozoan parasite called *Trypanasoma cruzi*. Antibodies to T. *cruzi* cross-react and bind with antigens on nerve and heart muscle. Therefore, infected individuals may suffer heart and nerve damage owing to immune-mediated inflammation.

Other examples of antigenic mimicry include rheumatic fever, multiple sclerosis, diabetes, and rheumatoid arthritis. Some susceptible children develop rheumatic fever after infection with certain strains of group A β-hemolytic streptococci (S. *pyogenes*). Rheumatic fever is an inflammatory disease characterized by fever, joint pain, and heart disease. Cross-reactive antibodies to the cell-wall M-protein of streptococci have been detected, which bind to cardiac muscle. Other strains of streptococci may cause the formation of cross-reactive antibodies to the basement membrane of glomeruli, thereby causing glomerulonephritis. The deoxyribonucleic acid (DNA) polymerase of Epstein-Barr virus (EBV) shares antigenic similarity with myelin basic protein (a component of nerve tissue) and may be involved in the development of multiple sclerosis.

Beta cells of the pancreas, which supply insulin, also make a protein called **glutamine acid decarboxylase (GAD).** A section of this protein resembles a portion of coxsackievirus. It has been proposed that a person at risk for diabetes could be infected by a coxsackievirus and recover. However, B cells and T cells have been programmed to remember epitopes of the coxsackievirus and years later are triggered to again respond to coxsackie. Immune-mediated damage occurs to the look-alike GAD and its home, the beta cells. Beta cells are destroyed, and type I diabetes is the result.

Killed M. *tuberculosis* in complete Freund's adjuvant causes arthritis if injected into rats. T cells can be isolated from these rats that are specific for heat shock protein-60 (HSP-60) of the *Mycobacterium*. If these cells are given to a normal litter mate, the recipient rat will develop arthritis as well. A clone of T cells specific for HSP-60 has been isolated from a human rheumatoid arthritis patient. Therefore, it has been suggested that autoantibodies cross-reactive to HSP-60 are involved.

Loss of Immune Regulation

Loss of normal immune regulation is a factor in the development of autoimmune disease. An immune-mediated destruction of RBCs or platelets may occur after infection with M. *pneumoniae*. A clone of B cells develops that produces cross-reactive antibody to the *Mycoplasma* organism and an antigen on RBCs and platelets. Fortunately, in most cases of **autoimmune hemolytic anemia** or **thrombocytopenia,** antibody production is suppressed or the clone of B cells is eliminated so that disease manifestations are of short duration.

Another example of loss of immune regulation in autoimmune disease is EBV infection of B cells and control of antibody production by T cells. EBV causes infectious mononucleosis and Burkitt's lymphoma. EBV may also be a factor in development of rheumatoid arthritis (RA). In EBV, if infected B cells are placed into tissue culture, they will proliferate and produce antibodies. Some of these antibodies are autoantibodies. A characteristic difference in the amount of secreted antibody can be seen if T cells and B cells from healthy donors are compared with lymphocyte cultures from patients with RA. In cultures from normal donors, B cells infected with EBV produced antibody for about 10 days, and then antibody production declined. In T-cell and B-cell cultures from RA patients, B cells continued to produce antibodies for several days longer. A possible explanation is that T-cytotoxic/suppressor cells in RA patients are not as effective in regulating antibody production as T cells from normal patients. This was confirmed by incubating normal T cells with RA B cells and vice versa. Normal T cells with RA B cells suppress antibody production, whereas incubation of RA T cells with normal B cells fails to halt antibody production (Fig. 12–13).

Loss of lymphocyte regulation as a factor in autoimmune disease can also be demonstrated with lymphoid tumors. Autoimmune hemolytic anemia can occur in some patients with chronic lymphocytic leukemia. The autoimmune disease **myasthenia gravis** may be associated with a tumor of the thymus. The **fas protein** has an important role in lymphocyte apoptosis. A defect in fas or the mechanism in stimulating fas production may result in failure to eliminate self-reactive T cells or B cells. This phenomenon has been demonstrated in the *lpr* strain of mice. These mice have a defect in their fas gene and develop autoimmune disease accompanied by lymphocyte proliferation. The defect in the fas gene can be traced to insertion of a DNA sequence derived from an endogenous retrovirus. Some investigators have suggested that a similar mechanism may occur in **systemic lupus erythematous (SLE).**

Genetic Factors

Gender, hormones, and histocompatibility genes have been implicated as factors in autoimmune disease. RA and SLE are autoimmune diseases that occur much more frequently in women than in men. SLE most frequently affects young women in their child-bearing years when female sex hormones are at their highest. Oral contraceptives that contain female sex hormones aggravate symptoms of SLE. If male New Zealand black mice (NZB) are neutered before puberty and given estrogen, they develop SLE. NZB are an inbred strain of mice in which females normally develop SLE symptoms.

A predisposition to inherit autoimmune diseases can be seen in families. An increased incidence of **Hashimoto's disease,** which is characterized by antithyroid antibodies is seen in certain families. **Pernicious anemia** is a disease in which autoantibodies are found to intrinsic factor and the parietal cells of the stomach that make this factor. Intrinsic factor is necessary for normal vitamin B_{12} absorption and the production of new blood cells. Pernicious anemia tends to be more prevalent in families and persons of Scandinavian or African American descent.

Links between specific histocompatibility genes and autoimmune diseases have been found. One of the strongest correlations between HLA type and autoimmune disease is ankylosing spondylitis. Ankylosing spondylitis is a chronic inflammatory disease involving attachment sites of ligaments to bone. Those inheriting the MHC class I gene, HLA-B27, have a much higher probability of developing ankylosing spondylitis than the general population. More than 90 percent of caucasian patients with ankylosing spondylitis have HLA-B27. Seven percent of the general population has this gene. Association between the inheritance of MHC class II genes and autoimmune diseases has also been found. HLA-DR4 is associated with the juvenile form of rheumatoid arthritis. HLA-DR3 and HLA-DR4 are associated with type I diabetes. Certain combinations of HLA genes have also been associated with autoimmune disease. The combination of HLA-A1, HLA-B8, and HLA-DR3 is associated with increased risk of developing diabetes, myasthenia gravis, and SLE. Difficulties in associating a particular MHC allele and disease susceptibility are

T-SUPPRESSOR CELLS AND AUTO IMMUNITY

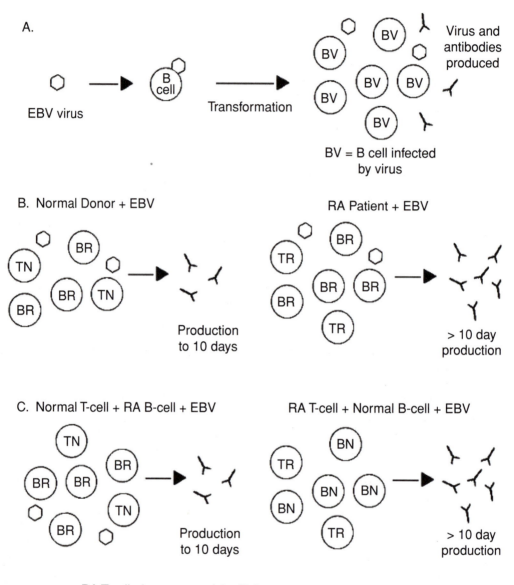

FIGURE 12–13. In panel A, Epstein-Barr virus (EBV) attaches to a B cell via CD21 and causes transformation and proliferation of infected B cells. Infection is followed by new virus production and production of antiviral antibodies and sometimes auto-antibodies. Circulating reactive T lymphocytes (T suppressor/cytotoxic T cells) also develop in the patient. In panel B, *in vitro* cultures of lymphocytes from normal and rheumatoid arthritis (RA) patients show differences in the amount of secreted antibody and duration of secretion. In panel C, Cultures of T cells from normal individuals, when incubated with EBV and B cells from patients with RA, showed similar antibody production patterns as seen with normal donors. T cells from patients with RA are not as effective at suppressing antibody production, because incubation of RA T cells with normal B cells results in extended antibody production. Bv, viral-infected B cell, Bn, normal B cell; Tn, normal T cell; BR = RA B-cell, TR = RA T-cell.

complicated by the genetic phenomenon of **linkage disequilibrium** in which two alleles are inherited together with a higher frequency than normal.

The reasons why the inheritance of certain histocompatibility genes leads to a greater incidence of autoimmune disease are not known. MHC molecules have an important role in processing and presenting antigen and therefore are a factor in the control of T-cell and B-cell recognition of antigen. MHC genes may also influence the selection of specific helper and cytotoxic T cells in thymic development. Clearly, many factors are involved in the development of autoimmune disease. These factors interact or may overlap in an unknown sequence of events to trigger production of autoantibodies. After deregulation and breakdown of tolerance occurs, many autoimmune diseases may occur in the same person. For example, the person with SLE may have RA, glomerulonephritis, autoimmune hemolytic anemia, and other related symptoms.

Autoimmune Diseases Involving Antibodies to Cell-Surface Antigens

Autoimmune diseases can be classified as either organ-specific or generalized. Generalized conditions, in which several different organs or cell types are affected, more often have a type III immunopathology and are discussed in the next section. In organ-specific conditions, antibody reactive against a defined tissue constituent provokes disease in the organ that expresses the antigen (Table 12–9).

Goodpasture's syndrome is unusual in that autoantibody of a single type produces disease at several sites. The antibody reacts with basement membrane protein. The organ most conspicuously involved is the glomerulus of the kidney. Antibody attaches to the basement membrane of glomerular capillaries and activates complement, provoking inflammation and altered vascular function. The resulting condition, called **antiglomerular basement-membrane (GBM) glomerulonephritis,** causes rapid deterioration of renal function (Fig. 12–14). The same antibody also binds to

TYPE II : ANTIBODY INTERACTS WITH SURFACE ANTIGEN

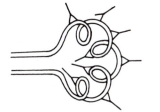
Anti-GBM attaches to
glomerular basement
membrane

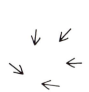
Complement
components

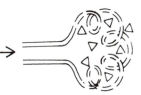
Complement provokes
acute inflammatory
damage to glomerulus

FIGURE 12–14. Circulating antibody to glomerular basement membrane (anti-GBM) adheres to the target tissue and initiates the complement cascade. Anaphylatoxic consequences of the complement cascade predominate, and the resulting cellular and vascular events cause inflammatory renal injury.

basement-membrane antigen in pulmonary capillaries, activating complement to cause lung damage that is primarily hemorrhagic rather than inflammatory. Basement-membrane protein is present in many tissues but is apparently more accessible to the antibody in glomeruli and lung than anywhere else.

Hematologic Conditions

Perhaps the most common type II condition is **autoimmune hemolytic anemia (AIHA),** in which antibody interacts with elements of the RBC membrane. The antibody may be IgM or IgG; complement activation may or may not contribute to shortened RBC survival. Sometimes other immune dysfunctions accompany the RBC autoantibody, but in many patients the autoantibody occurs as an isolated and apparently spontaneous event. Platelet antibodies are also common, producing the condition called **immune (or idiopathic) thrombocytopenic purpura (ITP),** in which antibody-coated platelets are removed from the circulation more rapidly than the bone marrow can replace them. **Autoimmune neutropenia** occurs much less often than AIHA or ITP, but has the same mechanism.

Endocrine Conditions

Thyroid cells and their products express many antigens, to which several different autoantibodies may develop. These induce functional or inflammatory changes in the gland and may cause enlargement of the gland (goiter), systemic hypothyroidism, or both. Hashimoto's thyroiditis is often associated with an autoantibody to thyroid peroxidase, whereas Graves' disease is associated with anti–thyroid-stimulating hormone (TSH) antibodies. Organ-specific antibodies have been identified that may depress glandular function in the adrenal glands, ovaries, or parathyroid glands. Often, however, autoantibodies to these tissues exist in the blood without causing endocrine hypofunction. In the insulin-dependent form of **diabetes mellitus (type I),** there may be antibodies against insulin-producing cells, against insulin receptors, or against insulin itself, but cell-mediated mechanisms are probably of greater pathophysiologic importance.

Antireceptor Antibodies

Antibodies against membrane receptors depress cellular functions in **myasthenia gravis** (acetylcholine receptors), in **insulin resistance** (insulin receptors), and in certain abnormalities of the autonomic nervous system (β_2-adrenergic receptors) (Fig. 12–7). Antireceptor antibodies have the opposite effect in the form of hyperthyroidism called **Graves' disease,** in which antibody is directed against receptors for the TSH secreted by the pituitary. Antibody to the TSH receptor crosslinks the membrane molecule; the underlying cell reacts as if TSH had engaged the receptor and responds by producing thyroid hormone. Production of thyroid hormone normally fluctuates in response to changing levels of TSH. In Graves' disease, the antibody to TSH receptor remains at a constant high level, and excessive production of thyroid hormone continuously occurs.

Autoimmune Diseases Involving Immune-Complex Formation

A large group of systemic, multiorgan diseases involve immune-complex reactions with autologous antigens. Sometimes called **collagen-vascular** or **connective-tissue** diseases, they are characterized by antibodies against such universally present constituents as single- or double-stranded DNA, nucleohistones, IgG proteins, phospholipids, and various cytoplasmic proteins. Clinical characteristics of these diseases are influenced by the specific disease syndrome, the genetic constitution of the patient, and the environmental events that the patient experiences. Frequent clinical findings are intermittent inflammatory episodes involving small or medium blood vessels, membrane surfaces, joints, or glomeruli. Table 12–10 lists some of the antibodies associated with this group of poorly understood conditions.

The classic example is **systemic lupus erythematosus (SLE),** which has an incidence of 15 to 50 per 100,000 population and a female-to-male ratio of 9 : 1. Patients often have arthritis, a butterfly-shaped skin rash over the face, fatigue, and fever at the time of diagnosis. The most consistent serologic findings in SLE are antibodies to nuclear antigens (ANA) and to DNA. During exacerbations, complexes that contain DNA, Ig, and complement are deposited on glomerular basement membranes and other sites of acute inflammation. Dysregulation of B-cell activity occurs with production of aberrant antibodies that form immune complexes with self constituents. Presence of high-titer ANA showing a homogeneous or speckled pattern by immunofluorescence assay are important for diagnosis (see immunofluorescence staining in Chapter 18).

Another common but poorly understood autoimmune disease is **rheumatoid arthritis (RA),** which has a less striking female-to-male preponderance (3 : 1) than SLE and tends to occur somewhat later in life. The conspicuous autoantibody in RA is called **rheumatoid factor,** which is IgG or IgM with specificity against the IgG Ig class. Deposits of antibody, IgG, and complement can be found in the membranes of inflamed joints. Many of the manifestations of RA can be explained by immune-complex deposition. Other tissues and organs may experience destructive changes in which antibodies do not seem to be implicated.

Other conditions in this category of connective-tissue disorders include **scleroderma, polymyositis, mixed connective-tissue disease, polyarteritis nodosa,** and other forms of arteritis. Demonstration of autoantibodies is useful in diagnosing these conditions, but the pathogenetic mechanisms remain unclear.

Treatments

With greater understanding of how normal immune responses and accompanying inflammation occur, new treatment modes for autoimmune disease are being developed. Autoimmune diseases have been treated principally with corticosteroids that suppress the entire immune system and have many toxic side effects. Cyclosporine is a drug useful for suppressing the immune response in patients receiving an organ transplant. It is somewhat more specific than corticosteroids in that its principal action seems to be suppression of lymphokines. An even better mode of treatment would be to selectively inhibit single lymphokines. IL-1 secreted by macrophages

TABLE 12–10. **Some Autoantibodies Associated with Systemic Diseases**

Antibody Specificity	Major Disease Associations	Methods of Detection	Comments
Nuclear Elements			
Native (double-strand) DNA	SLE	Immunofluorescence, ELISA (enzyme linked immunosorbent assay) counterimmunoelectrophoresis, others	Highly characteristic of SLE
Single- or double-strand DNA	SLE and other connective tissue diseases	Immunofluorescence, ELISA ELISA counterimmunoelectrophoresis, others	High titers in SLE Lower titers, less consistent occurrence in other diseases
Deoxynucleoprotein	SLE and drug-associated lupus	Immunofluorescence, ELISA latex particle agglutination	Cause of "LE cell" phenomenon
RANA	Rheumatoid arthritis, Sjögren's syndrome	Immunofluorescence, immunodiffusion	Reacts *in vitro* only with cells transformed by EBV
Cytoplasmic Elements			
Mitochrondria	Primary biliary cirrhosis, SLE	Immunofluorescence	Marker antibody, no pathogenetic role identified
Smooth muscle antigens	Chronic active hepatitis	Immunofluorescence	Marker antibody, no pathogenetic role identified
Noncellular antigens			
IgG	Rheumatoid arthritis, SLE, post-viral syndromes, otherwise normal elderly	Latex particle agglutination	Antibodies are called "rheumatoid factors" May be IgG or IgM Found in complement-activating complexes in affected joints
Phospholipids	SLE, many autoimmune and malignant diseases	Prolongation of prothrombin time test	Often called "lupus anticoagulant" Causes thrombotic tendency, not bleeding Common cause of "biologic false-positive" result in nonspecific tests for syphilis

DNA = deoxyribonucleic acid; RANA = rheumatoid arthritis-associated nuclear antigen; SLE = systemic lupus erythematosus.

promotes inflammation and has been detected in joints of patients with RA and in the pancreatic cells of persons with diabetes. The gene for the receptor of IL-1 has been isolated, and it may be possible to produce synthetic receptors, inject them into an RA joint, and thereby neutralize the macrophage-secreted IL-1. Another alternative is a monoclonal antibody to IL-1 or an inhibitor drug that can be injected into an inflammatory site.

Vaccination against the viruses associated with autoimmune disease may prevent more people from subsequently developing autoimmune disease. Measles vaccine has become readily available, and more children receive vaccination to measles along with polio, diphtheria, and tetanus. Measles has been proposed as a possible factor in the development of multiple sclerosis (MS). Patients with MS suffer progressive autoimmune damage to the myelin sheath surrounding nerve axons. The myelin sheath is an insulating material for electrical nerve transmission and therefore as myelin is subjected to immune destruction, nerve transmission is interrupted. If measles is a factor in the development of MS, then epidemiologists should begin to observe a decline in the number of new cases of MS.

Another treatment mode would be to suppress the T-cell responses to autoantigen. It is possible to isolate autoreactive T cells and use these as a "vaccine." T cells are recoverable from RA joint fluid or spinal fluid of patients with MS. These autoreactive cells can be grown in tissue culture, inactivated with gamma rays, and injected into the patient. Anti-idiotypic T cells are induced that suppress the autoimmune process. This vaccination procedure has been used to successfully prevent the development of experimentally induced autoimmune encephalomyelitis, arthritis, and thyroiditis. A better vaccination procedure would be to isolate the small peptides triggering autoimmune disease and then use them in a procedure similar to the desensitization therapy used for treatment of allergies. The peptides would block autoreactive T-cells or induce formation of cytotoxic/suppressor T cells. Monoclonal antibodies could also be used to destroy autoreactive T cells.

A novel experimental approach is to feed the patient large amounts of the antigen triggering the autoimmune disease. Encephalitis similar to MS can be induced in rats immunized with myelin in Freund's complete adjuvant. Feeding rats myelin-basic protein before immunizing with myelin induces tolerance and can reverse the paralysis in rats already experiencing autoimmune destruction of myelin. Exactly how oral suppression works is not known; however, a possible mechanism is that autoantigen presented to the immune system through the gut causes production of immunosuppressive CD8 cells or specific deletion of immunoresponsive T cells.

SUMMARY

1. Inflammation is a normal protective mechanism that works hand in hand with the immune system. Binding of antibody to antigen and activation of complement will trigger inflammation. Tissue injury and the presence of bacteria will trigger inflammation. Unregulated or misdirected immune processes can cause inflammatory disease and immunopathology.

2. Acute inflammation occurs rapidly after injury, is of short duration, and is characterized by the migration of neutrophils (PMNs) to the site of injury. Vas-

Continued on following page

odilation causes increased blood flow and permeability of the blood vessels. Local endothelial cells express cell adhesion molecules (P-selectin and intracellular adhesion molecules [ICAM-2]), which bind leukocyte function-associated antigen-1 (LFA-1) and CD15s on PMNs and thereby promote leukocyte migration into the affected tissues.

3. Leukocytes are attracted to a site by chemotactic factors. Exogenous chemotactic factors include bacteria and their products. Endogenous factors include the complement components and their breakdown products and various factors produced by injured cells, platelets and the leukocytes themselves. Leukotriene B_4, chemokines, and interleukins are examples of chemotactic factors. Increased activity and uncontrolled release of chemotactic factors can contribute to tissue damage and inflammatory diseases, such as septic shock or rheumatic fever.

4. Leukocytes and platelets secrete chemical mediators that initiate, maintain, and regulate the inflammatory process. Histamine and serotonin released from mast cells cause contraction of smooth muscle cells surrounding blood vessels. Therefore, vasodilation and increased permeability occurs. Leukotrienes and prostaglandins from arachidonic acid metabolism, kinins, and anaphylatoxic activity of complement components C3a and C5a are other mediators that promote chemotaxis and vasodilation. Cytokines such as interleukin-1 (IL-1), IL-6, and tumor necrosis factor-α (TNF-α) not only promote local inflammation, but affect tissues such as brain and liver to cause fever, fatigue, loss of appetite, and other accompanying symptoms of inflammation.

5. Chronic inflammation occurs if the injurious agent cannot be eliminated by acute inflammation. Macrophages infiltrate the inflammatory site several hours after the PMNs and phagocytose damaged tissue, microorganisms, and other debris so that healing can commence. Macrophages are potent sources of degradative enzymes and cytokines that will promote immune responses and healing. If the injurious agent persists, granuloma formation, further tissue damage, and weight loss can occur.

6. Hypersensitivities are inappropriate immune responses to antigen that can then cause tissue damage and even death. Immune-mediated diseases involving humoral responses are called immediate hypersensitivities because symptoms occur within minutes or hours after exposure to antigen. Delayed-type hypersensitivity (DTH) involves cell-mediated responses, and symptoms may not appear for several days. The Gell and Coombs classification system divides hypersensitivity reactions into four basic types.

    a. Type I immediate hypersensitivites occur when IgE attached to mast cells binds antigen (allergen) and stimulates release of inflammatory mediators such as histamine, eosinophil chemotactic factors of anaphylaxis (ECF-A), bradykinin, and platelet activating factor (PAF). Release of mediators at localized sites causes the clinical symptoms associated with allergens: hives, hayfever, edema, wheezing, diarrhea, and so on. Symptoms may also be generalized as with anaphylaxis, which, if inadequately treated, can be rapidly fatal. Skin testing and laboratory tests are available for identifying specific allergens. Therapies with blocking antibodies, antihistamine, steroids, or other agents are available.

b. Type II hypersensitivities result from damage initiated by binding of antibody to cell-surface antigen and subsequent lysis or anaphylatoxic actions of complement. Antibody may interfere with receptor molecules resulting in depressed activity of the cell. Antibody binding to red blood cell (RBC) surfaces results in intravascular or extravascular hemolysis, and therefore accurate blood typing and crossmatching of blood for transfusion purposes is critical. Hemolytic disease of the newborn (HDN) can occur if anti-D Rh antibodies cross the placenta and bind to Rh-positive fetal cells.

c. Type III hypersensitivities occur when soluble antibody and antigen form immune complexes that precipitate in various tissues. Deposition of immune complexes results in local accumulation of C3a and C5a and tissue damage. Immune deposits may form or be deposited in the kidney, lungs, joints, and blood vessels, and on blood cells and many other sites in the body.

d. In type IV delayed hypersensitivity disorders, antigen stimulates idiotype specific T lymphocytes to participate in direct cytotoxic activities or secrete lymphokines that activate macrophages and other cells to destructive actions. The tuberculin skin reaction is a classic example of type IV cell-mediated immune responses. Type IV tissue damage occurs in contact dermatitis, infectious diseases such as tuberculosis, and rejection of tissue grafts.

7. Autoimmune disorders result from a breakdown in immune tolerance. Autoantibodies can be found in normal individuals. These antibodies may be useful for disposal and clearance of defective or denatured molecules from the body and may also be important in regulating the immune response through the formation of anti-idiotypic antibodies and immune complexes.

8. Autoimmune diseases and formation of autoantibodies may occur because of exposure to altered or hidden antigen. Antigens on microbes may mimic normal cell components, resulting in destructive cross-reactive antibody formation. Examples include heart disease due to antibodies to *Trypanasoma cruzi* or *Streptococcus pyogenes*. Loss of immune regulation is another factor in development of autoimmune disease. A defective *fas* protein may result in failure to eliminate self-reactive T cells or B cells. Gender, hormones, and histocompatibility genes are also factors in development of autoimmune disease.

9. Autoimmune diseases can be classified as either organ-specific or generalized. Organ-specific includes diseases such as Goodpasture's syndrome in which autoantibodies react specifically with basement-membrane proteins. Hemolytic anemias are frequently the result of specific autoantibodies binding to RBC membrane antigens. Other autoimmune diseases are a result of autoantibody formation to membrane receptors on endocrine cells and muscle cells and to universally present constituents such as single- or double-stranded deoxyribonucleic acid (DNA), nucleohistones, immunoglobulins (Igs), phospholipids, and other proteins. Systemic lupus erythematosus is an example of a systemic, multiorgan autoimmune disease with widespread autoantibodies and immune-complex deposition.

Continued on following page

10. Treatments for autoimmune disorders include corticosteroids, which suppress many facets of the immune system and have many toxic side effects. Development of more specific drugs or inhibitors of lymphokines will provide better treatments. Vaccination procedures for cross-reactive microbes or autoreactive T cells and presentation of autoantigen to the immune system via the gut are treatment modes currently being developed.

REVIEW QUESTIONS

1. The characteristic cell type seen in acute inflammation is _____.
   a. lymphocytes
   b. monocytes
   c. neutrophils
   d. eosinophils
   e. mast cells

2. The first response in acute inflammation is _____.
   a. vasodilation
   b. vasoconstriction
   c. white blood cell (WBC) migration
   d. chemotaxis
   e. WBC adhesion

3. Important endothelial cell adhesion molecule(s) is/are _____.
   a. leukocyte function-associated antigen-1 (LFA-1)
   b. CD15s
   c. intercellular adhesion molecule-2 (ICAM-2)
   d. CD11a
   e. a and b

4. For polymorphonuclear neutrophils (PMNs) to accumulate at an inflammatory site, they must be first attracted to the site in a process called _____.
   a. cytokinesis
   b. cytotaxis
   c. chemotaxis
   d. chemotropism
   e. leukocytosis

5. Example(s) of endogenous chemotactic factor(s) is/are _____.
   a. C3a
   b. interleukin-8 (IL-8)
   c. staphylococcal toxin A
   d. a and b
   e. a, b, and c

6. Chemotactic factors that are characterized by the presence of closely spaced cysteine residues are _____.
   a. leukotrienes
   b. chemokines
   c. complement components
   d. interleukins
   e. prostaglandins

7. _____ release histamine.
   a. Eosinophils
   b. Neutrophils
   c. Erythrocytes
   d. Mast cells
   e. Smooth muscle cells

8. An important inflammatory mediator derived from the cyclooxygenase pathway of arachidonic acid metabolism is _____.
   a. leukotriene B_4
   b. prostaglandin
   c. kallekrein
   d. C-reactive protein (CRP)
   e. eosinophil chemotactic factor of anaphylaxis (ECF-A)

9. Angiogenic factors promote _____.
   a. growth of new blood vessels
   b. loss of appetite
   c. fevers
   d. fatigue
   e. phagocytosis

10. An example of an immediate hypersensitivity type I mediator is _____.
    a. histamine
    b. ECF-A
    c. C8
    d. a and b
    e. a, b, and c

11. _____ is a good example of a systemic autoimmune disease.
    a. Myasthenia gravis
    b. Multiple sclerosis
    c. Diabetes
    d. Rheumatoid arthritis
    e. Lupus erythematosus (SLE)

12. _____ binds to mast cells via _____.
    a. IgG . . . Fab
    b. IgA . . . secretory piece
    c. IgE . . . Fc receptor
    d. IgE . . . ICAM
    e. IgE . . . cyclic adenosine monophosphate (cAMP)

13. Common causes of anaphylactic shock include _____.
    a. insect venom
    b. penicillin administration
    c. exposure to poison oak
    d. a and b
    e. a, b, and c

14. Example(s) of type IV immune conditions include(s) _____.
    a. contact dermatitis
    b. lepromatous leprosy
    c. graft-versus-host disease (GVHD)
    d. a and b
    e. a, b, and c

15. Which of the following is *not* true concerning autoantibodies?
    a. They can be found in normal individuals.
    b. They are more frequently found in the elderly.
    c. Anti-idiotypic antibodies can be made to autoantibodies.
    d. Autoantibodies do not activate complement.
    e. Autoantibodies may be cross-reactive.

16. The autoimmune disease having the strongest correlation with inheritance of a specific HLA type is _____.
    a. diabetes
    b. SLE
    c. ankylosing spondylitis
    d. myasthenia gravis
    e. multiple sclerosis

17. Which of the following is *not* true concerning SLE?
    a. It is associated with a defective *fas* gene.
    b. Autoantibodies to nuclear antigens consistently occur.
    c. Affected patients often have arthritis.
    d. Self-reactive T cells or B cells fail to undergo apoptosis in animal models.
    e. It occurs more frequently in men than in women.

MATCHING QUESTIONS

Match the disease in column 1 to the type of hypersensitivity in column 2.

Column 1

18. poststreptococcal glomerulonephritis
19. hay fever
20. poison ivy
21. blood transfusion reaction
22. hives
23. Arthus reaction
24. rheumatoid arthritis

Column 2

a. Type I
b. Type II
c. Type III
d. Type IV

Match the autoimmune disease in column 1 to the affected tissue or cellular components in column 2.

Column 1

25. Diabetes
26. Pernicious anemia
27. SLE
28. Graves' disease
29. Myasthenia gravis

Column 2

a. acetylcholine receptors
b. DNA
c. Beta cells of the pancreas
d. parietal cells of the stomach
e. thyroid stimulating hormone receptors

ESSAY QUESTIONS

30. The ancient Greeks recognized four cardinal signs of inflammation. What are these signs of inflammation? Explain how and why they occur.

31. What types of test can be performed to identify specific allergens? How do these tests work?

32. What are the proposed mechanisms for development of autoimmune diseases? Provide an example for each in your discussion.

SUGGESTIONS FOR FURTHER READING

Ben-Baruch A, Michiel DF, Oppenheim JJ: Signals and receptors involved in recruitment of inflammatory cells. J Biol Chem 1995;270:11703–11710

Doherty PC, Allan W, Eichelberger M, Carding SR, et al: Heatshock protein and the gamma/delta T-cell response in virus infection: Implication for autoimmunity. Semin Immunopathol 1991;13:11–24

Gura T: Chemokines take center stage in inflammatory ills. Science 1996;272:954–956

Steinman L: Autoimmune disease. Sci Am 1993;269:107–114

Watanabe-Fukunaga R, Brannan CI, Copeland NG, et al: Lymphoproliferative disorders in mice explained by defects in fas antigen that mediate apoptosis. Nature 1992;356:314–317

Winter W, Atkinson M: Getting to the root of type I diabetes. Diabetes Forecast 1992;May:35–38

Wu J, Zhou T, He J, and Mountz JD, et al: Autoimmune disease in mice due to integration of an endogenous retrovirus in an apoptosis gene. J Exp Med 1993;178:461–468

REVIEW ANSWERS

1. c	6. b	11. e	16. c	21. b	26. d
2. b	7. d	12. c	17. e	22. a	27. b
3. c	8. b	13. d	18. c	23. c	28. e
4. c	9. a	14. e	19. a	24. c	29. a
5. d	10. d	15. d	20. d	25. c	

13 Transplantation Immunology

Transplantation introduces tissue from a donor into a recipient in whom it is expected to survive and to function permanently. This contrasts with transfusion, in which cells and proteins are expected to remain functional for only a limited time. Because the primary function of the immune system is to prevent the establishment of foreign cells, it is expected that overcoming immune differences is the major problem in tissue grafting. Problems of blood supply and incoming and outgoing connections are effectively addressed by surgical manipulation, but manipulation of immune events requires complex physiologic and pharmacologic intervention.

PRINCIPLES OF TRANSPLANTATION

Differences among individuals arise from differences in genetic composition. Each individual inherits a combination of major histocompatibility complex (MHC) alleles and therefore expresses unique self antigens. Immune defenses identify and react against non-self antigens; the greater the differences, the greater the immune response. Success in transplantation results from selection of the least immunogenic material, accompanied by strategies to modify the reactions that almost inevitably develop.

Types of Grafts

Grafted tissue is described according to the relationship between donor and host. Tissue removed from one site and introduced into another site in the same individual is an **autograft.** Tissue exchanged between different individuals with identical genetic composition is an **isograft.** In humans, this occurs only with monozygotic (identical) twins, but much experimental work makes use of inbred laboratory animals that possess exactly the same genes as all other members of the colony. When donor and recipient are of the same species but different genetic characteristics, the tissue is an **allograft.** A graft transplanted across species lines (e.g., from mouse to rat or from baboon to human is a **xenograft** or **heterograft.** Examples of these relationships are shown in Table 13–1.

TABLE 13–1. **Descriptive Terms Applied to Grafts**

Relation of Donor and Recipient	Noun	Adjective	Clinical Example
Tissue originates from the recipient	Autograft	Autologous, autogeneic	Frozen bone marrow infused after cytotoxic therapy Veins relocated during coronary artery bypass Skin taken from unburned site to cover raw burned area
Donor and recipient are different individuals with identical genes	Syngraft, isograft	Syngeneic	Kidney or marrow transplant in identical twins Experimental transplants with inbred animals
Donor and recipient are of same species but are genetically different	Allograft (homograft) is an older term)	Allogeneic, homologous	Human organ transplants from siblings, parents, or unrelated individuals
Donor and recipient are of different species	Xenograft (heterograft is an older term)	Xenogeneic, heterologous	Baboon heart transplant in human Heart valve from pig inserted into human heart

Nonimmunologic Problems

Autografts and isografts do not elicit immune rejection because no foreign genes that produce foreign antigens are involved. However, this does not guarantee that the graft will survive and function normally. Damage during removal, storage, and implantation may impair survival; there may be vascular problems at the recipient site that cause graft failure; or, the condition that damaged the original tissue may persist and damage the grafted tissue as well. Genetic predisposition to disease will affect grafts from an identical twin or syngeneic experimental animal just as it damaged the host's original tissue.

In humans, allografts are the major area for immunologic concern, inasmuch as xenografts are performed only rarely and with full knowledge that the effects will be temporary.

Antigens that Affect Allografts

HLA antigens, the MHC class I and class II products, exert major effects on allograft survival, but immune rejection occurs even when donor and recipient are HLA-identical. The nature, locations, and genetic determination of these additional immunogens remain subject to intense investigation. Until it becomes possible to identify these features and to circumvent their effects, transplantation immunology must concentrate on recognizing and matching HLA antigens and applying the most effective and least dangerous means of immunosuppression.

Class I Antigens

Class I HLA molecules consist of one polymorphic chain determined by alleles of the MHC and B_2 microglobulin that is the same on all human cells (see Chapter 3 for review). Because almost all nucleated cells express class I antigens, the antigens of the grafted tissue can be identified by testing white blood cells (WBCs) rather than cells from the organ itself. Class I antigens provoke both cellular and humoral immunity, but immune sensitization can be documented more easily in the humoral than in the cell-mediated arm of the system. The patient with preexisting or rapidly developing anamnestic antibodies against class I antigens of donor tissue may experience very rapid graft rejection. Early work in selecting donor-recipient pairs and predicting graft survival relied heavily on matching the class I antigens HLA-A and HLA-B.

Class II Antigens

Class II antigens (HLA-DR, HLA-DQ, and HLA-DP) are not present on all cells, not even on all lymphocytes. Methods for identification and classification were developed in the middle and late 1970s. Recognition of their importance in graft survival came relatively late, but it now appears that the HLA-DR series is the most significant HLA characteristic, followed by HLA-B and then HLA-A. Examination for class II characteristics requires enriched cell preparations. It is important to know whether the recipient's cells react with the potential donor's class II antigens. Cell-culture techniques, described in the text that follows, are used for detection of immune reactivity.

Non-MHC Antigens

The term **major histocompatibility complex** implies that other histocompatibility determinants also exist; non-MHC characteristics are receiving increasing attention. Animals are more suitable for experimental investigations than human beings. Strains of mice have been bred with identical MHC antigens but diversity in other respects. Transplantation within these mice has clearly demonstrated the presence of **minor histocompatibility (mH)** antigens. Antigens termed H-Y, present in male subjects but not in female subjects, affect survival or tissue grafted from male donor to female recipient mice. Other antigens, present in both sexes and determined by sites on several different chromosomes, also affect graft survival in these highly specialized circumstances. It is not yet clear how significant such antigens are in outbred strains of mice, let alone in human beings, but the inevitable immune attack on MHC-identical tissue indicates a definite role for these "minor" antigens.

Endothelial cells are also involved in the tissue events of rejection, and there is growing conviction that molecules associated with these cells determine antigenic distinctions among individuals. Except for HLA-directed events, immune activity against endothelial elements is the most consistent site of tissue damage in allotransplantation.

Types of Transplanted Tissue

Therapeutically effective tissue grafting began long before immunologic mechanisms were understood and for certain types of grafts, immunologic problems do not occur. The **cornea,** the clear part of the eye, has been successfully grafted since the 1940s. The cornea is transparent because it has no blood vessels. Because there are no blood vessels, engrafted corneal tissue lacks communication with immunologically active aspects of host tissue. No tissue typing or immunologic testing is necessary before the procedure, and no problems occur as long as the grafted tissue remains avascular. If blood vessels grow into the graft, however, the tissue loses its transparency and also its immunologic isolation. A vascularized cornea graft usually must be removed, and problems of inflammation and immune response seriously complicate replacement.

Bone and Skin

Bone grafting also has a long history independent of immunology. In most procedures, engrafted bone serves a largely mechanical function and is not expected to provide actively metabolizing elements. In addition, procedures for storing and sterilizing bone render the cells nonviable and the protein elements less immunogenic than in unmodified tissue. Transplanted bone, whether autologous or allogeneic, provides structural support and stimulates ingrowth and proliferation of the host's own tissues. Characteristically, the grafted material is degraded and eliminated when the healing process is complete. In bone grafting, the major concerns are sterility of the transplanted material and the vascularity and regenerative capacity of the recipient site. Innovative new orthopedic techniques now use viable autologous bone for permanent modification of structure and function.

Similar considerations apply to **skin grafting.** Autografts provide permanent repair of surface defects, but allografts and sometimes even xenografts can be useful temporary measures to cover extensively damaged surfaces. The goal is to protect against infection and protein loss and to encourage regeneration of damaged tissue; as healing progresses, the graft becomes unnecessary and the foreign tissue is sloughed off.

Renal Grafts

Kidneys provide the greatest opportunity for monitoring and manipulating immune events. Allografts from living donors are feasible because a person with two healthy kidneys can donate one kidney without adverse consequences. Most kidney grafts come from cadavers, however, and require careful attention to removal and preservation. The clinical condition of the recipient, the functional status of the donor organ, and many pharmacologic and clinical variables strongly influence success of renal transplantation. The best results are seen with grafts from HLA-identical sibling donors; the 10-year survival rate of these grafts is nearly 70 percent. With all the many variables that affect outcome, including nonrenal and nonimmunologic problems in the patient, the 10-year survival rate of cadaver grafts averages 20 percent or more. When the donor is a living relative (described as a "living-related" graft), long-term success is directly proportional to degree of HLA matching. For grafts of cadaver origin, controversy exists as to the significance of HLA matching and the relative importance of MHC class I versus class II products.

Bone Marrow and Heart

Bone marrow of autologous or homologous origin may be transplanted. Autografting is useful in patients treated with highly toxic anticancer regimens, which lethally damage hematopoietic tissue. Allogeneic marrow is used to replace marrow that harbors malignant or other disease that cannot be corrected medically. ABO blood groups need not be compatible for bone marrow allografts, but HLA matching, especially HLA-DR, is crucially important. (Bone marrow transplantation is discussed in more detail in a later section.)

The technical success of **heart transplantation** has created an imbalance between supply and demand. The major indications for cardiac transplantation are inflammatory or metabolic disease of heart muscle (cardiomyopathy) and coronary artery disease; 5-year survival rate in the several thousand procedures now on record is more than 50 percent. Practical considerations often make it difficult to do much preoperative matching, although it is desirable to match for the ABO blood groups and for HLA-A, HLA-B, and HLA-DR.

Liver Grafts

Success with **liver transplantation** has been variable. Suitable donors are hard to find because metabolic and circulatory problems often damage the liver during terminal illness, and traumatic injury precludes the use of many livers after serious accidents. When a suitable donor organ is found, little attempt is made to match antigens; it may be that the large mass of allogeneic tissue promotes a degree of immune tolerance. Graft and patient survival does improve with certain combinations of antigen matching and immunosuppression. In adults, the major indications for liver replacement are primary biliary cirrhosis, malignant tumors, inborn errors of metabolism, and cirrhosis from chronic active hepatitis. However, except for metabolic deficiencies and congenital deformities, there is substantial likelihood that the disease affecting the original liver will recur in the transplanted organ. Children are usually treated for defective development of the biliary tracts or inborn errors of metabolism. When the procedure is done before generalized deterioration has occurred, results can be very gratifying.

Problematic Procedures and Ethical Considerations

Procedures for transplanting **pancreas, other endocrine organs, lungs** (with or without the donor heart), and portions of the **intestines** are practiced less widely. These organs present complex problems in surgical and medical management, but no specific immunologic challenges unique to the tissue involved. Because immune dysfunction significantly affects insulin-dependent diabetes mellitus, attempts at transplanting pancreas to correct this condition carry a guarded long-term prognosis. For conditions other than diabetes, the usual alternative to transplantation is rapid progression of a known fatal process. In diabetes, the consequences of a difficult surgical procedure and a lifetime of immunosuppressive therapy must be weighed against the generally favorable clinical course and long life expectancy that accompany conventional therapy.

Organ transplantation can be lifesaving, but is also a very expensive proposition with many more potential recipients than donors. Ethical considerations become important in determining who should receive an organ transplant and how the physician should decide whether one patient is favored over another. Problems are further compounded by the buying and selling of body organs, particularly from poor countries such as India and the Middle East.

Human fetal tissue can also be used as a source of graft material and in fact is an excellent source because fetal cells grow more quickly, are multipotential, and less immunogenic. Should fetal tissue be used for transplantation? Does the mother who aborted her fetus have the right to donate that fetus to science or perhaps even sell it? Clearly difficult questions need to be resolved by society as the technical and immunologic problems of transplantation are overcome.

REJECTION PHENOMENA

More kidneys have been transplanted than all other types of organs. Immunologic mechanisms are universal, but the histologic details, the time sequence, and the clinical consequences of attempted grafting differ for different organs transplanted. For all vascularized grafts and in all donor-recipient pairs except monozygotic twins, the presence of transplanted tissue generates immunologic events that may lead to rejection. The events that accompany renal transplantation have been studied through several decades of biopsies from functioning grafts, examination of surgically removed failed grafts, and autopsies. The specific events described in this section summarize observations primarily from kidney transplantations. Table 13–2 outlines the forms that rejection may take.

Hyperacute Rejection

If the recipient already possesses antibodies against antigens of the donor tissue, irreversible damage can occur in the first minutes or hours after transplantation, an

TABLE 13–2. **Donor Tissue Rejection**

Type of Rejection	Time Sequence	Mechanism	Tissue Events	Prognosis
Hyperacute	Minutes to hours	Antibodies to HLA or ABO antigens	Fibrin, complement in vessel walls Thrombosis of small vessels Acute inflammatory cells	Irreversible
Accelerated	1 to 5 days	Antibodies to HLA or ? vascular antigens Previously sensitized T cells	Lymphocytes as well as neutrophils Fibrin, complement in vessels Thrombosis of small vessels	Irreversible
Acute	5 days to years	Newly developing cell-mediated immunity	CD4 and CD8 cells Many macrophages Damage to parenchymal and interstitial elements	Usually reversed by increasing immunosuppression
Chronic	Years	Probably not immune	Progressive narrowing of blood vessels, with tissue damage from inadequate blood supply	Gradual irreversible deterioration

event described as **hyperacute rejection.** Circulating antibodies combine with tissue antigens in complexes that activate complement in vessels of the transplanted tissue. This provokes intense acute inflammation with accumulation of neutrophils and their proteolytic enzymes, and aggregation of platelets with release of vasoactive and coagulation-promoting substances leading to small-vessel thrombosis and disseminated intravascular coagulopathy. Blood supply to the transplanted organ is irreversibly compromised, and the kidney undergoes ischemic necrosis.

HLA and ABO Antibodies

Hyperacute rejection is usually due to high-titered antibodies against class I antigens. The titer of such antibodies may wax and wane. Patients awaiting renal grafts are tested periodically for HLA antibodies, and there has long been the fear that transplantation could provoke anamnestic recurrence of antibody that had been identified previously, but was absent at the time of grafting. Until recently, a history of previous antibody contraindicated transplantation of a kidney with the corresponding antigens; however, accumulating data with current immunosuppressive strategies indicate relatively little danger from antibodies undetectable at the time of foreign tissue introduction.

Vascular endothelium expresses ABO antigens, and kidneys incompatible with the recipient's ABO agglutinins are susceptible to hyperacute rejection. This is a problem especially for group O patients, whose serum contains both anti-A and anti-B antibodies. Some successes have been reported in reducing the level of antibody by plasma exchange and then subsequent administration of immunosuppressive therapy to prevent their untimely reappearance. Kidneys are the tissue most susceptible to damage from ABO incompatibility; liver and bone marrow transplants have been successful across ABO lines.

Unknown Specificities

Patients with no detectable HLA or blood group antibodies may experience hyperacute rejection, more often with second grafts than with first. An unsuccessful graft seems to provoke antibodies that cannot currently be identified; specificity against vascular endothelium is a prime suspect.

Accelerated Rejection

Hyperacute rejection has an extremely rapid onset. The grafted kidney may become swollen and ischemic before the eyes of the surgeons, who must acknowledge defeat by removing the graft through the incision made to implant it. When failure occurs several days after the primary procedure, the process is sometimes called **accelerated rejection.** Lymphocytes as well as neutrophils are seen in the tissue, but the resulting thrombosis and tissue necrosis are essentially the same as in the hyperacute process. Accelerated rejection may reflect previously established cell-mediated immunity, because T lymphocytes already sensitized to the donor antigens require several hours to several days to produce their effects (compare with the tuberculin reaction). Some accelerated episodes involve both antibodies and cellular events through the mechanism of antibody-dependent cell-mediated cytotoxicity. The targets of accelerated episodes are characteristically class I antigens, although many researchers believe that activity against still-to-be-identified vascular endothelial components is also significant. Sensitive tests for preformed antibodies against HLA antigens have reduced the frequency of hyperacute and accelerated rejection episodes, but continued occurrence in 0.5 to 1 percent of transplantations indicates that the entire story has not yet been told.

Acute Rejection

The most common and prolonged problem with organ rejection seems to involve class II antigens and is largely cell-mediated. Susceptibility to this phenomenon, called **acute rejection,** begins within 1 week and remains as long as the graft persists. The antigenic stimulus is thought to be both parenchymal and nonparenchymal cells present in the transplanted organ. Dendritic cells and monocytes are non–organ-specific cells that express class II antigens and are present in grafted tissue along with organ-specific elements. Epithelial cells of the donor tissue may also be stimulated to express class II antigens in the recipient whose immune system is activated. Because rejection occurs even when donor and recipient are HLA-identical and have been shown to cause no mutual stimulation when lymphocytes are cocultured, at least some of the antigens involved must be additional to the known MHC determinants and are not detected by present typing procedures.

Importance of Matching Antigens

Since the earliest days of pretransplantation testing and post-transplantation immunomodulation, it has been difficult to determine the degree to which HLA matching affects graft outcome. Variables include whether donor and recipient are from the same kinship or population group; what antigens are identified and by what techniques; what other criteria are used for recipient eligibility; and how antibodies are sought and evaluated. In all circumstances, immunosuppression is crucial in promoting graft survival. Less suppression is required with less antigenic disparity, but some degree of immunosuppression is always needed. Declining function in an established graft often heralds impending rejection. Although infection and nonimmunologic vascular problems must be ruled out, intensifying the level of immunosuppression may reverse the functional deficit.

Tissue Events

Tissue undergoing acute rejection is heavily infiltrated by macrophages and both CD4-positive and CD8-positive T cells. Most have been recruited by lymphokines secreted after antigen has stimulated cells with receptors for specific antigens. Macrophages of both donor and host origin produce interleukin-1 (IL-1), which causes T-cell multiplication and generalized inflammatory activation. Stimulated host T cells produce other mediators, including interleukin-2 (IL-2) and interferon-γ which affect the number and the functional level of both lymphocytes and macrophages. Interferon-γ induces enhanced membrane expression of class I and class II antigens, which renders the donor cells more susceptible to recognition and attack by host lymphocytes.

Chronic Rejection

Because of progressive vascular failure and gradual tissue hypoxia, previously functioning grafts sometimes deteriorate months or years after transplantation. Proliferation of cells lining the blood vessels narrows the lumen and reduces the volume of blood entering the tissue. Deficient oxygenation causes impaired functioning, loss of cell and tissue elements, and progressive fibrous scarring. Immune activity does not seem to be the problem; after the process begins, intensifying immunosuppression does not reverse it. Reducing the immunosuppression may even improve graft function if there is concomitant toxic damage from the agents given (see later section on immunosuppressive drugs).

It is possible that growth factors from chronically stimulated platelets and IL-1 from activated macrophages combine to promote proliferation of endothelial cells. Proliferative changes are known to occur when vascular cells sustain such nonimmune insults as physical trauma or exposure to abnormal lipids in atherosclerosis. Chronic activation might also, or alternatively, be due to interaction of endothelial or other cell antigens with antibody present at levels too low to be detected. No specific vascular disease or cause for damage has been consistently associated with this deterioration of previously successful grafts.

TESTING BEFORE TRANSPLANTATION

Although some element of immune rejection inevitably affects allografts, survival and function of grafted tissue are improved by selection of suitable donor-recipient pairs. Suppression of the immune response is discussed in the next section.

Antigens of Donor and Recipient

Routine pregraft testing includes typing the recipient and the prospective donor for ABO blood group and for HLA-A, HLA-B, and HLA-DR antigens. ABO antigens are present on many cell types, and it is important that the transplanted tissue be compatible with these high-titered complement-binding antibodies. This puts group O recipients, who possess both anti-A and anti-B, at a disadvantage; only the 45 percent of the group O population can be suitable donors for most tissues. As discussed later in this chapter, bone marrow is an exception to the ABO rule, and some liver grafts have been successful across ABO lines.

Antisera for HLA typing is available from commercial sources and is often derived from the sera of women who have had multiple children (multiparous). HLA antibodies are produced as a result of alloimmunization during pregnancy. The mother is exposed to fetal antigens of paternal origin, and in response anti-HLA IgG antibodies are produced. These antibodies do not seem to harm the fetus because they are primarily absorbed by the placenta. Monoclonal antibodies have also been produced and are used to detect clinically significant HLA types.

Cross-reactivity of antibodies is a common observation and has led to the identification of shared epitopes among certain HLA types. These HLA types have been arranged into "cross-reactive groups," or CREGs. CREGs allow for greater latitude in donor-recipient HLA matching and, if antibody is present in a recipient, may predict potential problems with graft acceptance. Shared epitopes can also be found within an entire HLA family. For example, HLA-Bw4 and HLA-Bw6 are antigens with specific epitopes found to be associated with all HLA-B locus antigens. These antigens are referred to as "public" specificities. In contrast to public specificities, "private" specificities define very small groups of HLA antigens with shared epitopes. Antisera with antibodies to HLA-A9 also bind to cells expressing HLA-A23 or HLA-A24.

Microlymphocytotoxicity Testing

The most widely used technique for detection of HLA antigens is the **microlymphocytotoxicity test** originally developed by Terasaki and McClelland. Peripheral blood lymphocytes are obtained from the patient and incubated with antisera containing specific anti-HLA antibodies. After incubation, complement is added. In the presence of complement, antibodies that have attached to the cell surface will lethally damage the lymphocyte membrane (Fig. 13–1). Cell death can be observed by addition of a supravital dye such as eosin Y. Live cells will exclude the dye, whereas dead cells become swollen and stained. Class I antigen is easily detected on T cells or B cells. Class II HLA-DR antigens are expressed primarily on B cells; therefore, enrichment techniques for B cells are necessary. Peripheral blood lymphocytes can be separated using a density gradient solution such as Ficoll-Hypaque (Fig. 13–2).

LYMPHOCYTOTOXICITY
TESTING BY DYE EXCLUSION

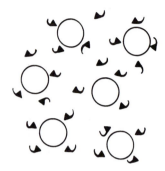 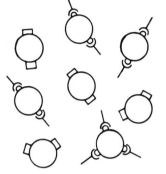 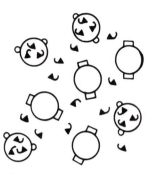

Viable lymphocytes
exclude dye molecules

Cytotoxic antibodies
damage cells of
appropriate specificity

Dye penetrates only
cells with which
antibody has reacted

FIGURE 13–1. When serum contains cytotoxic antibody specific for antigens on lymphocytes, the immune interaction causes cell damage that can be detected by observing that dye ineffective against normal cells is able to enter the injured cells.

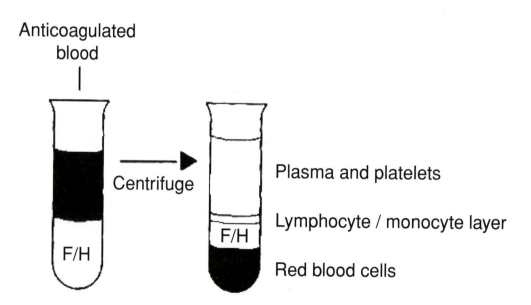

Anticoagulated
blood

Centrifuge

Plasma and platelets

Lymphocyte / monocyte layer

F/H

Red blood cells

F/H

Ficoll-Hypaque

FIGURE 13–2. Lymphocyte separation using Ficoll-Hypaque. Whole anticoagulated blood is layered over the density gradient and centrifuged. Lymphocytes and monocytes layer at their respective density in the gradient. Red blood cells and granulocytes have greater density and therefore settle to the bottom of the tube, whereas most of the platelets remain floating in the upper most layer.

B cells can be selectively isolated from the lymphocyte/monocyte layer by reacting T cells with sheep red blood cells (RBCs) and then centrifuging to remove the heavier T-rosettes. Separation can also be achieved by placing the lymphocyte suspension onto a nylon wool column. B cells adhere more easily to the fibers than T cells do. A novel approach using magnetic beads coated with IgM antibody is also used. B cells will attach to the antibody-coated beads through their Fc receptors.

Molecular Techniques for HLA Testing

Two-dimensional gel electrophoresis is a technique that has been applied extensively to the identification of beta chains of DR molecules. Lymphocytes are cultured in the presence of radioactively labeled methionine (35S), which is then incorporated into HLA molecules. Cells are subsequently harvested and lysed, and HLA molecules are immunoprecipitated with monoclonal antibodies specific for epitopes on the constant regions of the DR-beta chain. Immunoprecipitated molecules can be separated in one direction on a gel containing a pH gradient (isoelectric focusing). Further separation according to size and electrical charge occurs in a second dimension by rotating the gel 90 degrees. The now separated radioactively labeled immunoprecipitates can be visualized by exposing the gels to photographic film.

HLA typing can also be performed at the DNA level. Single-stranded DNA is prepared from patient's cells, and the DNA is cut by restriction enzymes. Because the enzymes recognize only certain nucleotide sequences, the DNA is cut into fragments of varying lengths and molecular weights. These fragments can be separated electrophoretically by charge and size. Fragments can be visualized by binding with a radioactively labeled or enzymatically labeled DNA probe. The DNA probe is single-stranded and has a complementary nucleotide sequence so that it will bind to the DR beta-gene region. Depending on their inheritance of DR beta genes, every individual will have a characteristic electrophoretic pattern of labeled fragments.

Choosing Among Donors

HLA matching influences graft survival, but the magnitude and significance of this effect are controversial. In selecting among potential living-related donors, the best matching gives the best results. Members of a single kindred posses only a limited number of haplotypes. If HLA-A, HLA-B, and HLA-DR antigens are the same, the entire chromosomal segment can be assumed to be the same, including genes that determine the class III products and unidentified aspects of the MHC. Unrelated donor-recipient pairs who share two, three, or four HLA antigens are much less likely to have shared alleles in the remaining portions of the MHC. The allotypes of the class III complement-related proteins can be determined if close MHC matching is essential, as, for example, for bone marrow transplants. The advent of highly effective immunosuppressive regimens has improved survival of mismatched kidney and other grafts, but the best match possible in each clinical circumstances is still desirable.

For kidney grafts, the Lewis blood group system influences outcome. Overall statistics are less favorable for Lewis-negative than for Lewis-positive patients who receive Lewis-positive kidneys. However, clinical circumstances usually preclude using Lewis types as a significant selection factor. If a Lewis-negative recipient needs regrafting after failure of the first graft, a Lewis-negative donor is definitely preferable.

The Sensitized Patient

Recipients with established immunity to histocompatibility antigens may experience hyperacute or accelerated rejection of grafted tissue expressing those antigens. Serum from patients awaiting transplantation is tested periodically for antibodies that could compromise graft survival. The **lymphocytotoxicity** procedure using patient serum against a panel of lymphocytes selected to express most of the significant HLA antigens is performed. Antibodies reactive against most or all of the cells on the panel carry a worse prognosis for successful transplantation than serum with limited reactivity or no antibodies. Some patients have antibodies that react with all allogeneic cells on the panel and with their own cells as well. These panreactive autoantibodies tend to be IgM, to have a low thermal optimum, and to react with class II antigens; their presence does not correlate with hyperacute rejection. Dangerous antibodies are those that are IgG and react at 37°C with class I antigens. Patients with these antibodies must await a donor organ that lacks the corresponding antigens.

Crossmatch Procedures

After a potential donor has been selected, suitability is confirmed by testing the recipient's serum in a lymphocytotoxicity assay against cells from the designated individual. This is done regardless of results in pretransplantation antibody screening panels. The patient whose serum reacts with panel cells but not the specific donor's cells is a suitable recipient; the patient whose serum is negative for the panel but cytotoxic for the specific donor should not receive the planned graft. In the past, it was customary to save serum samples that had been positive on screening procedures and to test the most highly reactive specimen against cells of the prospective donor. With current immunosuppressive therapy, even if a patient's serum has previous strong reactivity, good graft survival can occur with a negative crossmatch against the current donor.

Cellular Reactions

In selecting living-related donors, it is customary to use cell-culture tests against cells from the proposed donor, as well as serum testing. This is impractical for cadaver grafts because the culture procedure requires hours or days of delay that would damage an organ retrieved after death. The **mixed lymphocyte culture (MLC)** or **mixed lymphocyte reaction (MLR)** procedure tests the degree to which the donor's cells stimulate an immune response in the recipient's T lymphocytes. When cocultured with cells expressing foreign class II antigens, T lymphocytes undergo proliferation and activation. Lymphocytes are cultured in medium containing a radioactive DNA precursor (^{3}H thymidine). As stimulated cells undergo mitotic division, they incorporate the labeled thymidine. The amount of radioactivity in the cell can be measured and is proportional to the synthesis of new DNA and T-cell proliferation. Cytotoxic actions of host T cells against prospective donor target cells can also be measured. This is called the **cell-mediated lympholysis** test and is useful in measuring how much cell-mediated damage the patient can mount.

The One-Way MLC

When lymphocytes of different HLA phenotypes are cultured together, each proliferates after contact with foreign antigens on the other. The reaction significant for pretransplantation testing is recipient against donor; donor against recipient is not an issue because solid tissue grafts contain few, if any, donor cells that might react against recipient's antigens. In the **one-way MLC,** the donor cells are irradiated to abolish their proliferative capacity, but the antigens remain immunogenic and capable of provoking the recipient's cells to proliferate (Fig. 13–3).

The one-way MLC is used to select the donor whose cells provoke the least response in the recipient. MLC reactivity is to be expected whenever there is disparity of HLA-DR antigens, but some cells may be more immunogenic than others. Even when recipient and all potential donors are HLA-identical, the MLC results may differ for different stimulating cells. Negative results on the one-way MLC do not guarantee prolonged graft survival, but the likelihood of serious rejection problems increases with the degree of activity observed. Table 13–3 summarizes the usual battery of tests performed before transplantation.

MIXED LYMPHOCYTE CULTURE

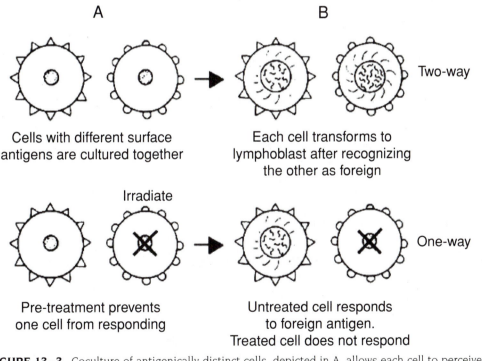

A

Cells with different surface antigens are cultured together

B

Each cell transforms to lymphoblast after recognizing the other as foreign

Two-way

Irradiate

Pre-treatment prevents one cell from responding

Untreated cell responds to foreign antigen. Treated cell does not respond

One-way

FIGURE 13–3. Coculture of antigenically distinct cells, depicted in A, allows each cell to perceive the foreign characteristics of the other. Cells that are immunocompetent undergo lymphoblast transformation (B). If, as shown in the lower drawings, one cell is prevented from responding, any blast transformation that occurs represents the response of the untreated cell to foreign antigens of the treated cell.

TABLE 13–3. **Pretransplantation Tests**

To determine antigens of donor and recipient
  ABO group
  (Lewis blood group, for kidney grafts)
  Class I antigens: HLA-A, -B
  Class II antigens: HLA-DR
  Family studies to distinguish haplotypes, in selecting living-related donors
To identify previous sensitization in recipient
  Periodic tests for lymphocytotoxic antibodies against a panel of cells
    Usually suspensions of peripheral-blood lymphocytes
    Sometimes separate suspensions of T cells and B cells
    If autoantibody is suspected, test at 37°C or inactivate IgM with a reducing agent
  Test recipient's serum for lymphocytotoxicity against lymphocytes of specific intended
      donor (lymphocytotoxicity crossmatch)
    Not considered necessary to retain and to test the most highly reactive of previous
      serum samples
To determine whether donor's antigens stimulate recipient
  One-way mixed lymphocyte culture with donor's cells inactivated

---

IMMUNOSUPPRESSION

As long as tissue that expresses foreign antigens remains in the host, there remains a risk of immune-mediated rejection. The risk is greatest in the first few years, but the need to suppress immune reactivity is lifelong. Ideal immunosuppression would eliminate reactions against the grafted tissue but leave all other immune actions intact. This ideal donor-specific immunosuppression has not been achieved. Strategies that prolong graft survival by reducing activity against the transplant also reduce the host's normal protective immunity. Immunosuppressive regimens rely heavily on pharmacologic agents, primarily drugs that impair cellular proliferation or alter inflammatory or membrane-associated reactions (Table 13–4). Other approaches to immunosuppression exploit immune events and products in an attempt to modulate immune reactivity.

Immunosuppressive Drugs

Immune reactivity requires that antigen-specific cells multiply, both during activation and as part of effector events. Agents that limit cell proliferation will limit immune activity; drugs that affect mitosis and cell division will have more destructive effects on rapidly proliferating populations than on stable populations of functioning cells. **Antiproliferative agents** are effective antitumor agents and, in somewhat smaller doses, are useful immunosuppressants. Unfortunately, these agents also damage populations of normal cells that have a high turnover rate, especially cells of the bone marrow and the lining of the gastrointestinal tract. The goal in administering cytotoxic agents is to use the smallest dose that eliminates unwanted antigraft activity. Characteristically, the dose will be high immediately after the procedure, with later reductions to a stable minimal level. Episodes of threatened rejection can be treated by increasing the dose or changing to more powerful but more dangerous

TABLE 13-4. **Immunosuppressive Drugs Used in Transplantation**

Drug	Action	Side Effects
Antiproliferative Agents		
Azathioprine	Interrupts DNA synthesis by inhibiting purine metabolism	Bone marrow depression Hepatotoxicity, hair loss
Cyclophosphamide	An alkylating agent Affects enzyme actions, nucleotide cross-linking	Depresses humoral immunity Bone marrow depression
Methotrexate	Folic acid antagonist Interferes with nucleotide synthesis	Gastrointestinal tract symptoms, liver damage, bone marrow depression
Anti-inflammatory Action		
Adrenal corticosteroids	Inhibits T-cell proliferation Reduces interleukin-2 (IL-2) production Reduces chemotaxis and activity of neutrophils and macrophages	Disturbs carbohydrate metabolism, bone metabolism, cardiovascular regulation Depresses wound healing, growth (in children), response to stress
Prevents Lymphocyte Activation		
Cyclosporine	Blocks proliferation of activated T cells; inhibits IL-2 production; depresses B-cell and macrophage actions by inhibiting production of lymphokines; modulates donor-tissue expression of class I and II antigens	Damage to kidneys Hyperplasia of gum tissue, hair growth Variable effects on liver, central nervous system, gastrointestinal tract

agents. Episodes of infection often require reduction in immunosuppressive intensity. Immunosuppressive drugs can also be used to treat autoimmune diseases.

Steroid Effects

Adrenal corticosteroids are powerful immunosuppressives that do not exert globally cytotoxic effects. Prednisone or prednisolone is routinely administered along with one or several cytotoxic drugs; the effects are additive, so that lower doses of each can be given. Corticosteroids exert a broad range of metabolic, anti-inflammatory, and anti-immune effects; high doses cause serious problems with infection, wound healing, hemodynamic balance, carbohydrate metabolism, and mineral regulation. Most patients routinely receive low or moderate doses, with high-dose therapy administered in response to acute rejection episodes. Corticosteroids affect cell-mediated immunity more than antibody production and infections that result from this type of immunosuppression often involve viruses, fungi, and intracellular microorganisms.

Actions of Cyclosporine

Since the mid-1980s, immunosuppression has been revolutionized by **cyclosporine.** This fungal metabolite exerts remarkable suppressive effects on helper T cells, thereby reducing both cellular and humoral responses to newly encountered antigens. Although B cells and suppressor and cytotoxic T cells are not directly affected, cyclosporine profoundly affects the activity of macrophages and other lymphocytes by reducing secretion of lymphokines. Cyclosporine interferes with activation of antigen-specific CD4 cells and prevents the secretion of IL-2 as well as the secretion of many T-cell products and expression of receptors for these lymphokines. Cyclosporine not only diminishes active rejection but may allow or encourage a state of specific immune tolerance by allowing the proliferation of antigen-specific suppressor cells. It is not toxic to hematopoietic precursors or to the alimentary tract, which is an advantage over most cytotoxic immunosuppressives. Unfortunately, it causes significant dose-related damage to the kidney; effects on the liver and nervous system are less severe but still potentially troublesome. Other immunosuppressive drugs in use include FK506 and rapamycin, which are agents chemically unrelated to cyclosporine, but have similar actions.

Despite its impressive therapeutic effects, cyclosporine has not made the immune problems of tissue transplantation disappear. It provides superior but nonspecific immunosuppression. Immunologic reactions to the transplanted tissue do continue, and normal immune actions against other foreign antigens are reduced. However, it has significantly improved graft survival in virtually all studies reported. With cyclosporine, imperfectly matched grafts give far better results than would previously be achieved. The survival of fully HLA-matched grafts has also improved. Most centers continue to observe better results with fully matched grafts than with mismatched grafts, but the overall consequence of cyclosporine use has been to make HLA matching less significant in selecting cadaver grafts.

Immune Manipulation

An approach to avoiding globally cytotoxic agents is administration of antibodies directed against effector lymphocytes. **Antilymphocyte globulin (ALG)** has proved unsuitable for long-term immunosuppression but works well for episodic treatment of acute rejection. A refinement is to use monoclonal antibodies against CD3, CD4, or the IL-2 receptor. Selective, shielded **irradiation** causes a rapid fall in circulating lymphocytes; this seems to diminish the intensity of response to antigens newly encountered at that time. It may become possible to induce antigen-specific tolerance through combinations of cyclosporine, irradiation, and selective exposure to the relevant antigens. Table 13–5 presents several categories of immunomodulating therapy.

Certain tissue can be engrafted as individual cells, rather than as solid tissue. Endocrine cells, like those of the pancreas or the adrenal or parathyroid glands, can perform their physiologic roles after injection as free cells. Experiments with aggregates of pancreatic islet cells in the portal vein of the liver or in the peritoneum have been performed. Survival of these cellular implants is improved over results with fresh cells if the cells are **cultured** *in vitro* for several generations. There is less class II antigenic activity in cultured than in fresh injected material, probably because culturing eliminates nonendocrine cells, such as lymphocytes and macrophages, which have potent expression of class II determinants.

TABLE 13-5. **Immunobiologic Manipulations Used in Transplantation**

Immunosuppressive Approach	Target Action	Clinical Efficacy
Depletion of Effector Cells		
Antilymphocyte globulin	Rapid, profound loss of T and B lymphocytes	Short-term use to reduce initial immune response or to reverse acute rejection
Monoclonal anti-CD3	Prompt fall in T lymphocytes; newly produced cells lose ability to recognize specific antigens	Short-term use to reverse acute rejection; antibodies often develop, which reduce later efficacy and mediate sensitivity reactions
Total lymphoid irradiation	Rapid, profound loss of T and B lymphocytes	Useful in pretransplant conditioning to induce tolerance to grafted antigens
Transfusion Therapy		
Donor-specific transfusion	Depresses antigen-specific immune response	Given before planned renal transplant from living donor
Random-donor transfusion	Seems to depress overall immune responsiveness; may serve to screen out hyperresponders	Given during support period before cadaver kidney grafting
Modification of Graft		
Culturing pancreatic or other endocrine cells	Eliminates "passenger" cells with strong class II antigens	In recipient also receiving antilymphocyte globulin, reduces response to foreign tissue

Transfusion Effect

A remarkable application of immunomodulation is the **transfusion effect.** Because preformed antibodies prejudice graft survival and because transfusion often stimulates antibodies, early workers tried to avoid transfusions to patients awaiting transplantation. By the mid-1970s, it became apparent that cadaver kidneys survived longer in recipients whose clinical state had made transfusion unavoidable than in those who had never received RBCs. Transfusion policy has come full circle; RBC transfusions are now a routine part of pretransplantation conditioning.

The transfusion effect is most striking in two situations: random blood transfusions given to a patient receiving a cadaver graft unmatched for HLA and pregraft transfusion from the specific individual who will donate a living-related graft. It is difficult to develop an optimum transfusion schedule, because the mechanisms for this graft-promoting effect remain unclear. RBC components are effective; leukocytes or platelet concentrates are not necessary or desirable. Benefit increases with increasing numbers of transfusions, up to about five or six in the weeks or months before transplantation.

BONE MARROW TRANSPLANTATION

Transplanting bone marrow has consequences different from those of most other grafts. A successful graft does not merely replace a defective organ; it introduces an active population of immunologically unique cells into a recipient with different constitution. Marrow grafts were initially used to treat aplastic anemia, global immunodeficiency syndromes, or leukemias refractory to other therapy. With increasingly successful transplantation techniques, the number of potential indications has broadened to include a variety of enzyme-deficiency conditions and hematologic dysplasias.

Donor Selection

HLA matching is more important for marrow transplant than for any other tissue. Until recently, only HLA-identical siblings were considered suitable donors, a restriction that made many patients ineligible for this form of treatment. Better immunosuppressive techniques now permit cautious use of one-haplotype matched relatives, opening the donor pool to parents and many additional siblings, and also use of HLA-matched unrelated individuals. Antibodies against donor ABO antigens can be removed by plasmapheresis; the profound immunosuppression used before marrow grafting prevents reexpression of the recipient's anti-A or anti-B.

Bone marrow is renewable; the donor loses only a finite number of aspirated cells, not the solid mass of an irreplaceable organ. Approximately 20 percent of functioning marrow is removed from an adult, and this can be regenerated within a couple of months. Because donation creates no permanent deficiency, marrow donors may be of varying size, age, and health status.

Autologous Donation

Autologous transplantation is practical because bone marrow can be collected and stored frozen for weeks or months with only moderate cell loss. Autologous marrow replacement is especially useful in treating nonhematologic malignancies. For such tumors as gonadal, breast, and certain lung cancers, permanent cure can be achieved by intensive radiation therapy and chemotherapy that destroys all traces of tumor. However, cytotoxic therapy of this magnitude also permanently destroys hematopoietic marrow. Provided the marrow does not harbor tumor cells, a generous hematopoietic specimen can be harvested before therapy begins. When the cytotoxic regimen is completed, the preserved hematopoietic elements are reinjected to replace blood-forming tissue destroyed by the ablative therapy.

Autologous marrow grafts can also be used to treat leukemia. If initial treatment produces complete blood and marrow remission, an aliquot of this restored normal marrow can be frozen for use if relapse occurs later. The relapse can be treated by intensive therapy intended to eliminate from the body every last lingering, malignant cell, and the nonmalignant autologous marrow can then be infused to reconstitute the system. Besides the problems of infection and bleeding that inevitably accompany marrow ablation, this procedure carries the risk that undetected malignant cells may be present in the marrow retrieved during apparent remission.

Hematopoietic Stem Cells

Use of monoclonal antibodies to tumor antigens has enabled marrow to be "cleansed" of malignant cells or monoclonal antibodies to early CD markers can be used to concentrate hematopoietic stem cells. Then only the cells necessary for reconstituting hematopoiesis are reinfused back into the patient. Hematopoietic stem cells carry CD34. A potential source of CD34-positive cells is the umbilical cord. These cells tend to have less immune reactivity and therefore are associated with less risk of rejection or graft-versus-host disease. Unfortunately, not enough cells are in cord blood to successfully treat adults; however, methods are underway to optimize stem-cell collection or expand CD34 populations *in vitro*. Use of stem cells for transplantation purposes leads to other exciting possibilities. With use of recombinant deoxyribonucleic acid (DNA) techniques, it is possible to correct genetic defects. Initial experiments to introduce a missing gene into stem cells of children suffering from adenosine deaminase (ADA) deficiency, a potentially fatal defect that cripples the immune system, have been partially successful. Other hematologic diseases involving single gene defects might be treatable with the latter technique. It has even been proposed that CD34 cells might be genetically engineered to be HIV-resistant. Stem cells are not infected with HIV; therefore, if stem cells were extracted from cord blood of babies born to HIV-positive mothers, treated, and then reinfused back into the child, the child should produce HIV-resistant T cells and macrophages and thus prevent neonatal development of AIDS.

Conditioning for Allogeneic Marrow Transplantation

Before a patient receives allogeneic marrow, it is necessary to eliminate all existing marrow elements and to destroy immune capability. In autologous grafting, post-graft immunosuppression is unnecessary, but the need to eliminate all hematopoietic elements remains. More intense and complete immunosuppression is needed for allogeneic marrow than for grafts of other tissue to avoid coexistence of residual host immunity along with activity derived from the transplanted allogeneic material. It is customary to use both radiation therapy and chemotherapy for several days before grafting is attempted.

The pregraft conditioning regimen leaves the patient with no immune, inflammatory, or hematologic resources. RBCs normally remain in the circulation for several months, so patients retain modest oxygen-carrying capacity after acute marrow destruction, but platelets and neutrophils drop to zero and remain absent until the grafted marrow establishes itself. This leaves the patient extremely susceptible to infection and bleeding. Prophylactic platelet transfusions are useful in preventing spontaneous bleeding, and potent antibiotics must be given to protect against infection. Neutrophils reappear within 2 to 4 weeks if the graft is successful, but platelets take much longer to achieve effective levels.

Graft-versus-Host Disease

The short-term risks of marrow transplantation are infection and bleeding. The most serious long-term complication of marrow transplantation is **graft-versus-host disease (GVHD),** in which immunocompetent cells from the donor recognize host antigens as foreign and attack the host tissues. GVHD can occur whenever viable T cells are transplanted into a recipient who is profoundly immunodeficient. Graft recipients who are only partially immunosuppressed retain the capacity to recognize and eliminate potentially aggressive donor T cells. For most transplantations, the goal is to preserve as much immune capacity as possible, but in bone marrow grafting, the recipient is deliberately and explicitly rendered unresponsive.

Because GVHD occurs after grafts from an HLA-identical sibling, it appears that HLA antigens are not the major target. Engrafted viable T cells initiate the process, but antibodies, macrophages, and natural killer cells may also have effector roles. GVHD can be either acute or chronic. Although chronic changes may follow acute manifestations, the processes are different, and either can occur independently.

Clinical Events

Acute GVHD begins in the first few weeks after transplantation and lasts for several months, affecting most severely the gastrointestinal tract and the skin, along with the liver. Intractable diarrhea, necrotizing skin lesions, and depressed hepatic function occur in the most severe cases, and susceptibility to infection increases. Immunosuppressive therapy is variably effective in reversing the process. Eliminating viable T cells from the grafted material has been attempted as a way to prevent acute GVHD, but this has not demonstrably prolonged patients' survival.

Of graft recipients who survive for 3 months or longer, up to 50 percent suffer from **chronic GVHD,** which causes gradual damage to skin, joints, and mucous membranes that resembles the changes seen in autoimmune collagen-vascular diseases. Indolent liver damage is common, but the most conspicuous problem is progressive loss of immune defense. The number of cytotoxic/suppressor T cells increases, and both humoral and cell-mediated functions decline, leaving the patient excessively vulnerable to both pathogenic and opportunistic organisms. The same agents used to treat autoimmune conditions are used, with varying degrees of success, for chronic GVHD.

Survival studies of leukemic patients treated with marrow transplantation indicate that patients who experience chronic GVHD have fewer disease recurrences than those without this immune complication. Leukemic complications, graft rejection, and inappropriate lymphoproliferative responses to viral infection occur more often when allografts have been treated to eliminate T cells than when unmodified grafts are used. An aphorism summarizing these observations is that allogeneic marrow exerts a "graft-versus-leukemia" effect.

SUMMARY

1. Transplantation of tissue into a recipient differs from transfusion in that a transplant is expected to survive and function permanently, whereas cells in a transfusion are expected to remain functional for only a limited time. Success in transplantation results from selection of the least immunogenic material and subsequent immune suppression to aid in acceptance of the graft.

2. Allografts are the most common type of transplanted tissue. Immune rejection occurs because of differences between the donor's and recipient's HLA antigens and other immunogens. Major histocompatibility complex (MHC) class I HLA-A and HLA-B antigens provoke both cellular and humoral immune responses, but class II HLA-DR antigens may be more significant in graft survival. In addition to MHC antigens, other histocompatibility determinants also exist (minor histocompatibility antigens), which can induce immune activity and graft rejection.

3. Many types of tissues can be transplanted with varying degrees of success. The cornea lacks blood vessels and communication with the immune system and therefore can be successfully grafted without matching tissue antigens. Allogeneic bone and skin may be transplanted for temporary repair purposes. Autografts of bone and skin can be used to provide permanent changes in structure and function. Kidney grafts from living donors and cadavers have been successfully performed. Autografting of bone marrow is useful in patients undergoing chemotherapy for cancer. Other organs are more problematic because of availability and prior condition of the donor organ. Ethical considerations concerning expense, limited availability, use of fetal tissue, and many other issues need to be resolved.

4. Rejection of transplanted tissue occurs in several different forms.
    a. With hyperacute rejection, circulating antibodies are already present in the recipient. These antibodies immediately combine with donor tissue antigens, activate complement, and induce acute inflammation. Hyperacute rejection is usually due to HLA class I incompatibility or ABO incompatibility. Sensitive tests for preformed antibodies are performed, but these tests may not detect all antibodies.
    b. Acute rejection is the most common problem. Prolonged cell-mediated immune activity against parenchymal and nonparenchymal cells occur. Parenchymal cells express MHC class I antigens, whereas donor dendritic cells and monocytes express class II antigens. Donor tissue becomes infiltrated by macrophages and CD4+ and CD8+ T cells, which secrete lymphokines that promote inflammatory processes.
    c. With chronic rejection, progressive vascular failure and gradual tissue hypoxia lead to graft deterioration months or even years after transplantation. Low-level immune responses and chronic stimulation of platelets and macrophages possibly contribute to endothelial cell proliferation and obstruction of blood vessels.

5. To enhance acceptance of transplanted tissue, pregraft testing is performed for ABO blood group and for HLA-A, HLA-B, and HLA-DR antigens. Testing procedures include the microlymphocytotoxicity test, which uses patient blood lymphocytes. Class I antigens can be detected on T cells and B cells. MHC class II HLA-DR antigens are expressed primarily on B cells. HLA typing of the beta chain of DR molecules can be performed by two-dimensional gel electrophoresis and deoxyribonucleic acid (DNA) probes.

Continued on the following page

6. The donor and recipient are tested for HLA type. Serum from patients needing transplants can also be tested for presence of antibodies by exposing a panel of lymphocytes selected to express most of the significant HLA antigens to patient serum and determining lymphocyte viability (lymphocytotoxicity assay). Suitability of the donor is then confirmed by testing the recipient's serum with cells from the donor in a lymphocytotoxicity assay. Suitability of a living-related donor is tested with serum in a lymphocytotoxicity assay and with the mixed-lymphocyte culture procedure.

7. Immunosuppression is needed as long as donor tissue continues to express foreign antigen. Immunosuppressive regimens rely heavily on pharmacologic agents that impair cellular proliferation or alter inflammatory reactions. Adrenal corticosteroids are powerful immunosuppressives, but high doses cause problems with infection, wound healing, fluid balance, carbohydrate and mineral metabolism. Cyclosporin is a better immunosuppressive agent with fewer side effects than corticosteroids.

8. HLA matching is more important for marrow transplants than for any other tissue. Bone marrow includes immunologically active cells from the donor and therefore graft-versus-host disease may occur. Autologous transplantation is especially useful for treating nonhematologic malignancies when intensive chemotherapy or radiation may destroy the marrow. Hematopoietic stem cells express CD34; therefore, techniques for identification, isolation, and concentration are being developed. Development of techniques for expanding stem cell numbers *in vitro* could lead to exciting possibilities such as use of stem cells from umbilical cord blood, correction of genetic defects in stem cells with recombinant DNA techniques, and resistance of genetically engineered stem cells to HIV and other diseases.

REVIEW QUESTIONS

1. Tissue exchanged between individuals of the same species, but with differing genetic characteristics is called _____.
   a. autograft
   b. isograft
   c. allograft
   d. xenograft
   e. heterograft

2. Which type of graft(s) will not elicit immune rejection?
   a. Autograft
   b. Isograft
   c. Allograft
   d. Xenograft
   e. a and b

3. Relative importance of HLA antigens for graft survival is _____.
   a. HLA-A > HLA-B > HLA-DR
   b. HLA-DR > HLA-A > HLA-B
   c. HLA-DR > HLA-B > HLA-A
   d. HLA-B > HLA-A > HLA-DR
   e. HLA-B > HLA-DR > HLA-A

4. The cornea is considered an immune-privileged site because _____.
   a. it is avascular
   b. it lacks communication with the immune system
   c. allografts are not rejected
   d. it temporarily covers damaged surfaces
   e. a, b, and c

5. Chronic rejection is characterized by _____.
   a. development of HLA antibodies
   b. previously sensitized T cells
   c. progressive narrowing of blood vessels
   d. macrophage damage to parenchymal and nonparenchymal tissues
   e. thrombosis of small vessels

6. HLA antibodies for typing purposes are derived from _____.
   a. sera of multiparous women
   b. commercially developed monoclonal antibodies
   c. male volunteers
   d. a and b
   e. a, b, and c

7. HLA antigens with "public" specificities _____.
   a. have shared epitopes that can be found within an entire HLA family
   b. include HLA-Bw4 as an example
   c. HLA-A9 as an example
   d. a and b
   e. a and c

8. The microlymphocytotoxicity test requires _____.
   a. lymphocytes
   b. antisera containing specific anti-HLA antibodies
   c. complement
   d. eosin Y
   e. all of the above

9. Which is *not* required for the mixed-lymphocyte culture test?
   a. donor B cells
   b. recipient T cells
   c. ^{3}H thymidine
   d. cell-culture media
   e. detector for radioactively labeled cells

10. Risks involved with bone marrow transplantation include _____.
    a. infection and bleeding
    b. graft-versus-host disease (GVHD)
    c. subsequent ABO antibody incompatibility
    d. a and b
    e. a, b, and c

MATCHING QUESTIONS

Match the characteristics in column 1 to the type of rejection in column 2.

Column 1

11. Transplanted tissue infiltrated
    with macrophages and T cells
12. Activated complement in blood vessels
13. Occurs within days to years
14. Presence of preformed antibody
    to HLA or ABO antigen
15. Lymphokine-mediated inflammation

Column 2

a. hyperacute
b. accelerated
c. acute
d. chronic
e. a and b

ESSAY QUESTIONS

16. Corneal transplants are commonly performed. Contact lenses may be worn for days. Heat valves made with glutaraldehyde-treated (fixative) valve material from pigs can be used for human heart valve replacement. Why are these materials not rejected?
    •

SUGGESTIONS FOR FURTHER READING

Armitage JO: Bone marrow transplantation. N Engl J Med 1994;330:827–838

Chao NJ, Schmidt GM, Niland JC, et al: Cyclosporine, methotrexate, and prednisone compared with cyclosporine and prednisone for prophylaxis of acute graft-versus-host disease. N Engl J Med 1993;329: 1225–1230

Hansen JA, Anasetti C, Martin PJ, et al: Allogeneic marrow transplantation: The Seattle experience. In: Terasaki PI, Cecka JM, eds. Clinical Transplants 1993. Los Angeles: UCLA Typing Laboratory, 1994: 193–209.

Mach B, Tiercy JM: Genotypic typing of HLA class II: From the bench to the bedside. Hum Immunol 1991;30:278–284

Milford EL: Immunological testing for renal transplantation. In: Rose NR et al, eds: Manual of Clinical Laboratory Immunology, 4th ed. Washington, DC: American Society for Microbiology, 1992:825–839

Niederwieser D, Grassegger A, Aubock J, et al: Correlation of minor histocompatibility antigen-specific cytotoxic T lymphocytes with graft-versus-host disease status and analyses of tissue distribution of their target antigens. Blood 1993;81:2200–2208

Noreen HJ: Crossmatch tests. In: Zachary AA, Teresi GA, eds. ASHI Laboratory Manual, 2nd ed. Lenexa, KS: American Society for Histocompatibility and Immunogenetics, 1990:307–320

Sullivan KM: Graft-versus-host disease. In: Forman SJ, Blume KG, Thomas ED, eds. Bone Marrow Transplantation. Oxford, England: Blackwell Scientific Publications, 1994:339–362

Thompson C: Umbilical cords: Turning garbage into clinical gold. Science 1995;268:805–806

REVIEW ANSWERS

1. c	6. d	11. c
2. e	7. d	12. e
3. c	8. e	13. c
4. e	9. a	14. a
5. c	10. d	15. c

14 Cancer Immunology

NATURE OF CANCER

Cancer is not a single disease but includes a large number of diseases characterized by abnormal, unregulated growth of cells. **Neoplasm** is a term often used in place of cancer and it means new uncontrolled growth of cells derived from one's own tissues. The abnormal tissue resulting from this uncontrolled growth is called a **tumor.** A **benign tumor** is usually confined to a single site, whereas cells from a **malignant tumor** are invasive and capable of spreading to adjacent or even distant sites in the body. Any cell type in the body may become cancerous, with over 200 different types of cancer being described. Cancer that originates from epithelial cells are called **carcinomas.** Those that originate from connective tissues are referred to as **sarcomas.** With advances in medical science, better hygiene, vaccines, and antibiotics, the number of deaths from infection has declined in the Western world. Cancer has therefore become much more important and is the second leading cause of death, surpassed only by heart disease.

Cancer cells are altered or mutated self cells, which no longer observe normal growth-regulating mechanisms and may occur frequently in the body. Lewis Thomas postulated that one of the primary duties of constantly circulating lymphocytes may be recognition of cancer cells and prevention of tumor growth—a theory called **immune surveillance.** Certainly if the immune system can recognize and reject grafted tissue, it should be capable of rejecting tumor cells. The existence of immune surveillance is suggested by the increased incidence of tumors in thymectomized animals or clinically by the association of increased cancer risk with chemotherapy and other immunosuppressive conditions. This chapter briefly examines causes of cancer, properties of cancer cells that enable and disable immune recognition, and immunodiagnostic and immunotherapeutic techniques.

Causes of Cancer

Carcinogens

Malignant tumors have been described in pictures and writings from ancient civilizations. Bone cancer (osteosarcoma) has been observed in Egyptian mummies. Manuscripts from the Middle Ages refer to "cancer families" and "cancer villages," which suggests inherited or environmental causes of cancer. The English physician, Sir Percival Pott, observed in 1775 that young men in their 20s who had been chimney sweeps as boys had a high rate of death due to cancer of the scrotum. He suggested that exposure to chimney soot might be the cause. Years later, the coal tars in soot have indeed been identified as **carcinogens.**

Humans are exposed to many chemicals and physical agents that can cause cell mutations and transformation into tumor cells. Some **chemical carcinogens,** such as polycyclic hydrocarbons (tar), tobacco smoke, benzene, and asbestos, are known mutagens. Other chemicals can be converted into mutagens with enzymatic activity by the liver. **Physical carcinogens** include ionizing radiation and ultraviolet light. Ionizing radiation can cause DNA damage through breakage or crosslinkage of nucleotides, and ultraviolet light induces the formation of thymine dimers. Deletion of nucleotides and the formation of highly reactive free radicals owing to ionizing radiation exposure can cause further damage to chromosomal DNA. Malignant transformation of cells appears to involve multiple steps with **initiation** leading to changes in the DNA of the cell, followed by **promoters** that stimulate cell division and malignant transformation.

Identification of an agent as a carcinogen is sometimes very difficult. **Epidemiology** is the study of disease occurring among various populations and the control of these diseases. From epidemiologic studies, associations between environmental factors and the incidence of different types of cancer have been established. Proving that a particular agent is the cause of cancer is more problematic. Animals may be exposed under controlled conditions to the agent, but such bioassays are complex in design, expensive, and time-consuming. The amount of carcinogen administered is critical. The route of exposure should mimic as closely as possible the exposure route of humans. The experiment must last through the life span of the animal.

Because of the problems involved with long-term bioassays, numerous short-term tests have been developed. These tests are based on the concept that carcinogens are also mutagens and will cause genetic alterations. Microorganisms or cells in tissue culture are used in these tests, and changes in DNA structure, chromosome damage, or changes in cell behavior are considered to be indicators of carcinogenicity. The **Ames test** uses an enzyme-deficient strain of *Salmonella typhimurium*. This strain is unable to grow on a medium that is deficient in histidine. However, on exposure to a carcinogen, the bacteria may undergo mutation and be converted to a strain capable of making their own histidine and therefore capable of growing on deficient media. Short-term assay using bacteria or tissue culture cells have made carcinogen testing much simpler and more rapid. However, they are not perfect. False-positive and false-negative results may be obtained. Negative results do not establish safety of an agent, and positive results may require more extensive testing in long-term animal bioassays to confirm carcinogenicity.

Viruses

The first evidence that a virus could cause cancer came from experiments by Peyton Rous in 1910. Rous prepared cell-free extracts from chicken sarcomas and injected them into healthy chickens. The healthy chickens developed the same type of sarcoma. Later experiments demonstrated the presence of ribonucleic acid (RNA) virus responsible for the tumor formation. Virally infected cells can be grown in tissue culture, and identification of a virus capable of causing tumor formation is confirmed by an **in vitro transformation assay.** When normal cells are grown in tissue culture, the cells attach to the bottom of a petri dish and grow until they contact another cell. Normal cells observe **contact inhibition** and form an organized single layer of confluent cells. Malignant cells do *not* observe contact inhibition and grow over each other to form disorganized, multilayered clumps. If normal fibroblasts are infected with a **tumor-causing virus,** some of the cells undergo malignant transformation. The original shape of the cell type is altered, cell division occurs, contact inhibition is lost, and disorganized cell growth is easily observed.

Virally transformed cells can be injected into appropriate test animals. This procedure has been very useful in detecting a large number of human tumor viruses. Both DNA- and RNA-containing viruses are associated with cancer. DNA viruses randomly integrate into the host cell chromosomal DNA, thereby interfering with normal cell transcription and causing the production of proteins that induce malignant transformation. Epstein-Barr virus (EBV) is a DNA virus causing Burkitt's lymphoma. The human papillomaviruses are DNA-containing viruses that can cause warts in the lower layers of the epidermis and mucosal epithelium and are linked to cancer of the cervix.

Most RNA viruses replicate in the cytoplasm and do not induce malignant transformation. However, retroviruses produce reverse transcriptase and can transcribe their RNA into DNA, which is then inserted into the host cell DNA. Retroviruses can be transmitted from generation to generation within certain species of higher animals. RNA tumor viruses can be grouped by their ultrastructural morphology, nucleic acid sequences, displayed antigens, and biologic activities into four types: A, B, C, and D. Type C is the most important as a cause of human malignancies. Human T-cell leukemia virus type I (HTLV I) is found in patients with Sézary T-cell leukemia and can be transmitted by breast-feeding, sexual intercourse, blood transfusions, and needle sharing. A second human T-cell leukemia virus (HTLV II) has been found in patients with a variant of hairy cell leukemia. Human immunodeficiency virus (HIV) is a related virus originally called HTLV III because it also infects T lymphocytes. As with HIV infection, leukemia due to HTLV I or II may take years to develop. Retroviruses may contain **oncogenes** (cancer genes) or, on insertion into host DNA, may activate host cell oncogenes. A persistently infected cell undergoing proliferation is more susceptible to mutational events, which can accumulate and eventually result in malignant transformation.

Hormones

Hormones are associated with certain types of cancer. Hormones are protein messengers secreted into the bloodstream and transported to cells at another site in the body. Responsive cells have membrane receptors that bind the hormone. Tumor cells derived from tissues that normally do not secrete hormones may develop the ability to secrete large amounts of a certain hormone and thus cause disease in another tissue. Tumor cells may also express hormone receptors not found in the original tissue and thereby gain altered function or growth responses. Many hormones also have profound effects on cell differentiation. For example, if the thyroid gland is removed from a tadpole, the tadpole cannot enter metamorphosis to become a frog. Similarly, cancer can be considered a disorder of differentiation characterized by immature cells that continue to proliferate and fail to respond to external homeostatic signals. Endometrial cancer, which is cancer of the cells lining the uterus, is related to prolonged exposure to the hormone estrogen in the absence of progestogens. Endometrial cells divide in response to estrogens. Progestogens can reduce or inhibit mitotic activity of these cells. Conditions in which high levels of estrogen occur and can predispose women to develop endometrial, ovarian, and breast cancer include diabetes, obesity, and having never birthed a child. The anticancer drug, **tamoxifen,** is particularly useful because of its antiestrogenic effects.

Cancer of the prostate in men is influenced by the hormone testosterone. Testosterone controls mitotic activity in the prostate. Dogs have a high incidence of prostatic carcinoma, and estrogen has been found to enhance the effect of testosterone in these animals by increasing the number of testosterone receptors. In human men, the relation between testosterone and estrogen in prostate cancer has not been well studied. Moreover, differences in testosterone and estrogen levels are seen in different races. Young black men have higher levels than young white men, and black Americans have the highest rate of prostate cancer in the world. Reasons for the high testosterone and estrogen levels in the black population are not known. Clearly, hormones are related to cancer, and increased levels or disturbances in normal balance may be important factors in cancer causation.

Genetic Aspects of Cancer

It is evident from the previous paragraphs that many different agents are capable of causing cancer. Most of these agents share an important biologic property: they damage or alter DNA. Cancer is the result of multiple genetic changes. There are well-characterized genes and chromosomal changes associated with certain types of cancer. Certain cancers tend to occur more frequently in families indicating a hereditary factor. Individuals with an inherited deficiency in the ability to repair lesions in their DNA have an increased incidence of cancer. Laboratory mice can be bred that have a high incidence of cancer.

Oncogenes

After the discovery of oncogenes in tumor viruses, it was suggested that oncogenes might also be found in normal cells and that viruses acquired these oncogenes from the genome of an infected cell. The oncogene hypothesis of cancer has been confirmed. Cellular oncogenes are referred to as **proto-oncogenes** (*c-onc*) to distinguish them from their viral counterparts (v-*onc*). Many different oncogenes associated with different retroviruses have been identified. Each of these oncogenes contains the information for membrane, cytoplasmic, or nuclear proteins that have the potential for inducing malignant transformation. The virus associated with a particular tumor can be isolated and injected into normal cells that will become tumorous. The original experiment by Rous in 1911, who described a transmissible sarcoma in chickens, demonstrated transmission of a tumor-causing virus. The oncogene carried by this virus was later isolated and given the three-letter abbreviation *src* (*sr* for sarcoma, *c* for chicken). Other oncogenes are also usually designated by three-letter abbreviations referring to their origin.

In normal cells, proto-oncogenes are generally expressed in relatively low levels and have defined roles in growth, differentiation, and healing processes. The c-*sis* proto-oncogene contains the information for a protein called platelet-derived growth factor (PDGF). Fibroblasts require PDGF to undergo mitosis in tissue culture, and it is probably necessary for normal healing to occur. The proto-oncogene *erb* B contains the information for a cell membrane receptor of epidermal growth factor (EGF). The interaction of EGF with its membrane receptor induces proliferation of skin and breast epithelial cells. The protein products of proto-oncogenes *src*, *abl*, and *ras* are found in the cytoplasm of cells and serve as messengers to transfer signals from the cell membrane to the nucleus. Products of other proto-oncogenes are nuclear in location and may play an important role in controlling cell division.

Cancer occurs when the proto-oncogenes become altered or overexpressed. A retrovirus may introduce numerous copies of an oncogene, resulting in overproduction of the oncogene product controlling cell replication; or, increased receptors are made that cause the cell to begin replicating. A cell that normally does not make a proto-oncogene product is now induced to produce this protein, resulting in cancerous change. The oncogene carried by a retrovirus may also undergo mutation or, when inserted into the host DNA, is now in a position to cause uncontrolled cell proliferation. Carcinogens such as ionizing radiation may cause mutations in proto-oncogenes resulting in a cancer cell.

Tumor Suppressor Genes

Proto-oncogenes promote normal cell proliferation, whereas tumor suppressor genes inhibit growth. The existence of **tumor suppressor genes** was suspected in experiments in which normal cells were fused with tumor cells and grown in tissue culture. The resulting hybrid cells lost their cancerous characteristics. However, hybrid cells are frequently genetically unstable and as normal chromosomes were lost on subsequent mitoses, the hybrid cells reverted back to cancerous cells. These experiments showed that normal cells were donating genetic information capable of suppressing tumor characteristics.

Inactivation or mutation of tumor suppressor genes has been observed in human cancers, and several of these types of genes have been isolated (Table 14–1). *p*53 is a tumor suppressor gene. Mutations in *p*53 are the most common genetic change associated with cancer. More than 51 types of human tumors with mutations in *p*53 have been identified and include cancer of the bladder, brain, breast, cervix, colon, esophagus, larynx, liver, lung, ovary, pancrease, prostate, skin, stomach, and thyroid. The importance of *p*53 in preventing cancer is illustrated in a line of genetically altered mice that produce no *p*53 protein. These "knock-out" mice (their *p*53 genes have been knocked out) look perfectly normal

TABLE 14–1. **Some Oncogenes and Tumor Suppressor Genes**

Oncogene	Gene Product/Function
sis	Growth factor, form of platelet-derived growth factor (PDGF)
erb A	Receptor for thyroid hormone
erb B	Receptor for epidermal growth factor (EGF)
fms	Receptor for colony-stimulating factor (CSF-1)
neu	Protein related to EGF receptor
abl	Signal transduction, tyrosine kinase
ras	Signal transduction, guanosine triphosphatase activity
src	Signal transduction, tyrosine kinase
fos	Component of gene transcription factor AP1
jun	Component of gene transcription factor AP1
myc	Transcription factor necessary for cell activation and proliferation
APC	Suppressor of adenomatous polyposis
DCC	Suppressor of colon carcinoma
NF1	Suppressor of neurofibromatosis
p53	Nuclear protein involved in regulation of cellular proliferation
bcl-2	Suppressor of apoptosis

when born, but after several weeks they begin to form tumors and by 6 months they all have tumors or have died.

How does *p53* suppress tumors? The *p53* gene carries the information for a nuclear protein involved in the regulation of cellular proliferation. A complex interaction of proteins called **cyclins** and their associated kinases have been identified in the cell cycle. *p53* binds to cyclin-dependent kinases and can halt the cell cycle before the cell is committed to division. This is an important function because it gives the cell time to repair DNA before dividing and thus prevents occurrence of mutated cells. *p53* may also be necessary for normal programmed cell destruction (apoptosis) and therefore help suppress growth of unwanted cells.

p53 may be useful for prognostic and therapeutic purposes. Mutated forms of *p53* can be correlated with more aggressive tumors, metastasis, and lower survival rates. Specific carcinogens have been found to cause mutations in the *p53* genes. Identification of *p53* as an important tumor suppressor gene opens up a new area of possible cancer therapy. If a normal copy of *p53* could be incorporated into tumor cells, it might stop further growth of these cells. Mutant forms of *p53* proteins could be used as vaccines to trigger an immune response in a person with a *p53*-associated tumor. Investigations of the *p53* tumor suppressor gene are an example of the progress made in understanding cancer at the molecular level, which will lead to improvements in treatment and detection of tumors.

Genes Associated With Apoptosis

Genes that regulate apoptosis have also been identified. If cells that are supposed to die do not undergo apoptosis, these cells will form an abnormal cell population. Oncogene *bcl-2* is an anti-apoptosis gene that was first identified in B-cell lymphomas. Expression of *bcl-2* prevents programmed cell death by apoptosis and allows unregulated growth of B-lymphoma cells. Under normal situations, *bcl-2* probably has important roles in regulating cell survival of selected B cells and T cells during maturation.

Cancer Cell Behavior

Many terms are used to differentiate normal cell behavior from that of cancer cells. In a normal adult, cell replication occurs to replace cells lost by wear and tear or injury. Replacement cells should be identical with the original cells. In response to increased work demands, some cells may increase in size. This is called **hypertrophy.** It is possible to "build up" muscles and cause hypertrophy by training with weights. Heart muscle may undergo hypertrophy in response to continued high blood pressure.

Hyperplasia is an increase in the number of cells in a tissue or organ. Anemia or loss of blood may cause hyperplasia in the bone marrow. Elderly men may develop hyperplasia of the prostate gland. Hyperplastic cells are normal cells, but they are replicating at an increased rate and cause enlargement of the prostate. Hyperplasia can be a premalignant cell change. The change from normal cells to neoplastic tissue is a sequence of tissue alterations referred to as **metaplasia, dysplasia, carcinoma in situ,** and finally **invasive carcinoma.** Metaplasia is recognized microscopically as a replacement of one type of differentiated tissue by another. An example of metaplasia is replacement of normal, ciliated epithelial cells lining the bronchus of a smoker by multilayered, flattened squamous epithelial cells. The cells are normal, but not at this location, and they do not function to move mucus and entrapped debris along the respiratory tract. Dysplasia is the presence of abnormal cells. Normal tissue boundaries are observed, but the cells and their nuclei are enlarged, more immature cells are present, and cell products may be disrupted. The metaplastic squamous epithelium previously referred to becomes dysplastic as more and more cell irregularities occur. Carcinoma in situ is literally cancer at the site. Dysplastic cells are now cancer cells. They may or may not have begun to grow outward, which occurs with invasive carcinoma.

Neoplastic or cancer cells display variable size and shape, referred to as **pleomorphism.** The nuclei of cancer cells may be larger and may stain darker and exhibit a variety of abnormal mitotic figures. Tissue organization and structure are lost because the cells no longer respond to contact inhibition. Continued growth of neoplastic cells may lead to invasion of surrounding normal tissue. Tumor cells produce **proteases,** which can digest collagen and other components of connective tissue and thus enhance their invasiveness. As the tumor grows outward and becomes larger, a greater blood supply is needed. Tumor cells produce **angiogenic factors,** which promote then ingrowth of new blood vessels. Growth of tumor cells drains nutrients from the rest of the body and contributes to the weight loss and wasting seen in cancer. Tumor necrosis factor-alpha (TNF-α) produced by macrophages aids in killing of tumor cells, but also is a factor in the wasting and cachexia seen in cancer and AIDS.

Metastasis

Not all tumor cells are invasive. **Benign** tumors generally exhibit a slower growth rate and are encapsulated by connective tissue. The capsule inhibits invasion or **metastasis** of the tumor cells. Metastasis refers to the ability of malignant tumor cells to "break away" from the primary site of origin, enter the bloodstream or lymphatic system, and cause tumor formation elsewhere in the body. Even though the primary tumor can be removed surgically, all the secondary sites where tumor cells have migrated and become hidden often cannot be eliminated. Cancer would be a less devastating disease if metastasis could be prevented.

Some tumors are more metastatic than others. Metastases occur more commonly with large tumor masses. Different types of tumor cells show preferential sites of metastasis, and the tumor cells in a primary tumor differ in their ability to break away and establish a secondary tumor. After tumor cells detach from a primary tumor, they must infiltrate into adjacent tissue and migrate through the wall of a local lymphatic or blood vessel. While circulating, the tumor cells must evade destruction by immune cells and emerge at a new site. For subsequent growth to occur, the tumor cells must then be capable of producing angiogenic factors. Each of these steps requires a different set of control mechanisms, which are not well understood. Some tumor cells are less adhesive and detach more readily from the primary tumor. Others produce greater quantities of proteases, which break down the extracellular matrix and basement membrane of the blood vessel and thus enhance invasiveness.

Metastatic tumor cells have mechanisms for immune evasiveness. Tumor cells can avoid immune detection and destruction while growing locally and while migrating in the circulation. Once in the circulation, these cells may aggregate with other metastasizing tumor cells and become trapped in a capillary. Another mechanism by which tumor cells become fixed at a site is by inducing the formation of fibrin. The tumor cells become enmeshed in a fibrin clot and are attached to the vessel wall. Tumor cells have surface receptors that may help them identify suitable sites for growth and aid in the preferential metastasis of certain tumors to specific organs.

TUMOR IMMUNITY

Does the immune system have a role in recognizing and eliminating cancer cells? The answer is a resounding yes. Understanding how the immune system is able to perform this function, understanding why it sometimes fails, and developing ways to manipulate it to improve its efficiency against cancer are the goals of the emerging discipline of tumor immunology.

Tumor Antigens

Cancer cells do form tumor antigens, and two types have been identified: **tumor-specific antigens (TSAs)** and **tumor-associated antigens (TAAs).** TSAs are unique antigens found on specific tumor cells and do not occur on other cells in the body. TAAs may be expressed on normal cells but at very low levels or may be fetal antigens that are expressed during early development and then reexpressed in a cancer cell in adulthood. For the immune system to rid the body of tumor cells, TSA or TAA must be recognized and a humoral or cell-mediated response generated. Although a few tumor antigens have been shown to induce the production of antibodies, most tumor antigens induce a cell-mediated response. A cell-mediated response can be shown by transplanting tumor cells into syngeneic mice. These mice have identical major histocompatibility complexes (MHCs) and other cell antigens except for the tumor antigen. The rejection of tumor cells by these mice demonstrates the presence of tumor-specific or **tumor-associated transplantation antigens (TATAs)** (Fig. 14–1).

The experiment can be modified to demonstrate an **anamnestic** or memory response to a TATA. If a chemically induced tumor is removed from a mouse and cells from the tumor are later injected into the same animal, intense immune activity and

CELL MEDIATED RESPONSE TO TUMOR
ASSOCIATED TRANSPLANTATION ANTIGENS (TATA)

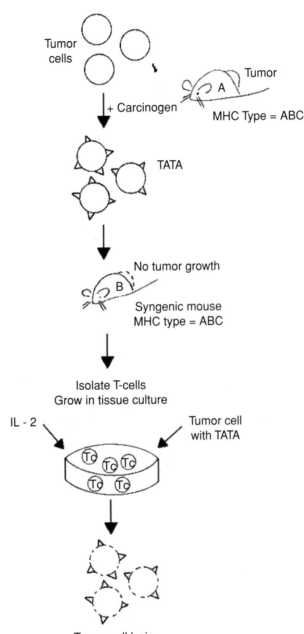

FIGURE 14–1. A tumor cell line, if injected into mouse A, causes formation of a tumor. Exposure of these tumor cells to a carcinogen can induce expression of a TATA. Subsequent injection of these cells into mouse B results in no tumor growth because the TATA is immunogenic. Note that mouse B is a syngeneic mouse to A and therefore has identical major histocompatibility complex (MHC) molecules. Mouse B rejects the tumor cells because of the presence of TATA. Development of a cell-mediated response is shown by isolation of cytotoxic T cells (CTLs) from mouse B, a growth of CTLs in tissue culture with the addition of interleukin-2, and lysis of tumor cells expressing TATA by the cultured CTLs.

no recurrence of the tumor is seen. A probable explanation is that the immune response to the initial tumor was too slow or deficient, but on reexposure to TATA, a memory response is generated that can destroy the tumor cells. Chemicals and other carcinogens cause unique TSAs to be produced on different cell types. One type of carcinogen does not cause the production of the same TSA in all affected cell types. This is unfortunate because many cancers are associated with a particular carcinogen (e.g., radiation, asbestos, and cigarette smoke). If a specific TSA was associated with one carcinogen, it might be possible to vaccinate a person exposed to a particular carcinogen and prevent development of cancer or development of metastases. For example, if cigarette smoke caused the production of a unique TSA, that TSA could be isolated, purified, and used as a vaccine (Fig. 14–2).

Unlike carcinogens, oncogenic viruses cause production of TSA unique to the virus being carried in the tumor cell. Polyomavirus (PV) causes malignant transformation and the production of a specific TSA in cancer cells. If syngeneic mice are injected with killed cells from a PV-induced tumor, the recipient mice are protected from subsequent injection of live cells from any PV-induced tumor. Therefore, it is possible to vaccinate against some virally induced tumor antigens. PV-TSA has been purified, the viral gene has been isolated, and a genetically engineered recombinant form of the TSA has been produced. Recombinant TSA or vaccinia virus genetically engineered to express the PV-TSA gene can be injected into a mouse. This mouse will subsequently reject implanted live PV-transformed tumor cells. (Vaccinia is a nonpathogenic virus related to the smallpox virus.)

DIFFERENCES IN TUMOR SPECIFIC ANTIGENS
INDUCED BY CARCINOGENS AND VIRUSES

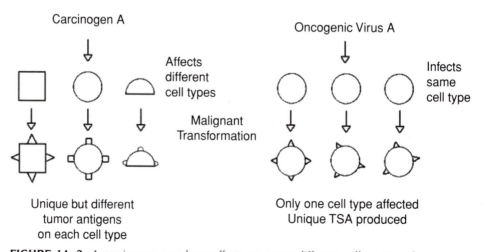

FIGURE 14–2. A carcinogen may have effects on many different cell types and may cause the formation of unique, but different, tumor antigens on each cell type. Furthermore, the same carcinogen may not cause formation of the same tumor antigen in each patient. On the other hand, viruses can only bind and infect a cell type expressing certain surface proteins. Therefore, usually only one cell type is infected, and the presence of virus in the host cell causes incorporation of unique viral antigens (TSAs) in the host cell membrane.

The PV phenomenon does not always occur with other viruses. For example, all oncogenic RNA viruses do not produce species-specific TSA. These viruses may cause production of antigens shared by other related viruses. Furthermore, viral tumor antigens may also be normal differentiation antigens; therefore, vaccine development for oncogenic viruses will be difficult.

Tumor-Associated Antigens

Most TAAs are not unique to tumor cells, but are also found on normal cells. These antigens may be expressed in very low concentrations on normal cells, but at much higher levels by tumor cells. Increased numbers of receptors for growth factors have been found on cancer cells and may be considered TAAs. Epidermal growth factor receptors (EGFr) are overproduced in a variety of tumor cells. Hepatocyte growth factor receptors (HGFr), members of the fibroblast growth factor family have been observed in human stomach carcinoma cell lines. The genes for many of these growth factors and growth factor receptors are proto-oncogenes. On mutation or cancerous transformation of the proto-oncogene to an oncogene, the oncogene product may be produced in too high a quantity resulting in abnormal cell function and proliferation. Because these proteins are normally present, there is no immune response to the tumor with TAA. Another theory is that there is an immune response that eliminates tumor cells that express strong tumor antigens; therefore, only the weakly immunogenic tumor cells survive.

It is possible to purify a growth factor receptor or its gene and prepare a vaccine. The TAA may be presented to the immune system combined with adjuvant or the gene inserted into a vaccinia virus, and a recombinant TAA is produced that is immunogenic. Because the TAA is present in such high numbers on the tumor cells, these cells should be preferentially destroyed by the immune system. Such experiments have been conducted in mice and may be possible in humans in the future.

Oncofetal Tumor Antigens

Fetal antigens are antigens produced by fetal cells during early stages of development. These proteins generally disappear as differentiation and cell maturation progress. Very small amounts of fetal antigens may continue to be produced by certain cells through adulthood. On malignant transformation, cancer cells may produce large quantities of fetal antigens, which are then called **oncofetal tumor antigens.** Presence of increased quantities of fetal antigens in the adult can be used to detect and monitor cancer growth.

Carcinoembryonic antigen (CEA) and **alphafetoprotein (AFP)** are oncofetal tumor antigens associated with certain types of cancer. Elevated levels of AFP in the serum are found in most patients with liver cancer and is also associated with cancer of the pancreas and testes. CEA is a membrane glycoprotein normally found on fetal gastrointestinal and liver cells. Increased levels of CEA can be detected in serum of adults with colon, lung, and bladder cancers. CEA and AFP can be found in healthy adults, so their presence is not absolutely diagnostic of cancer and other tests are necessary to confirm a diagnosis. After a tumor is identified and removed, CEA or AFP levels can be monitored and any increase in antigen level interpreted as further tumor growth.

Immune Responses to Tumor Cells

Malignant tumors removed surgically are often observed as being surrounded by lymphocytes and signs of inflammation. In experimental animals, tumor antigens can be shown to induce cell-mediated and sometimes even humoral immune responses. Some human tumors are very immunogenic and have tumor antigens that can be recognized by T cells or B cells. In animal studies, tumor antigens induced by ultraviolet rays or oncogenic viruses are generally more immunogenic than chemically induced tumor antigens. Other tumor antigens may be poorly immunogenic and escape immune detection.

Cytotoxic T Lymphocytes and Natural Killer Cells

Cytotoxic T lymphocytes (CTLs), which can recognize specific tumor antigens, have been identified in human and animal cancers, and their ability to recognize and specifically kill a tumor cell can be measured in an *in vitro* assay. Tumor cells are labeled with chromium-51 (^{51}Cr) and incubated with the CTLs. Release of ^{51}Cr into the medium is indicative of tumor cell lysis and specific killing by the CTLs. Cytotoxic T lymphocytes can also be maintained in tissue culture and their numbers expanded with the addition of IL-2. It is possible to reinfuse these specific CTLs and observe regression of tumors in animals and humans. It is also possible to manipulate the way in which CTLs recognize tumor cells. CTLs must be stimulated not only by antigen plus MHC but also by the costimulatory molecule B7 binding with CD28 and CTLA-4 on the CTL. It has been suggested that a cancer cell that lacks surface B7 will not deliver a sufficiently stimulatory signal to a CTL. However, by transfecting B7 into cancer cells they can be made highly susceptible to CTL killing. If these B7-modified cancer cells are injected into mice, they are rapidly destroyed; in addition, unmodified cancer cells become susceptible to CTL killing as well.

Natural killer (NK) cells are another population of lymphocytes capable of killing tumor cells. NK cells do not express membrane-bound immunoglobulin (Ig), T-cell receptors, or CD3. They do not require prior sensitization or immune memory for activation. These cells spontaneously recognize tumor cells and kill them. NK cells are large, granular lymphocytes that originate in the bone marrow and circulate in the peripheral blood. These cells are not processed through the thymus, and nude mice that lack a thymus do have NK cells. Cytotoxic lymphocytes and NK cells kill tumor cells by both **antibody-dependent** and **independent processes.** Antibody-dependent processes depend on Fc receptors on NK cells or CTLs binding to antibody-coated tumor cells. The antibody-independent process is mediated by the presence of **perforins.** The granules of NK cells contain perforin and granzymes (cytotoxins). On contact with tumor cells, the granules of NK cells mobilize toward the surface and released perforins form a tubular complex that is inserted into the cancer cell membrane. Lymphotoxin (TNF-β) and other destructive enzymes in the granules are injected through the pore in the cell membrane, resulting in tumor cell lysis.

The importance of NK cells can be seen in the beige mouse mutation. This mouse strain has normal B cells and T cells, but severely depressed NK-cell function and a high incidence of spontaneous tumor formation. Nude mice that have no T cells have normal NK cells and no increase in incidence of tumors. Humans who have Chédiak Higashi syndrome have depressed NK activity and an increased incidence of tumors of lymph nodes.

NK cells are also active against bacteria, fungi, and virally infected cells. They are responsive to interleukins and interferon-gamma (IFN-γ). Macrophages produce IL-12 and TNF-α, which by itself has potent antitumor activity and which also stimulates IFN-γ production by NK cells. IFN-γ enhances NK activity by promoting the rapid differentiation of pre–NK cells and further activates macrophages. Cytokines may be useful in treatment of some human cancers. IFN-α has been successfully used in the treatment of hairy cell leukemia and Kaposi's sarcoma.

Immune Evasive Mechanisms of Tumor Cells

Even though the immune system is capable of destroying tumor cells, life-threatening cancer still occurs. This suggests that the immune system is ineffective or that tumor cells have mechanisms for evading the cytolytic activities of immune cells. Some types of tumor cells make mucoproteins that mask tumor antigens. The mucoproteins themselves are normal secretory products and therefore do not induce an immune response, but do provide a protective coat preventing tumor antigen recognition.

Blocking Antibodies

Ironically, humoral antibodies to tumor antigens are not necessarily cytotoxic. They may be **blocking antibodies** that do not activate complement, but cover tumor antigens and prevent CTLs from binding and killing tumor cells. This phenomenon can be demonstrated by injecting serum from a tumor-bearing animal into another animal with the same tumor. Instead of inhibiting growth, the tumor of the second animal grows even faster. This activity is called **immune enhancement.** Similar effects can also be seen *in vitro.* Blocking antibodies can be added to cultures of tumor cells and CTLs. Cytotoxic activity is blocked. Serum from healthy persons or those with other types of tumors have no effect.

Antigenic Modulation

Even if complement-fixing, cytotoxic antibodies are produced, they may be ineffective because of a phenomenon called **antigenic modulation.** Tumor cells can shed tumor antigens. The released antigens can then bind to antibody and form immune complexes that prevent binding of antibody to cell surfaces and cell killing. Immune complexes can also inhibit antibody-dependent cell killing by binding to Fc receptors on NK cells or macrophages. Furthermore, tumor cells can alter their expression of tumor antigen. In the presence of antibody, certain tumors can stop making tumor antigens and begin making new antigen when antibody is no longer present.

Influence of MHC

Cytotoxic CD8+ T lymphocytes recognize antigen associated with MHC. Therefore, any alteration in expression of MHC class I may profoundly affect CTL anticancer activities. Malignant transformation of tumor cells is often associated with reduction or even complete loss of MHC class I. The type of MHC expressed may also influence antigen recognition. If mouse tumor cells with a high density of a MHC marker called H-2D and a small amount of a marker called H-2K are injected into healthy mice, these mice have a high incidence of metastases. Similar tumor cells, but those expressing equal amounts of H-2D and H-2K, produce fewer metastases.

INFLUENCE OF MHC ON METASTASIS

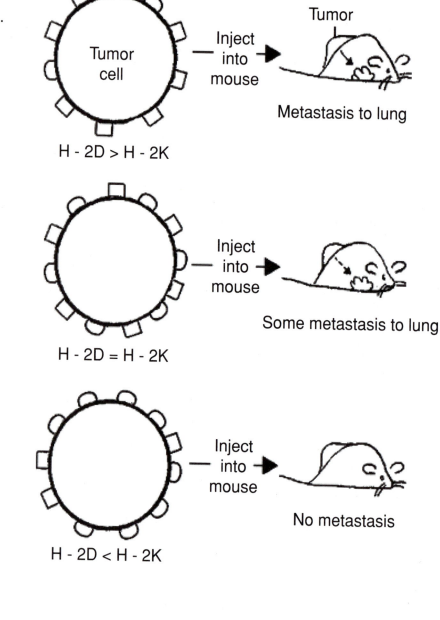

A.

Tumor cell

Inject into mouse

Tumor

Metastasis to lung

H - 2D > H - 2K

B.

Inject into mouse

Some metastasis to lung

H - 2D = H - 2K

C.

Inject into mouse

No metastasis

H - 2D < H - 2K

☐ = H - 2D

⬠ = H - 2K

Treatment of tumor cells with different interferons was found to modify the amount of H-2D and H-2K produced. Treatment with IFN-α and IFN-β caused increased production of H-2D and therefore more metastases, whereas IFN-γ increased the amount of H-2K and fewer metastases were seen. Tumor cells with increased H-2K on their surfaces were observed to be more immunogenic and therefore produced fewer and smaller metastases (Fig. 14–3).

CANCER IMMUNOTHERAPY

The immune system is capable of destroying cancer cells. If the various immune mechanisms could be enhanced or supplemented in a patient with cancer, a new and better treatment mode could be developed. Much progress has been made in cancer immunotherapy, but this area of medical science is still in its infancy. Methods that use the immune system in treatment of cancer can be broadly classified into two categories: those that nonspecifically stimulate the immune system and those techniques that are tumor-specific.

Nonspecific Immune Stimulants

The most widely used, nonspecific stimulant of the immune system is the **bacille Calmette Guérin (BCG).** BCG is an attenuated strain of *Mycobacterium bovis* used in some circumstances for vaccination against tuberculosis. Injection of BCG into tumor nodules of patients with melanoma has led to shrinkage of the injected tumors and occasionally of neighboring nodules. Unfortunately, this technique does not affect distant metastases. The effectiveness of BCG is related to tumor size, ability of the patient to form an immune response to BCG and tumor antigens, and close contact between BCG and the tumor cells. BCG activates macrophages, stimulates production of IFN-γ and IL-1 production, and promotes CTL activity.

Another bacterium, *Corynebacterium parvum*, has also been used as a nonspecific stimulant. However, both C. *parvum* and BCG can cause complications. Lesions at the site of injection may occur with hypersensitivity and toxic reactions. Purified cell-wall preparations can be used without the side effects of the whole bacteria. Levamisole is an antihelminthic drug that stimulates phagocytosis and lymphocyte activity. Azimezone and isoprinosine are mitogens that can activate lymphocytes in the absence of antigen and have also been used in nonspecific cancer treatment. Dinitrochlorobenzene is a chemical that causes localized hypersensitivity reactions and, when painted onto skin tumors, regression of tumors is seen. The localized hypersensitivity reaction also causes destruction of tumor cells.

FIGURE 14–3. Panel A shows that when tumor cells expressing greater amounts of H-2D than H-2K are injected into syngeneic mice, tumor formation with a high incidence of metastases occurs. If the expression of H-2D and H-2K on the same tumor cell line is altered so that equal amounts are present, tumor formation occurs but incidence of metastases decreases. Tumor cells with increased quantities of H-2K compared with H-2D when injected into syngeneic mice produced tumors, but no metastases. These tumor cells are evidently more immunogenic and are eliminated before they can establish lung metastases.

Cytokines and Cytokine-Activated Killer Cells

The use of cytokines is an exciting area of immunotherapy research. Cloning of the various cytokine genes has resulted in recombinant sources for production of large amounts of cytokines. Treatment with different interferons has been attempted with breast cancer, multiple myeloma, and malignant lymphomas. Complete or partial regression of hairy-cell-type lymphocytic leukemia has been achieved with IFN-γ. TNF-α and TNF-β are toxic for cancer cells *in vitro* and therefore may be useful for cancer treatment. However, *in vivo* application of cytokines is complicated by their multiple functions and effects on multiple cell types.

Of the various interleukins, only IL-2 has shown success as an anticancer agent. IL-2 can be added to NK cells or CTLs in tissue culture and promotes proliferation of these cells. If these lymphokine-activated cells are injected into a tumor, they cause tumor cell destruction and regression of the tumor. Thus, these cells are called **lymphokine-activated killer cells (LAK cells).** To enhance the specificity of these cells, the cancer patient's own lymphocytes can be obtained. Tumors often contain infiltrating lymphocytes that are presumably there to help promote antitumor activities. The tumor and associated lymphocytes are removed. The lymphocytes are isolated and placed into tissue culture. With the addition of IL-2, the lymphocytes proliferate and form an effective army of **tumor-infiltrating lymphocytes (TIL cells).** These cells are then injected back into the patient to fight any residual tumor cells. Positive responses have been shown in trials with patients with melanoma, colon, rectal, and kidney cancer. However, side effects of this therapy are often severe. A further modification of TIL cells can be performed to enhance antitumor activities. TIL cells can be genetically engineered to carry the gene for TNF-α. These cells will then have enhanced cytolytic capabilities against tumor cells.

Interleukins have also been directly administered to treat various cancers. Use of IL-2 has resulted in some success in patients with melanomas. A major difficulty with the use of interleukins and other cytokines is the complexity of interaction and the multiple activities of these immune messengers. When administered alone, IL-2 causes fever, chills, nausea, weight gain, rashes, endocrine abnormalities, and psychological changes. It can also cause anemia, decreased platelets, and damage to the lung. Localized administration and use of interleukins in combination with other immunotherapeutic agents or traditional chemotherapy may provide better treatments in the future.

Specific Immune Stimulants

Monoclonal Antibodies

Monoclonal antibodies (Mabs), which are specific for tumor antigens, can be produced. Administration of Mabs to a patient with cancer should then promote specific binding of antibody and lysis of the tumor cells via complement activation or antibody-dependent cytotoxicity. It is also possible to produce Mabs to growth factors or growth factor receptors. Because tumor cells produce increased quantities of growth factors or receptors, Mabs directed against these proteins would slow tumor cell proliferation without affecting normal cells.

Mabs can also be linked with a toxin to form an **immunotoxin.** The Mab is now a specific carrier that binds and kills only cancer cells, leaving normal cells unharmed. Treatment of experimental tumors in mice with immunotoxins has shown some success, and clinical trials in humans are in progress. Difficulties that need to be solved include uptake of the toxin and subsequent activity in the tumor cell. Of course, the tumor antigen must be unique to the tumor cell and readily available for binding by the Mab. A further difficulty encountered is that Mabs are usually made in mouse hybridomas. Thus, the Mab is of mouse origin and foreign to humans. The mouse Mab quickly triggers an immune reaction in the human and is eliminated. This problem can be partially solved with genetic engineering techniques. It is possible to produce a **chimeric immunoglobulin** that consists of mouse binding sites, but a human Fc portion. A chimeric antibody should thus be less immunogenic than a pure mouse Mab.

Other combinations of chimeric antibodies are possible. For example, one binding site of the Mab may be specific for the tumor antigen and the other for a CTL marker. This antibody would specifically bind to a cancer cell and bring cytotoxic lymphocytes into contact with the tumor cell. Another combination antibody consists of a binding site specific for the tumor antigen with the other binding site specific for a toxin, cytotoxic drug, or radioactive compound. When this **hybrid** or **bifunctional antibody** is administered to a patient with cancer, the antibody binds to the tumor cells, and when the cytotoxic agent is administered, it also becomes bound to the tumor cell by the second binding site of the Mab.

Mabs are also useful for cancer diagnosis and image localization. They are used in sensitive immunoassays (ELISA, immunoblot) for detection of tumor antigens shed into the blood. CEA, AFP, human chorionic gonadotropin, prostatic and many other tumor markers can be detected in the blood and aid in the diagnosis of cancer. Mabs tagged with fluorescent dyes can be used to identify leukemia or lymphoma cells, and the number of fluorescent tagged cells can be enumerated with a fluorescence-activated cell sorter. Mabs may be tagged with radioactive labels and administered to a patient. They bind to tumor antigens, and, wherever they become localized, they can be detected by their radioactive emissions. With the use of different types of scanning instruments or computed tomography (CT scans), tumors can be identified and localized very accurately.

Tumor Cell Vaccines

Various approaches for developing tumor vaccines are in progress. If mice are vaccinated with tumor cells that have been inactivated by treatment with drugs or radiation, growth of the same type of tumor is inhibited. To increase the effectiveness of the tumor cell vaccine, immunoadjuvants such as BCG are injected with the inactivated tumor cells. Tumor cells can be made more immunogenic by prior treatment with neuraminidase or glutaraldehyde. Neuraminidase strips off protective sugar molecules from the surface of the tumor cells, revealing tumor antigens. The mucoproteins themselves can be targets for vaccine production. If peptides from the mucoproteins or mucins coating tumor cells can be isolated and identified, a vaccine using these peptides could be produced.

Discovery of B7 as a necessary costimulatory molecule for T-cell activation has led to a novel immunotherapy for cancer. Tumor cells lacking B7 may escape immune recognition, even though they carry specific tumor antigen. A mouse melanoma cell line lacking B7 was genetically manipulated to produce B7 on its cell membrane. When the genetically engineered melanoma cells were implanted into normal mice, tumors initially formed, but rapidly regressed within 2 to 3 weeks. Furthermore, if mice already having the same melanoma were injected with the B7-engineered cells, these mice also showed regression of tumors. The B7-engineered cells served as a vaccine to enhance recognition of tumor antigens and induced a cytotoxic immune response against the tumor cells.

Many different approaches to cancer immunotherapy are possible. Use of immune-enhancing agents such as BCG or cytokines show promise and combined together or with traditional chemotherapy may provide alternative modes of cancer treatment. Production of LAK cells or TIL cells is a very labor-intensive procedure and requires individualized patient cell cultures. Use of Mabs requires detection and identification of TSAs, and they are useful only with the types of tumors that produce unique antigens. However, expanded use of Mabs in diagnosis of tumor will allow earlier and more sensitive detection of cancer. With early detection, cancer is a more treatable and curable disease. The potential for using a person's own immune system to fight cancer is a tantalizing proposition, and therefore tumor immunotherapy will continue to be a field of intense interest and research.

SUMMARY

1. Cancer cells are altered or mutated cells that are unregulated and, if malignant, are capable of tumor formation and metastasis. Cancers that originate in epithelial tissues are called carcinomas; those originating in connective tissues are referred to as sarcomas. Cancer cells may frequently occur in the body, but are eliminated by the immune system through immune surveillance.

2. Humans are exposed to many different carcinogens. Malignant transformation of cells due to carcinogen exposure involves multiple steps with initial changes in DNA followed by promoters that stimulate cell division and malignant transformation. Epidemiologic studies may establish an association between a carcinogen and cancer; however, proving that a particular agent is the cause is more problematic. Various causes of cancer include chemical and physical carcinogens, viruses, hormones, and genes.

   a. Both ribonucleic acid (RNA) and DNA-containing viruses can cause malignant transformation. If normal fibroblasts are infected with a tumor-causing virus in *in vitro* culture, the cells change shape, proliferate and lose contact inhibition, and will display disorganized cell growth.

   b. Hormones affect cell differentiation, and tumor cells may acquire the ability to secrete hormones and express new hormone receptors or increased quantities of receptors, thereby gaining altered function or growth responses.

   c. Cancer is the result of multiple genetic changes. Specific genes and chromosomal changes are associated with certain types of cancers. Familial inheritance patterns occur with certain types of cancers. Inbred mice strains with high incidences of cancer can be produced. Proto-oncogenes can become altered or overexpressed. Retroviruses may introduce these oncogenes into normal cells. Loss or mutation of tumor suppressor genes such as p53 is associated with cancer. Mutation of genes regulating apoptosis (*bcl*-2) have also been correlated with increased cancer occurrence.

3. Tumor formation is a sequence of events that can be observed as increasing aberrant cell behavior. Hypertrophy may be followed by hyperplasia, which then may be followed by metaplasia, dysplasia, carcinoma in situ, and finally invasive carcinoma. Malignant tumor cells are less adhesive. They secrete proteases that enhance invasiveness and angiogenic factors that promote ingrowth of new blood vessels.

4. Cancer cells form tumor antigens, which have been classified as tumor-specific antigens (TSAs) and tumor-associated antigens (TAAs). Chemicals and other carcinogens cause TSA formation in different cell types. Unfortunately, one type of carcinogen does not cause the production of the same TSA on all affected cell types. Viruses cause unique TSA production, and, because viruses only infect one cell type, it may be possible to vaccinate against virally induced tumor antigens. TAAs are not unique to tumor cells, but are also found on normal cells. They may be receptors for growth factors or fetal antigens reexpressed in greater quantity.

5. Immune responses to tumors do occur. Malignant tumors are often surrounded by lymphocytes and signs of inflammation. These lymphocytes may be cytotoxic T lymphocytes (CTLs) or natural killer (NK) cells. CTLs and NK cells kill tumor cells by antibody-dependent and antibody independent processes. Tumor cell lysis by T cells or NK cells can be quantitated with the chromium-51 release assay. Costimulatory molecule B7 enhances CTL killing. Cytokine secretion by lymphocytes and macrophages further aids in tumor cell killing.

6. Unfortunately tumor cells have immune-evasive mechanisms. Tumor cells can make mucoproteins that mask tumor antigens. Blocking antibodies that do not stimulate complement or antibody-dependent cell cytotoxicity can cover tumor antigens and prevent immune recognition. Tumor antigens may be shed, and then they neutralize cytotoxic antibody. Tumor cells can modulate their expression of tumor antigen and produce altered or decreased quantities of antigen and major histocompatibility complex (MHC).

7. It is possible to use the immune system in treatment of cancer. Nonspecific immune stimulants include local injection of bacille Calmette Guérin vaccine (BCG) or *Corynebacterium parvum* to enhance phagocytic and lymphocytic activity. Cytokines produced in large quantities by recombinant DNA techniques can be used as chemotherapeutic agents. Lymphokine-activated killer cells (LAK) or tumor-infiltrating lymphocytes (TIL) produced *in vitro* can be injected into tumor sites and will cause shrinking of tumors.

8. Specific immune stimulants include monoclonal antibodies (Mabs) to tumor antigens. Monoclonal antibodies may be modified with a linked toxin or bifunctional Fab sites to bind tumor antigen and CTLs. To prevent inactivation of mouse origin Mabs, chimeric Mabs with human Fc can be made. Mabs are used in immunoassays for cancer diagnosis and can also be used in image localization techniques.

9. Tumor cell vaccines are possible using neuraminidase to better reveal tumor antigens. Tumor cell mucoproteins can be targets for vaccine production. Tumor cells can be genetically manipulated to produce B7 and render them more immunogenic.

REVIEW QUESTIONS

1. Cancer of the bone is referred to as _____.
   a. osteosarcoma
   b. osteocarcinoma
   c. giant cell tumor
   d. myeloma
   e. adenocarcinoma

2. Which of the following is *not* a carcinogen?
   a. tar
   b. nicotine
   c. thymidine
   d. benzene
   e. ultraviolet light

3. The term meaning transmission and occurrence of disease in various populations is _____.
   a. pathology
   b. pathogenesis
   c. epidemiology
   d. oncology
   e. histology

4. The Ames test detects _____.
   a. possible carcinogen activity
   b. presence of retroviruses
   c. presence of oncofetal tumor antigens
   d. presence of natural killer (NK) cells
   e. tumor suppressor genes

5. Most retroviruses associated with human malignancies are type _____.
   a. A
   b. B
   c. C
   d. D
   e. E

6. The proto-oncogene _____ contains the information for a cell membrane receptor of epidermal growth factor.
   a. *erb*-B
   b. c-*sis*
   c. c-*abl*
   d. c-*src*
   e. p53

7. An increase in the number of cells in a tissue or organ is called _____.
   a. hypertrophy
   b. hyperplasia
   c. metaplasia
   d. dysplasia
   e. angiogenesis

8. Tumor cells that are metastatic show which of the following characteristics:
   a. less adhesive
   b. produce proteases
   c. produce angiogenic factors
   d. a and b
   e. a, b, and c

9. Most tumor antigens induce _____.
   a. humoral immune responses
   b. cell-mediated immune responses

10. CEA (carcinogenic embryonic antigen) is an example of a _____.
    a. oncofetal tumor antigen
    b. tumor-associated antigen
    c. tumor-specific antigen
    d. carcinogen
    e. proto-oncogene

11. A costimulatory molecule that enhances recognition of tumor cells is _____.
    a. p53
    b. B7
    c. CD28
    d. alphafetoprotein (AFP)
    e. epidermal growth factor receptor (EGFr)

12. Which of the following is *not* necessary for NK cells to kill tumor cells?
    a. perforins
    b. granzymes
    c. tumor necrosis factor (TNF)-β
    d. Fc receptor
    e. interferon-γ

13. Which of the following is *not* necessary to produce tumor-infiltrating lymphocyte (TIL) cells?
    a. tumor-associated patient lymphocytes
    b. *in vitro* culture conditions
    c. interleukin-2
    d. BCG
    e. c and d

ESSAY QUESTIONS

14. What are the differences between tumor specific and tumor associated antigens? Which are carcinogen or virally associated? What are the immune implications of these tumor antigens?

15. Describe the various mechanisms that tumor cells use to evade the immune system.

SUGGESTIONS FOR FURTHER READING

Aaronsen S: Growth factors and cancer. Science 1991;254:1146–1153

Brooks CG, Georgiou A, and Jordan RK, et al: The majority of immature fetal thymocytes can be induced to proliferate to IL-2 and differentiate into cells indistinguishable from mature natural killer cells. J Immunol 1993;151:6645–6656

Feldman M, Eisenbach L: What makes a tumor cell metastatic? Sci Am 1988;259:60–85

Harris CC: p53: At the crossroads of molecular carcinogenesis and risk assessment. Science 1993;262: 1980–1981

Moul JW, Sesterhenn IA, Connelly RR, et al: Prostate-specific antigen values at the time of prostate cancer diagnosis in African-American men. JAMA 1995;274:1277–1281

Townsend S, Allison J: Tumor rejection after direct co-stimulation of CD8 and T-cells by B7-transfected melanoma cells. Science 1993;259:386–370

Weinberg RA: Tumor suppressor genes. Science 1991;254:1138–1146

Zur Hausen H: Viruses in human cancers. Science 1991;254:1167–1173

REVIEW ANSWERS

1. a 6. a 11. b
2. c 7. b 12. d
3. c 8. e 13. d
4. a 9. b
5. c 10. a

PART
III
LABORATORY APPLICATIONS

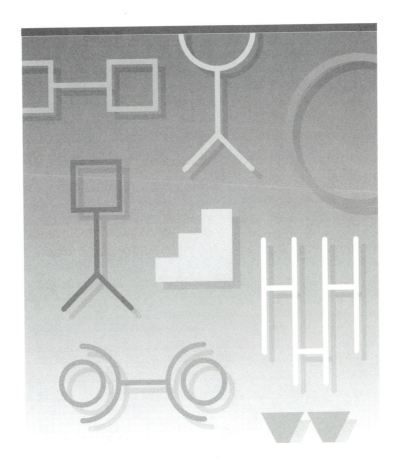

15 General Laboratory Principles

Using antibodies of suitable specificities, immune-mediated reactions can be exploited to measure innumerable materials. Ingenious applications of antigen-antibody interactions have long been used in analysis of chemical, physical, and clinical phenomena. With the availability of monoclonal antibodies, the amount of information obtainable through immunologic testing has expanded enormously. Measurement of immune complexes formed by antibody combining reversibly with antigen is a subdiscipline of immunology called **serology.**

END POINTS

The end point of a test must signal occurrence or magnitude of the event under investigation. The simplest form of observation is enumeration: counting, weighing, and measuring. Magnification, fixation, denaturation, or staining of the target material often facilitates observation and quantification, but these manipulations distort evaluation of dynamic events. It is important that an end point reflect the interaction under study in a specific and unambiguous fashion, free of positive or negative artifacts. In immunologic tests, the fundamental concerns must be specificity of antigen-antibody recognition and stability of the reactants and the resulting complexes. These chapters cannot describe procedures for developing, concentrating, purifying, and evaluating reagent antibodies; the laboratory worker must scrutinize the credentials of reagent antibodies before accepting results based on them. Biologic materials such as antibodies, enzymes, or proteins of any kind must be continuously monitored for expected potency, purity, and behavior.

The exquisite specificity of antibody and antigen interactions has led to the development of a variety of immunologic assays. These assays can be classified into three types of techniques. **Primary binding tests** directly measure the immune complexes formed in *in vitro* systems. **Secondary binding tests** detect and measure the consequences of immune complex formation. These include phenomenon such as precipitation, agglutination and complement activation or cell lysis, cytotoxicity, and toxin neutralization. **Tertiary binding tests** occur *in vivo* and include observation of inflammation or measurement of the protective effects of antibody. Tertiary tests are much more complex than primary or secondary binding tests and are affected by the health status and responses of the host.

Tests that use immune binding interactions often have end points common to other laboratory tests, such as measuring transmitted, reflected, or scattered light; measuring physical properties like color, size, viscosity, or pressure; observing and quantifying movement; and quantifying electrical charge or radioactivity. Some procedures use techniques that directly reflect properties of the immune reactants.

Antigen-Antibody Binding

The union between antigen-binding (Fab) sites of antibody and individual epitopes of antigen is the primary phenomenon on which all immune events depend. Primary immune tests are best conducted with a pure preparation of antibody and a preparation of soluble antigen that expresses only one active epitope. In a soluble system of this nature, union of antigen and antibody produces no readily detectable event, so the reactants must be manipulated to provide an indicator.

A classic procedure for demonstrating formation of soluble antigen-antibody complexes uses an agent, such as ammonium sulfate or polyethylene glycol, which precipitates the combined complex but leaves the uncombined reactants in solution. More recent techniques label individual reactants with radioisotopes, fluorescent dyes, or enzymes that allow distinction between bound and unbound material. These techniques are discussed in Chapter 18.

Association of Antigen and Antibody

The union of Fab site and epitope is a result of **noncovalent bonds.** These bonds are much weaker than the covalent bonds that join amino acids into polypeptides or sulfur-containing moieties into disulfide bonds. Distance between the reacting materials markedly affects noncovalent bonds. Infinitesimally small differences in proximity significantly alter the strength of association, which is why reciprocal configurations of antigen and antibody are so important. If the shapes fit together in a perfect lock-and-key relationship, all parts of both molecules have optimal proximity, so affinity is maximal. Shape changes induced by altered structure or by physical modification significantly diminish these bonds.

The attraction between the two molecules depends not only on configurational fit, but also on intrinsic properties of the antibody. The strength of the binding forces between Fab site of an antibody molecule and its corresponding epitope is denoted by the term **affinity.** Conventionally produced antiserum is called **polyclonal** because it contains immunoglobulin (Ig) molecules synthesized by a variety of individual cells. The Igs all may react with a specific antigen, but bind at different epitopes and exhibit different affinities. Binding of antibody to antigen at one site increases the probability of binding at a second site. The cumulative total of all attractive forces between antigen and the antibody molecules in a specimen is described as the **avidity** of the serum.

Forces of Attraction

Many physical forces influence affinity of Fab sites for antigen. Conspicuous among these are **van der Waals forces,** in which the presence of electrical fields in one molecule modifies electron distribution in another molecule, creating a reciprocal electrical field with attraction of opposite charges. **Electrostatic forces** depend on the attraction of opposites that occurs when molecules exist in ionized form at the pH of the medium, for example, NH_3^+ and COO^-. **Hydrogen bonding** depends on attraction between electropositive and electronegative atoms in the reactive site. **Hydrophobic bonds** arise from the properties of amino acids, which expel molecules of solvent water as they approach one another, generating an increment of energy that keeps the amino acids close to one another. The primary determinant of affinity is the molecular structure of the Fab site; the attractive forces previously described vary in strength with changes in pH, in tonic strength of the medium, in temperature, and in the nature of the solvent. Therefore, in *in vitro* testing the environment of the antigen and antibody reaction is often manipulated, or the incubation time can be lengthened so that optimal binding conditions occur. An example is the use of low-ionic-strength saline or overnight incubation at 4°C to enhance binding.

Consequences of Interaction

To detect the primary interaction, it is necessary to know the precise starting concentrations of antigen and antibody and to correlate the disappearance of free material with the consequent increase in combined product. Relative concentration of antigen and antibody do not affect the primary immune event. However, the concentrations of antigen, antibody, and combined complexes may affect the means of detecting the reaction.

Some measuring techniques lose accuracy or sensitivity at different concentrations. **Precipitation** is the end point most significantly affected by the starting concentration of antigen and antibody. Strictly speaking, precipitation is a secondary binding phenomenon, but many antigens can be studied only in macromolecular form and macromolecules often form precipitates after combination with antibody. Various conditions influence precipitation, and the conditions at which maximum precipitation occurs is referred to as the **zone of equivalence.**

Precipitation and Equivalence Zone

Phenomena

When soluble antibody reacts with soluble antigen, the resulting immune complexes vary in size. The simplest complex is union of two separate hapten molecules with the two Fab sites of an Ig monomer. If a single antigen expresses the same epitope at several sites, one epitope may combine with the Fab site of one Ig monomer, whereas another may bind with the Fab of a separate molecule. Two or more antibody molecules now form a complex that contains both antigen and antibody. Very small complexes tend to remain in solution, undetectable by visual inspection. If numerous antigens and Fab sites combine, this generates a lattice of alternating antigens and antibodies that becomes too large to remain in solution. A **precipitate** forms, which is the result of soluble antibody and antigen interacting in the formation of an insoluble immune complex. The size of the complex determines whether or not the precipitate becomes visible.

Excess of Antigen or Antibody

If antigen in preparations of varying concentration is added to multiple aliquots of antibody at a single concentration, precipitation characteristically occurs in the middle concentration range. Little visible precipitate accumulates at low concentrations of antigen or with highly concentrated antigen. The specificity of epitopes remains the same, and epitopes continue to combine with Fab sites, but the size of the resulting immune complexes reflect concentration of the reacting materials (Fig. 15–1). With dilute antigen there is **antibody excess,** and lattice formation is minimal because individual monomers compete for the few antigen epitopes available. When the number of multivalent antigen sites and bivalent antibody molecules is approximately equal, lattice formation is optimal and visible precipitation occurs. As antigen concentration increases to a state of **antigen excess,** lattice formation again declines because relatively few antigen macromolecules succeed in simultaneously binding several different antibody molecules. The relative concentration at which there is maximal lattice formation and minimal residual uncombined material is the **zone of equivalence** (Fig. 15–2).

Detecting Reactions

In experimental settings, absence of a visible end point occurs more frequently with antibody excess than with antigen excess. When concentrated or unmodified antibody is tested against an undiluted preparation of antigen, no reaction is seen. However, if the antibody is diluted before addition to the same antigen, precipitation promptly develops. Inhibition of visible end point by excess antibody is often called the **prozone phenomenon.** The reverse situation, failure to obtain a positive result until antigen is diluted occurs much less frequently. Some workers use an analogous term, **postzone phenomenon,** to describe inhibition by antigen excess.

ANTIGEN-ANTIBODY PROPORTIONS
AFFECT PRECIPITATION

A. Maximum precipitation at equivalence of antigen and antibody   B. In antibody excess, precipitates do not form   C. In antigen excess, precipitation is scanty, may be difficult to detect

FIGURE 15–1. Precipitation is greatest when antigen and antibody are present in approximately equal concentrations (A). At less than optimal proportions (B and C), antigen-antibody reactions occur, but produce much less visible precipitate.

PRECIPITIN CURVE

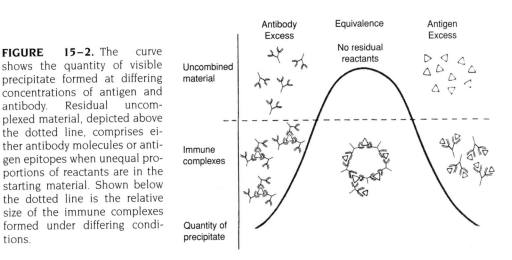

FIGURE 15–2. The curve shows the quantity of visible precipitate formed at differing concentrations of antigen and antibody. Residual uncomplexed material, depicted above the dotted line, comprises either antibody molecules or antigen epitopes when unequal proportions of reactants are in the starting material. Shown below the dotted line is the relative size of the immune complexes formed under differing conditions.

It is important to remember that absence of visible end point does not mean absence of immune reactivity. It is possible to demonstrate that free antibody and free antigen have united to form immune complexes by showing reduced levels of unbound molecules. This requires removal of the complexed materials, so that remaining free reactant can be measured. In prozone, uncomplexed antibody molecules are the residual reactant. With antigen excess, the suspending medium will contain unbound antigen but no antibody molecules.

Agglutination

Formation of an antigen-antibody complex characteristically alters the physical, chemical, or immunoreactive state of the starting materials. Precipitation of insoluble immune complexes is the simplest such end point. Analogous to precipitation is **agglutination,** in which a lattice forms between soluble antibody and an antigen present in particulate form (Fig. 15–3). When Fab sites of several antibody molecules combine with antigens present on several particles, the resulting lattice brings the particles together into readily detectable clumps called **agglutinates.** Although this end point is affected by variables of antibody activity, particle composition, reaction conditions, and properties of the suspending medium, the size of the agglutinates reflects, in a crude fashion, the magnitude of the antigen-antibody reaction. Proportions between antibody and antigen are much less critical for agglutination than for precipitation.

Applications of Agglutination

Agglutination is a more sensitive indicator system than precipitation, generating visible reactions at much lower antibody concentrations. It is often useful to convert a test system from precipitation to agglutination to exploit this increased sensitiv-

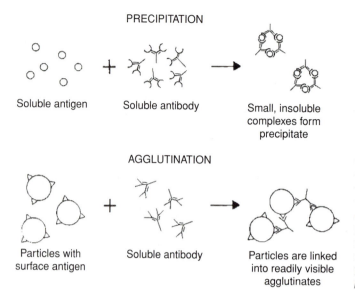

PRECIPITATION

Soluble antigen   Soluble antibody   Small, insoluble
complexes form
precipitate

AGGLUTINATION

Particles with
surface antigen   Soluble antibody   Particles are linked
into readily visible
agglutinates

FIGURE 15–3. As shown in the *lower panel*, agglutination involves particulate antigens, which are much larger than soluble molecules. When a lattice develops, the resulting complexes are larger and more easily detected than the macromolecules that constitute the precipitation end point (*upper panel*).

ity. A known preparation of either antibody or antigen can be attached to inert particles, which are then tested against the unknown in soluble form. A combination of soluble unknown and solid-phase reagent forms agglutinates that give a readily detected end point. Soluble antigen and soluble antibody can also be manipulated to inhibit previously demonstrated agglutination, a variant procedure called **agglutination inhibition.** Laboratory tests based on precipitation are discussed in detail in Chapter 16 and those based on agglutination in Chapter 17.

Complement as Indicator

Complement activation is a secondary phenomenon that is different from agglutination or precipitation. Complement-activating antibody must unite with its antigen before the first component of complement (C1) enters the recognition phase of the classical pathway. Complement activation, which can be documented in several different ways (see Chapter 19), then serves as the indicator that the antigen-antibody reaction has occurred.

Measuring Reactants

Demonstrating disappearance, inactivation, or consumption of starting materials are other methods to determine that antigen and antibody have combined. The antibody molecules do not disappear, but if their Fab sites have combined with antigen, no reactive markers remain to be measured. Antigenic material does disappear in a functional sense because binding with Fab sites prevents interaction with other molecules of the same antibody. However, molecules, cells, or particles may have numerous different epitopes so that antigenic material fully combined with antibody of one specificity may remain accessible to antibodies that recognize other configurations.

Bioassays

Measurements of physiologic events initiated by reaction of antigen with antibody are considered **tertiary tests**. Complement activation is a secondary event, but the phagocytic or inflammatory changes that follow in the living host are tertiary manifestations. Early immunologic tests used tertiary effects as end points because techniques to detect and demonstrate the initiating events were lacking. Examples of these observations include the skin changes used to demonstrate combination of cell-bound IgE with its antigen and opsonic enhancement of phagocytosis in the presence of antibody to a specific organism. **Biologic assays** in laboratory use include skin tests to demonstrate tuberculin-type cell-mediated immunity, several kinds of allergy tests, and administration of virulent organisms as a challenge to immunity induced in experimental animals.

MANIPULATING END POINTS

The remainder of this chapter describes, in general terms, some ways to enhance end points. If an immune reaction does not spontaneously generate a detectable secondary phenomenon, there is no immediate way to determine whether or not the reaction has occurred (Fig. 15–4).

Labeling Proteins

Proteins are complex molecules that can undergo independent interactions involving different parts of the molecule; material can often be added to or removed from a protein without affecting its remaining attributes. Antigens or antibodies can be labeled in ways that leave immune reactivity intact. Chemical stains are labels for denatured proteins; stains are useful in identifying location or intensity of an immune reaction after it has occurred but are unsuitable for ongoing reactions. How-

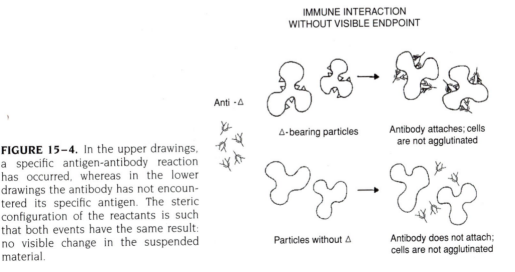

IMMUNE INTERACTION
WITHOUT VISIBLE ENDPOINT

Anti -Δ

Δ-bearing particles

Antibody attaches; cells are not agglutinated

Particles without Δ

Antibody does not attach; cells are not agglutinated

FIGURE 15–4. In the upper drawings, a specific antigen-antibody reaction has occurred, whereas in the lower drawings the antibody has not encountered its specific antigen. The steric configuration of the reactants is such that both events have the same result: no visible change in the suspended material.

DETECTING AN END POINT

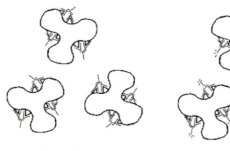

Antibody attachment
produces no
visible end point

Labeled antibody can
be detected by radio-
activity, fluorescence, etc.

FIGURE 15–5. Labeling the antibody molecules makes it possible to demonstrate that antigen-antibody attachment has occurred in circumstances that produce no detectable secondary phenomenon.

ever, attaching a radioactive, enzymatic, or fluorescent label marks the protein without interfering with reactivity (Fig. 15–5). The bond must be firm enough that label does not detach but gentle enough that the target protein is not altered. The labels most commonly used are radioisotopes, fluorescent compounds, and enzymes.

Major Forms of Labeling

Radioisotopes used as labels must emit levels of radioactivity susceptible to prompt and precise quantification but harmless to laboratory workers. Sometimes a radioisotope is substituted for an element in the natural molecule, such as iodine-125 (^{125}I) in thyroid studies or cobalt-51 (^{51}Co) in vitamin B_{12}; more often, an unrelated radionuclide is conjugated to the native compound. Most commonly used for proteins is ^{125}I, which binds to the amino acid tyrosine without affecting chemical or immunologic reactivity. Provided all molecules are uniformly labeled, measuring the amount of radioactivity directly quantifies the amount of labeled protein present.

Fluorescence labeling is comparable, but uses a different physical principle for the end point. Compounds called **fluorochromes** experience excitation after absorbing light at certain wavelengths. Excitation causes the substance to emit light at a different wavelength, detectable with appropriate optical equipment. Fluorochromes can be bound to soluble proteins or to proteins on cells or other biologic surfaces.

Another approach is labeling proteins with **enzyme** molecules, for measurement in multistage assays. The indicator enzyme must retain activity when conjugated to the immunologically reactive proteins. Once the enzyme-labeled material has completed its immune activities, substrate for the enzyme is added to the system; the still-active enzyme acts on substrate to generate a measurable product. The concentration of product is directly proportional to the amount of enzyme, which is proportional to the amount of labeled immune reactant present (Fig. 15–6). Enzyme labeling avoids the problems of radioactive waste disposal or of maintaining expensive equipment to measure radioactivity or fluorescence.

Overcoming Solubility

Measurement may be easier if proteins undergo alteration of physical state. Small individual molecules may be invisible in suspension but are readily observed if aggregated into a multimolecular mass. Another approach is to convert soluble mole-

ENZYME AS INDICATOR

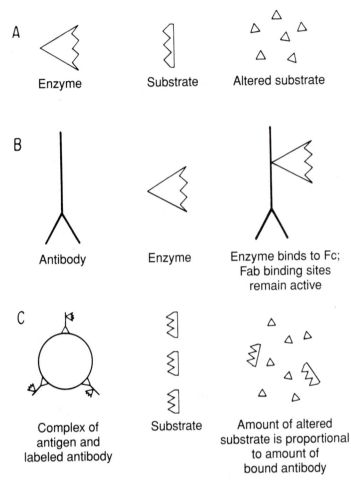

FIGURE 15–6. *Panel A shows* the effect of active enzyme on its substrate. Enzyme can be linked to an antibody molecules without altering the activity of either protein (*panel B*). When substrate is added to a system containing enzyme-labeled antibody (*panel C*), alteration of the substrate occurs at a level proportional to the number of enzyme-labeled antibody molecules present.

cules into solid phase by adsorbing them to an inert carrier surface. Tanned red blood cells (RBCs), latex particles or tiny beads, the walls of tubes, plates, or wells are useful for this purpose.

Antibodies to Antibodies

Antibodies against antibodies open an entirely new way to study immune events. Antibodies are proteins, and proteins are excellent antigens. Proteins from one species stimulate antibody formation when injected into members of another species. Early researchers injected whole human serum into rabbits, goats, and other animals, producing serum with a wide but unpredictable range of antihuman protein activity. Antihuman serum is often called **Coombs' serum,** in recognition of work done in the 1940s by Coombs and his coworkers in England. Subsequent refinements in processing antigen and in purifying and concentrating antibodies have allowed preparation of highly specific antibodies targeted against individual proteins and fractions of proteins. Especially important in analytic procedures are antisera against individual classes and subclasses of Igs, against light chains, heavy chains and portions thereof, and against the effector and regulator proteins of the complement system. Anti-idiotype antibodies are the ultimate refinement. They react with the antigen-specific recognition site of individual antibodies.

Antiantibody antibodies, called **antiglobulins,** have numerous uses. The earliest antiglobulin procedures were used in RBC serology to induce visible agglutination after attachment of nonagglutinating antibody to surface antigens of RBCs (Fig. 15–7). Antiglobulin antibodies can be used to identify immune precipitates dispersed in fluid, gel, or solid media. Fluorescence-labeled antiglobulins localize attachment of antibodies to various tissue sites in microscopic sections and to the surface of individual cells. Radiolabeled or enzyme-labeled antiglobulin antibodies are used in receptor-ligand assays for a wide variety of substances.

Separation Techniques

Nature rarely provides materials in purified, concentrated form. Biologic specimens contain numerous components; specific assays attempt to measure individual constituents. It may be necessary to separate antigens from a diverse mixture, to isolate antibodies from a multispecific serum, or to separate materials so that individual elements can be quantified. Many techniques for separating molecules are based on physical properties, including such procedures as ultracentrifugation, molecular sieving, and dialysis. **Electrophoresis** separates proteins according to their migration through an electrical field. The size, shape, and net charge of a protein determine the rate and direction at which it travels through a charged medium (see Fig. 6–4). Movement can be modified by altering the suspending medium or the duration, direction, and intensity of the current.

Antigen-antibody reactions can perform highly targeted separation procedures. Diverse mixtures can be separated by introducing an antigen or antibody that complexes with a single material. The resulting complex usually has different properties from the remaining materials and can be separated by physical manipulation, such as precipitation, filtration, or differential mobility. Antibody can be used to capture an antigen, or antigen can be introduced to isolate a specific Ig. Centrifugation and filtration are simple methods used to separate immune complexes that have precipitated or agglutinated (Fig. 15–8). Adsorption is the separation procedure used in **affinity chromatography.** The reagent is immobilized on a solid-phase preparation, and the mixed solution is passed across the system. If concentrations and flow rate are appropriate, the immobilized agent captures its target material. The depleted ef-

AGGLUTINATION OF ANTIBODY - COATED CELLS

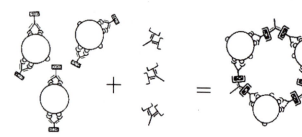

Antiglobulin serum reacts
with Fc of antibody

FIGURE 15–7. Combination of antibody with cell-surface antigens may leave the cells coated with antibody, but freely suspended in the medium. Antibody against the Fc portion of the coating antibody links the bound immunoglobulin molecules and brings the underlying cells together into visible agglutinates.

AGGLUTINATION USED TO
SEPARATE MIXED ANTIBODIES

FIGURE 15–8. Particles that express a single antigen can be used to separate a mixture of antibodies of different specificities. The relevant antibody will link the particles into agglutinates, which can be removed from the medium by centrifugation; uncombined antibody remains in the supernatant fluid. The bound antibody can be harvested from the agglutinated material by subsequent manipulation.

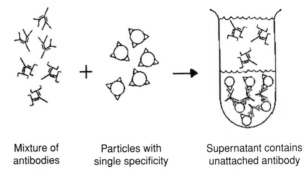

Mixture of
antibodies

Particles with
single specificity

Supernatant contains
unattached antibody

fluent or the captured material can be subjected to further manipulation for isolation, concentration, or quantification (Fig. 15–9).

Inhibiting an Indicator Reaction

Formation of soluble antigen-antibody complexes can be demonstrated through removal of material needed for an indicator reaction that has previously been standardized. Assays of this sort, called **neutralization** or **inhibition,** are useful end points in microbiology and in studying soluble antigens and antibodies. For example, under appropriate culture conditions, a virus may consistently infect and kill cells. To demonstrate whether serum contains antiviral antibody, one aliquot of virus is incubated with the test serum and another with a control serum known to be negative for viral antibody. Test and control materials are then inoculated into preparations of sensitive cells. If the virus incubated with the negative serum continues to kill the cells but incubation with test serum renders the virus harmless, the presence of antivirus antibody can be inferred (Fig. 15–10).

ADSORPTION USED TO
SEPARATE MIXED ANTIGENS

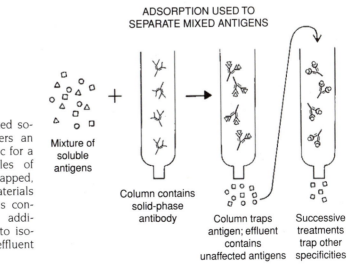

FIGURE 15–9. When a mixed solution of antigens encounters an immobilized antibody specific for a single constituent, molecules of that antigen remain trapped, whereas the unaffected materials remain in solution. Columns containing antibodies against additional solutes can be used to isolate other material from the effluent fluid.

Mixture of
soluble
antigens

Column contains
solid-phase
antibody

Column traps
antigen; effluent
contains
unaffected antigens

Successive
treatments
trap other
specificities

VIRUS NEUTRALIZATION DEMONSTRATES
PRESENCE OF ANTIBODY

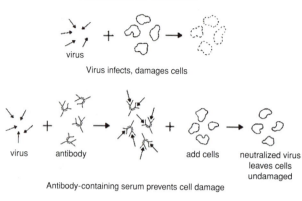

virus

Virus infects, damages cells

virus   antibody   add cells   neutralized virus
                                                    leaves cells
                                                    undamaged

Antibody-containing serum prevents cell damage

FIGURE 15–10. The upper panel shows the damage that a virus inflicts on target cells. In the lower panel, incubation with antibody-containing serum neutralizes the virus and prevents it from damaging indicator cells added to the incubated mixture.

Inhibitory assays are useful when the test material is in soluble form or when an antibody reacts preferentially with nonparticulate forms of the antigen. Many antibodies react more rapidly with soluble antigen than with the same material on a cell surface—a property that can be exploited to demonstrate presence of the soluble material in a test solution. The indicator system uses agglutination, at predetermined intensity, of antigen-coated particles. If incubation with the test material abolishes the agglutinating activity of the antibody, presence of soluble antigen has been demonstrated.

SUMMARY

1. The exquisite specificity of antibody and antigen interactions has led to the development of a variety of immunologic assays. Measurement of immune complexes formed by antigen-antibody binding is a subdiscipline of immunology called serology.

2. Noncovalent bonds are formed between Fab sites and epitopes. Strength of these binding forces (affinity) is dependent on reciprocal configuration, that is, how closely the shapes of antigen and antibody fit. Polyclonal antiserum contains immunoglobulins (Igs) synthesized by a variety of individual cells. These Igs all may react with a specific antigen, but bind at a different epitope.

3. Other physical forces that affect affinity of Fab sites for antigen include van der Waal forces, electrostatic forces, and hydrogen and hydrophobic bonds. These forces can be influenced by changes in pH, tonicity, temperature, and nature of the solvent. Therefore, *in vitro* assay conditions can be manipulated to enhance binding conditions.

4. Very small antigen-antibody complexes tend to remain in solution; however, if numerous antigens and Fab sites combine, a lattice is formed and can often be seen as a precipitate. If the amount of antibody is greater than antigen (prozone) or if antigen concentration exceeds the amount of antibody (postzone), lattice formation declines and precipitates may not be visible. Precipitation is greatest when antigen and antibody are present in approximately equal concentrations (zone of equivalence).

5. Agglutination occurs when a lattice forms between soluble antibody and antigen in particulate form. Agglutination is a more sensitive indicator system than precipitation generating visible reactions at much lower antibody concentration. Soluble antigen or antibody detectable by precipitation can be converted to agglutination reactions by attaching antigen or antibody to inert particles.

6. Bioassays detect antigen-antibody reactions in a living host. Inflammation or delayed hypersensitivity responses to allergens or tuberculin are examples of bioassays.

7. Other types of end points can be used to detect antigen-antibody binding besides precipitation or agglutination. Antigen or antibody can be labeled in ways that leave immune reactivity intact. Radioactive, fluorescent, or enzymatic labels can be attached to antigen or antibody. Immune-complex formation is then detected by the presence of one of the latter labels.

8. Formation of an antibody against another antibody is a technique to detect immune-complex formation. Coombs' serum or antihuman globulin can be used to induce visible agglutination of red blood cells (RBCs) coated with nonagglutinating antibody. Fluorescence-labeled antihuman serum can localize immune complexes deposited in tissue sections.

9. Antigens or antibodies can be used to separate mixtures of materials. An antigen reacted with a mixture of antibodies binds to only the relevant antibody. If the antigen is large enough, the antigen-antibody complex may be separated from the rest of the antibodies by centrifugation. Antigens or antibodies adsorbed onto a solid phase can be used to separate mixtures in a procedure called affinity chromatography.

REVIEW QUESTIONS

1. Polyclonal antibody demonstrates _____ avidity for antigen than monoclonal antibody.
   a. greater
   b. lesser

2. Serology is the detection and measurement of _____.
   a. antibodies
   b. antigens
   c. precipitins
   d. immune complexes
   e. adsorbents

3. Tertiary binding tests _____.
   a. can detect delayed-hypersensitivity reactions
   b. are affected by the health status of the host
   c. occur *in vitro*
   d. a and b
   e. a, b, and c

4. _____ can be used to separate immunoglobulins from other serum proteins.
   a. Electrophoresis
   b. Ammonium sulfate
   c. Restriction enzymes
   d. a and b
   e. a, b, and c

5. The strength of the binding forces between a Fab site and its corresponding epitope is called _____.
   a. affinity
   b. avidity
   c. proximity
   d. hydrophobicity
   e. electrostatic association

6. Lattice formation between _____ and _____ results in precipitation.
   a. soluble antigen . . . soluble antibody
   b. insoluble antigen . . . soluble antibody
   c. soluble antigen . . . insoluble antibody
   d. insoluble antigen . . . insoluble antibody

7. Maximum precipitation occurs _____.
   a. when antibody concentration is greater than antigen concentration
   b. when antigen concentration is greater than antibody concentration
   c. when antigen and antibody concentration are approximately equal
   d. at the zone of equivalence
   e. c and d

8. End points that are used to detect antibody binding to antigen include
   a. presence of fluorescence
   b. presence of radioactivity
   c. enzymatic reactivity
   d. complement-induced cell lysis
   e. all of the above

9. Coombs' serum is _____.
   a. antihuman serum
   b. antihuman IgM
   c. antihuman IgG
   d. made in a rabbit
   e. all of the above

10. Which of the statements below is *incorrect* concerning antigen-antibody binding?
    a. Hydrophilic interaction maximizes hydrogen bonding of water molecules.
    b. Ionic bonds between oppositely charged residues are important.
    c. Antigen to antibody binding is reversible.
    d. A large number of bonds are needed to form a strong interaction.
    e. In an aqueous environment, noncovalent interactions are extremely weak and depend on close structural complementarity between antibody and antigen.

ESSAY QUESTION

11. A substance called protein A can be isolated from *Staphylococcus aureus*. Protein A has the unique capability of binding to IgG. For what type of laboratory application(s) could protein A be used?

SUGGESTIONS FOR FURTHER READING

Arevalo JH, Taussig MJ, Wilson IA: Molecular basis of cross-reactivity and the limits of antibody-antigen complementarity. Nature 1993;365:859–863.

Gosling JP: A decade of development in immunoassay methodology. Clin Chem 1990;36(8):1408–1427

Gosling JP: Introduction to immunoassay. In: Gosling JP, Basso LV, eds: Immunoassay: Laboratory Analysis and Clinical Applications. Boston: Butterworth-Heineman, 1994:1–30

REVIEW ANSWERS

1.	a	6.	a
2.	d	7.	e
3.	d	8.	e
4.	d	9.	e
5.	a	10.	b

16 Laboratory Procedures Based on Precipitation

The union of soluble antibody with its specific antigen forms an immune complex that may or may not be apparent as a visible end point. An end point that may be observed and measured is precipitation of insoluble immune complexes. Many factors affect precipitation of the immune complex. The relative concentration of antigen and antibody is the most significant, but the solvent medium is also important.

PHYSICAL ASPECTS OF PRECIPITATION

As the Fab sites of one or more antibody molecules join several molecules of antigen, a lattice is formed that incorporates both participants. Whether the lattice becomes a visible precipitate is dependent on the initial state of antigen and antibody, the medium in which they are suspended, and the size of the immune complex that evolves.

Equivalence

When antibody molecules greatly outnumber antigen molecules, many antibody molecules remain uncombined, and each antigen unit binds to so many antibody molecules that little crosslinking occurs. Complexes containing far more antibody than antigen are usually too small to precipitate. As antigen and antibody approach equivalent concentrations, the number and size of immune complexes increase to levels that form visible precipitates. If antigen concentration continues to increase, the reverse phenomenon occurs; individual antibody molecules become so saturated with antigen that small or incomplete lattices form. The curve relating concentration and precipitation is parabolic, with maximum precipitation occurring at the point of equivalence (see Fig. 15–2). Analytic techniques exploit this quantitative relationship by controlling concentration of the known reagent material and measuring precipitation as a reflection of the unknown reactant.

Soluble antigen and soluble antibody that diffuse toward one another through an inert medium create their own zone of equivalence. As solutions of the materials diffuse from highly concentrated starting locations, precipitate forms where optimum concentration is achieved. Early immunologists layered solutions directly on each other, generating a ring of precipitate called a **precipitin line** at or near the interface (Fig. 16–1). A precipitin ring at a fluid interface is easily disrupted and is difficult to observe and to quantify. Current precipitation methods incorporate the materials in a supporting medium such as agarose gel or cellulose acetate, or they measure the precipitated material as it is dispersed in the medium.

Modifying Conditions

The nature of the supporting medium and the physical properties of the reactants affect diffusion. From a well cut into a gel, a solution diffuses outward in a 360-degree arc (Fig. 16–2). In the same gel, smaller molecules diffuse more rapidly than larger ones. The viscosity, molecular size, hydration, and chemical composition of the gel affect the rate of diffusion. When solutions of antigen and antibody are simultaneously placed in suitably located wells, the outwardly moving molecules encounter each other, and immune complexes precipitate at the equivalence zone

PRECIPITIN RING WITH
ONE-DIMENSIONAL DIFFUSION

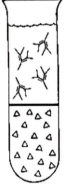 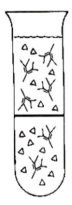 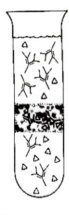

FIGURE 16–1. From left to right, antigen and antibody molecules in the layered solutions are shown diffusing toward one another. Where proportions are optimal, a ring of visible precipitate forms, usually at or near the interface between the solutions.

Solutions of antibody and antigen are layered

Molecules diffuse across interface

Precipitin ring forms where equivalence occurs

MOLECULES DIFFUSE
THROUGH A GEL

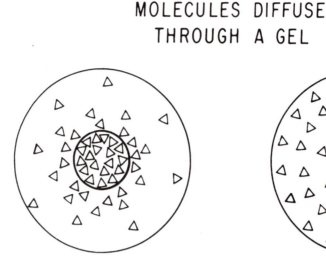

Molecules begin to diffuse
from well into gel

Eventually, molecules are evenly dispersed throughout gel

FIGURE 16–2. (*Left*) The diagram shows molecules in a highly concentrated solution beginning to diffuse from a central well into the surrounding gel. (*Right*) With the passage of time, all parts of the gel contain equal numbers of solute molecules.

(Fig. 16–3). The size and intensity of the precipitin line reflect the quantity of precipitated immune complex. If the materials diffuse from wells of equal size, the precipitin line will be arc-shaped, concave to the well from which diffusion was slower. Higher molecular weight or lower concentration may slow diffusion rate (Fig. 16–4). Diffusion can be accelerated or slowed by modifying the supporting medium or by altering such physical conditions as electrical charge or temperature.

Antigen   Antibody

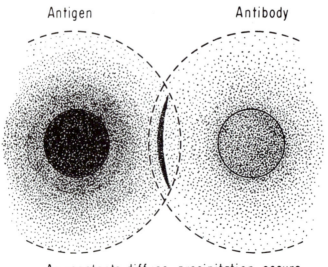

As reactants diffuse, precipitation occurs
where equivalence is reached

FIGURE 16–3. When solutions of antigen and antibody are placed in adjacent wells, molecules diffuse into the surrounding gel in all directions. Where the molecules encounter one another in optimal proportions, precipitation occurs, and a precipitin line is seen between the two wells.

MOLECULAR SIZE AND CONCENTRATION
AFFECT DIFFUSION RATE

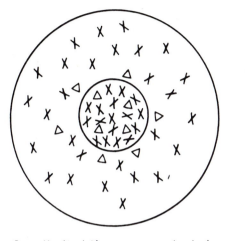

In a limited time, concentrated material moves farther than less concentrated material

In a limited time, smaller molecules move more rapidly than larger ones

FIGURE 16–4. If the central well contains a mixture of materials (*left*), the more concentrated material travels through the gel more rapidly. In a mixture of small and large molecules (*right*), the smaller molecules reach the periphery more rapidly than the larger ones.

Significant Variables

Different materials diffuse at different rates. Proteins vary in size, charge, substituted side groups, and three-dimensional configurations, all of which affect their physical and immunochemical properties. All antibodies are immunoglobulins (Igs). Despite differences in size and valence, they share many physical characteristics. On the other hand, antigenic materials embody a wide range of size, chemical composition, and reactive characteristics. Further variation may occur if reagents undergo changes in state. With some techniques, reagent properties are deliberately manipulated, but sometimes physical alterations occur unexpectedly and produce results that do not reflect true analytic conditions. The nature and location of a precipitin end point must be evaluated in light of these considerations.

Immunodiffusion Techniques

Diffusion is a dynamic process. Equilibrium is reached when solute molecules are uniformly dispersed throughout the medium. After antigen and antibody meet at the zone of equivalence, molecules continue to diffuse and to change the concentrations of both reactants. This can cause the quantity of precipitate to diminish or to disappear. Therefore, tests based on precipitation in gels must be read within a realistic time frame.

Analytic techniques that exploit diffusion can be classified as single or double.

In **single diffusion,** the supporting medium contains one reactant at a uniform concentration, so only the added unknown manifests changing concentrations. Usually, antibody is uniformly distributed, so diffusion of antigen molecules determines the location and intensity of the precipitate. An example of simple diffusion is called **radial immunodiffusion,** in which antibody is uniformly distributed in the gel and antigen is added to wells cut into the gel. In **double diffusion,** the gel is inert, and both antigen and antibody molecules travel through the medium.

DOUBLE DIFFUSION

The earliest immunodiffusion procedure to be widely used was developed by Ouchterlony and continues to bear his name. Although it has been largely replaced by more rapid and quantitative techniques, it remains an important investigative tool.

Ouchterlony Double Diffusion

In the simplest double-diffusion system, antigen and antibody solutions are placed into wells that have been cut into an immunologically inert gel. As antigen and antibody diffuse radially, a precipitin line forms where the migrating molecules meet. Appearance of a precipitin line indicates that antigen and antibody of complementary specificity are present. The density of the precipitin line reflects the amount of immune complex formed.

Most Ouchterlony plates have a central well surrounded by wells equidistant from the central well and from each other; material diffusing from the central well encounters the molecules diffusing from each of the peripheral wells. If the central well contains antibody and all circumferential wells contain the same antigen, lines of identical shape form between the central well and all surrounding wells. If the peripheral wells contain the same antigen at differing concentrations, the density of the precipitin arcs reflects the starting quantities of antigen (Fig. 16–5). If the peripheral wells contain different antigens, lines form only where antibody and antigen have the same specificity. If the central well contains several antibodies, each recognizing a different antigen, the appearance and location of the precipitin lines will reflect the specificity of antigens present in the surrounding wells (Fig. 16–6).

Ouchterlony double diffusion is a qualitative technique best suited to demonstrating specificity of antigen or antibody. Materials that give a "reaction of identity" have the same immunologic specificity, whereas a preparation that generates additional arcs with varied shape and location demonstrates the presence of antigen-antibody complexes with different properties. Absence of precipitation indicates that the unknown lacks any material reactive with the reagent in use.

Counterimmunoelectrophoresis

Spontaneous diffusion through a gel characteristically takes hours. Applying an electric current increases the rate of diffusion and induces movement that is linear rather than radial. In a suspending medium of constant properties, the speed and direction of migration vary with the composition of the protein. The net charge of

DOUBLE DIFFUSION DEMONSTRATES CONCENTRATION

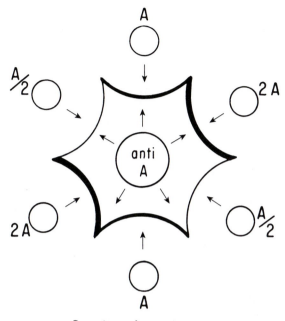

FIGURE 16-5. With a constant antibody level, the quantity of precipitate is proportional to the concentration of antigen. The peripheral wells shown at right contain a single antigen at different concentrations. The precipitin arcs for the lowest concentration, A/2, are half as dense as those for A, which in turn are half as dense as those for the doubled concentration shown as 2A. Arrows indicate direction of diffusion.

Density of arc is proportional to concentration

SHAPE AND LOCATION OF ARCS INDICATE SPECIFICITY

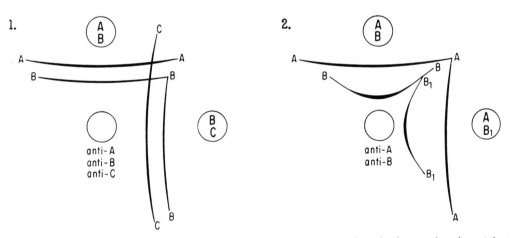

FIGURE 16-6. In both panels, the center well contains a mixture of antibodies, and each peripheral well contains two antigens. In *panel 1*, the crossed arcs for A/anti-A and C/anti-C indicate that the two antigens are unrelated. The perfectly matched B/anti-B arcs constitute a "reaction of identity" for the B antigen in each of the two wells. In *panel 2*, the A/anti-A arcs give a reaction of identity. The spur extending beyond the junction of the two B/anti-B arcs indicates "partial identity" of the B antigens present in the two wells.

many antigen preparations and antibody solutions causes them to migrate in opposite directions. **Counterimmunoelectrophoresis (CIEP),** also called **countercurrent immunoelectrophoresis** and **electroprecipitation,** exploits this phenomenon.

In CIEP, the reagent material and the unknown are placed in side-by-side wells. Most procedures use a known antibody to determine whether or not antigen is present in the material under investigation. The supporting gel and buffered pH are selected so that the antibody, which has a small net negative charge, moves toward the cathode while the antigen migrates toward the anode (Fig. 16–7). If antigen is present in the test material, a precipitin line forms between the two wells at a location determined by the concentration of antigen. Absence of a line indicates absence of the antigen. Counterimmunoelectrophoresis is often used to demonstrate presence of microbial antigens in the body fluids of a patient in whom infection is suspected. Cultures require one or more days before microbial growth can be detected, whereas documenting microbial antigens takes only 1 hour or so and is not affected by antibiotics or by viability of the organisms. Success of the procedure depends on knowing which organisms are likely to be present and having available identifying antibodies of high specificity and affinity.

Immunoelectrophoresis

Immunoelectrophoresis (IEP) is a two-stage procedure in which proteins are first separated by electrophoresis and then allowed to diffuse toward a preparation of precipitating antibody. First, a mixture of proteins such as serum is placed into a small well cut into a gel, and an electrical current is applied. Each protein migrates at its own rate and direction, generating individual protein bands distributed along the gel strip (Fig. 16–8, step 1). Antibody is then placed in a trough parallel with the line of separated proteins. Diffusion occurs from the trough and from the concentrated collections of individual protein molecules (Fig. 16–8, steps 2 and 3). The

COUNTERIMMUNOELECTROPHORESIS

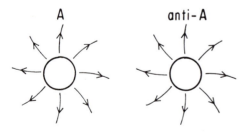

A   anti-A

Unmodified reactants diffuse
slowly and radially

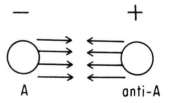

A   anti-A

Electric current speeds movement, imparts direction

FIGURE 16–7. In counterimmunoelectrophoresis, an electrical current passing through the gel affects the speed and direction of protein migration. Antigen and antibody molecules move more rapidly and more directly toward one another (*right*) than they would in simple diffusion (*left*).

IMMUNOELECTROPHORESIS

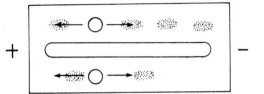

$+$ $-$

Electrophoresis separates antigens

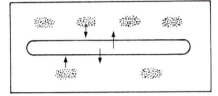

Trough contains mixture of antibodies

FIGURE 16–8. The upper panel depicts migrated proteins of two different serum specimens, separated by electrophoresis. The middle panel shows the trough from which the selected antibodies diffuse outward. The lower panel shows the precipitin arcs formed from antigen-antibody binding reactions. The migrated protein bands are invisible in the native gel, so only the precipitin arcs reveal the existence and location of reactive material. The upper serum sample contains several proteins that react with the reagent antibodies; the lower specimen contains only one. The fact that the arcs are in different locations indicates that the two specimens contain reactive proteins of different compositions.

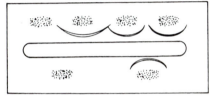

Arcs form where antibody meets
corresponding antigen

trough may contain antibody of a single specificity or a mixture expected to react with several of the electrophoretically separated proteins.

Immunoelectrophoresis is often used for qualitative or semiquantitative demonstration of proteins in serum, urine, or cerebrospinal fluid. If the antibody trough contains a mixture of antibodies, numerous precipitin bands form that identify individual proteins, such as albumin, transferrin, α-antitrypsin, or various classes of Igs. Failure to develop an expected band suggests a protein deficiency. Bands of abnormal location, shape, or intensity indicate abnormalities of protein composition or concentration.

In other applications, the antibody trough may contain a single antibody. A common example is antibody to an Ig light-chain isotype. A precipitin line forms at any site where there are Ig molecules with that light chain. An abnormal precipitin arc develops if the fluid contains unpaired light chains, which often occurs in multiple myeloma (see p. 231).

Immunofixation Electrophoresis

Proteins that have been separated by migration can be exposed directly to antibody, rather than by diffusion. In **immunofixation electrophoresis (IFE),** antibody is layered onto the gel on which proteins have migrated. Combination occurs more rapidly, and results are more sharply defined than when antibodies diffuse from a trough. However, only one antibody can be used per strip, and proportions of antigen and antibody are less flexible. IFE with an antibody of known specificity is often used to determine whether antigenic material with characteristic migration properties is present in a specimen. With addition of antibody onto the gel strips, immune complexes will precipitate at the site of the migrating antigen. Nonprecipitated proteins are washed away, leaving only precipitated immune complexes that can then be stained or labeled (Fig. 16–9).

IFE is useful in demonstrating antigens present at low concentrations, because the antibody is highly specific and electrophoretic migration leaves the antigenic material isolated and fully accessible. This method is often used to demonstrate abnormal proteins in spinal fluid or proteins present in serum at low concentrations, such as complement degradation fragments or other abnormal immune products. IFE is largely replacing immunoelectrophoresis for detection of abnormal proteins in serum or urine of patients with diseases such as multiple myeloma. IFE-staining patterns are easier to read and interpret than the precipitin arcs formed with IE. Furthermore, the amount of stain or label associated with an IFE band can provide a semiquantitative measurement of antigen (see Fig. 11–5).

Western Blotting

The **Western blot (WB)** procedure is conceptually similar to IFE, in that a specific protein in a complex mixture of proteins or antibody to a given protein can be identified. The first step in Western blotting is electrophoretic separation of the complex antigenic material. This is often a mixture of proteins or glycoproteins prepared from virus or other microorganisms. The separated components are transferred from the initial gel to a nitrocellulose medium by "blotting" from one surface to another. The term "Western blot" is a scientific joke. Transfer of electrophoretically separated material from one surface to another was developed by Dr. Edward Southern, who transferred fragments of deoxyribonucleic acid (DNA). DNA transfer thus became

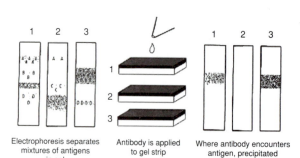

IMMUNOFIXATION ELECTROPHORESIS

Electrophoresis separates mixtures of antigens in gel

Antibody is applied to gel strip

Where antibody encounters antigen, precipitated complex can be stained

FIGURE 16–9. (*Left*) The migration patterns of three different protein mixtures designated 1, 2, and 3 are shown. The protein bands would not be visible without further manipulations. In the center, a single antibody (anti-B) is applied to each strip. The strips are then stained to show protein precipitated at those sites where antibody complexes with antigen. (*Right*) The results show that serum 1 had a small amount of B antigen, serum 2 had none, and serum 3 had a large amount. To test for A, C, or D antigen, additional strips would have to be treated with the corresponding antibody.

known as "Southern blotting." A later application of the technique was to transfer ribonucleic acid (RNA); this was dubbed "Northern blotting." Transfer of migrated proteins was named for one of the two remaining compass points, to become Western blotting.

Procedure and Interpretation

In Western blot procedures, the proteins are separated in one medium and then blotted onto a nitrocellulose support where antigen-antibody complexes can be demonstrated. The test is done to determine if a serum contains one or more antibodies to any of the antigenic bands. For each antibody present, immune complexes form at the site where the individual antigens have been blotted onto the nitrocellulose. After unbound proteins are washed away, the strip is labeled to reveal the presence and intensity of precipitated immune complexes. The test is most often used to detect antibodies against organisms of complex antigenic composition. Material from a purified preparation of microorganism is blotted to the support medium after electrophoretic separation. If the serum contains antibodies to any of the antigens, immune complexes precipitate in bands at characteristic locations. The location of stained bands reflects the specificity of the antibody (Fig. 16–10).

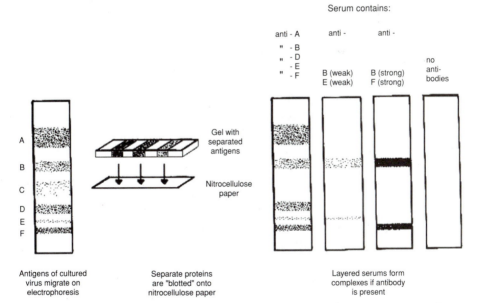

FIGURE 16–10. The first step in Western blot testing is electrophoretic separation of a protein mixture into bands of individual antigen (*left*). (*Middle*) "Blotting" the proteins onto nitrocellulose leaves each antigen in a distinctive location. The strips on the right show staining patterns achieved when four different serums are reacted with the separated antigens. The serum on the left contains moderately strong antibodies to five of the six antigens present. The second serum generates weak precipitin bands against two antigens. The next serum contains much stronger antibody against the B band and also strong activity against F. The last serum contains no antibodies against any of the antigens in this preparation.

The most familiar application of Western blotting is to identify antibodies to human retroviruses, especially those involved in AIDS. These viruses provoke a range of antibodies against well-characterized antigens. The number and location of precipitated bands indicate the presence of specific host antibodies to HIV antigens and confirm infection.

Antigens or slight antigenic differences between microorganisms can also be detected by Western blot and are often called **immunoblot** procedures. An example is the differentiation of closely related strains of *Staphylococcus aureus*. If extracts from different patient isolates undergo electrophoresis, are blotted, and are then reacted with polyclonal antisera, the different strains of S. *aureus* will show slightly different band patterns. Matching of immunoblot patterns from patient isolates can be used to trace transmission of a specific S. *aureus* strain from one patient to another.

SINGLE DIFFUSION

Single-diffusion procedures may use spontaneous or electrically modified movement through the medium. Because concentration of one reactant remains constant, the position and nature of the precipitation reaction reflect the quantity of the other reactant.

Single Radial Diffusion

In **radial immunodiffusion (RID),** antibody is uniformly distributed in the supporting gel, and antigen diffuses outward from a single well. The proportions between antigen and antibody change continually as the diffusion front moves radially; antigen-antibody complexes form at the zone of equivalence. After a predetermined interval, the radius of the precipitin ring is measured as an indication of antigen concentration. If the initial amount of antigen was small, the ring will be small. The more material initially present in the well, the greater the distance the material must travel to reach the zone of equivalence (Fig. 16–11).

With the Mancini End Point Method of measurement, once equivalence is reached, the diameter of the precipitin ring is measured. The square of the diameter is directly proportional to the concentration of antigen. A standard curve is constructed from the size of rings produced by reference preparations of known concentrations. By plotting concentration on the X axis versus the diameter squared on the Y axis, the concentration of the unknown antigen can be determined by comparison. Complete diffusion may take as long as 72 hours, but quantitative calculation is possible from observations taken at a fixed interval after loading the well. Using an alternative technique, the Kinetic Method, ring diameter may be measured as early as 6 hours after addition of antigen and compared with high and low standard preparations. Qualitative results are reported as either abnormally low or high.

RID allows simple, accurate measurement of relatively low protein levels. It is used to quantify serum levels of Igs or haptoglobin. A specific example of the use of RID is to quantitate serum IgE levels in patients with suspected allergies. Unfortu-

RADIAL IMMUNODIFFUSION

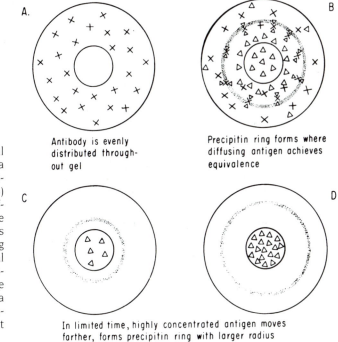

FIGURE 16–11. (A) Radial immunodiffusion starts with a single antibody evenly dispersed throughout the gel. (B) Antigen placed in the well diffuses radially, forming a visible ring wherever equivalence is reached. The radius of the ring formed after a limited interval is proportional to concentration of the antigen because diffusion is more rapid from a solution that is highly concentrated (D) than from one that is less concentrated (C).

A.

Antibody is evenly distributed through-out gel

B

Precipitin ring forms where diffusing antigen achieves equivalence

C

D

In limited time, highly concentrated antigen moves farther, forms precipitin ring with larger radius

nately, RID is affected by a number of artifacts. If proteins polymerize or form aberrant complexes, the resulting macromolecular aggregates diffuse more slowly than the native protein. This makes the precipitin ring smaller and causes underestimation of total concentration. Conversely, low-molecular-weight variants of normally polymerized proteins migrate faster and give falsely high results. Abnormally reactive serum constituents such as rheumatoid factor, which has intrinsic reactivity with IgG, may create misleading precipitation patterns. Other sources of error include underfilling or overfilling wells, nicking the wells, or using dehydrated gel preparations.

One-Dimensional Electroimmunodiffusion

In **one-dimensional electroimmunodiffusion** (also called **rocket electrophoresis** or **Laurell's rocket procedure**) electric current stimulates movement of antigen through an antibody-containing gel. Mixtures of proteins can be examined without special preparation because the reagent antibody incorporated in the medium reacts only with its target antigen. Electrical stimulation causes the antigen to move through the gel, thereby causing the zone of equivalence to change continually, relative to the fixed concentration of antibody incorporated in the medium. Precipitation occurs at the leading edge of the band, leaving reduced quantities of antigen in the trailing material. As antigen is depleted, the zone of equivalence moves more and more toward the center, giving a pointed (rocket-shaped) contour to the resulting precipitin line (Fig. 16–12).

Antigen concentration is proportional to the distance the rocket travels. Absolute values are calculated from a standard curve constructed with preparations of known concentrations. Rocket electrophoresis is especially useful for measuring materials too concentrated for receptor-ligand assays (see Chapter 18) but below the accuracy threshold for light-scattering (see next section) or other analytic techniques. Examples include alphafetoprotein in amniotic fluid and Igs in cerebrospinal fluid.

Variations of the rocket technique provide comparison of protein behavior and allow identification of abnormal protein derivatives or contaminating proteins. In the **fused-rocket technique,** separate antigen preparations are placed side by side. If the elements in both materials are the same, the rocket curves fuse in a manner analogous to the "reaction of identity" on an Ouchterlony plate (see earlier section on Ouchterlony double diffusion). In **crossed immunoelectrophoresis,** the materials in the mixture are separated by initial electrophoresis in an immunologically inert medium; the separated proteins are then subjected to electrical stimulation at a right angle to the original current to carry them into an antibody-containing gel where rockets can form.

ROCKET ELECTROPHORESIS

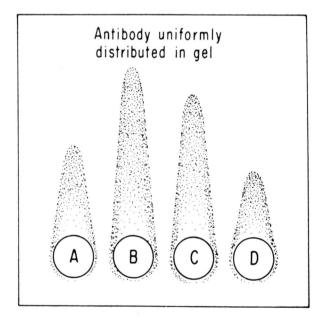

Antibody uniformly
distributed in gel

A   B   C   D

Migrating antigen forms
precipitin arcs

FIGURE 16–12. In rocket electrophoresis, the precipitin arc is shaped by an electrical current, which causes the antigen to move in a single direction through the antibody-impregnated gel. Height of the rocket reflects the relative concentration of antigen; absolute quantities must be extrapolated from comparison with controls of known concentration. Relative concentrations, in the example shown, are $B > C > A > D$.

TECHNIQUES THAT MEASURE LIGHT

When immune complexes precipitate out of solution, the behavior of light traveling through the medium is affected. The concentration, size, and shape of the immune complexes will affect light transmission. The physics of these interactions is exceedingly complex, and quantitative relationships are confounded by different rates of formation and dissipation at differing concentrations of antigen and antibody. In biologic systems, relationships are further confused by materials such as dispersed lipids or abnormal pigments that independently absorb or scatter light.

Nephelometry and **turbidimetry** are photometric techniques widely used in laboratory analysis. Turbidimetry measures changes in light transmission; nephelometry measures light scatter at one or more defined angles. Both techniques can be used to measure immune-complex formation in a fluid medium. Most procedures introduce a monospecific antibody into the antigen-containing test material. The resulting immune complexes alter the behavior of light transmitted through the fluid in a measurable fashion. Generally, the greater the concentration of immune complexes, the greater the turbidity or light scatter. If the physics of the instrument and the properties of the individual antigen-antibody system are carefully controlled, the technique allows accurate quantification at microgram or milligram levels of proteins such as complement components and their degradation products, serum Ig isotypes, abnormal Igs, and variant immune products, such as C-reactive protein.

SUMMARY

1. Binding of Fab sites with soluble antigen results in lattice formation and precipitation that may or may not be visible. Visible precipitation of the lattice usually occurs when antibody and antigen concentration are equivalent. Layering antigen and antibody solutions one on top of the other will generate a ring of precipitate called a precipitin line.

2. When solutions of antigen and antibody of matching specificity are simultaneously placed into wells cut into a gel, the molecules diffuse away from the wells and form a precipitate at the equivalence zone. Size and intensity of the precipitin line are indicative of the quantity of precipitated complex. Therefore, measurement of the precipitate can be used as an assay procedure. Formation of the precipitin line is dependent on physical properties of the supporting gel (viscosity, molecular size, hydration, chemical composition), concentration of antigen and antibody and their diffusion rates. These factors must be considered when interpreting or designing assays using precipitation as an end point.

3. Ouchterlony is one of the simplest and oldest immunodiffusion procedures. Antibody is usually placed in a central well surrounded by several wells containing antigen. Antigen and antibody diffuse radially, and a precipitin line forms only between those wells containing antigen and antibody of the same specificity (reaction of identity). Presence of additional precipitin arcs with varied shape and location demonstrates immune complexes with different properties.

Continued on the following page

4. With counterimmunoelectrophoresis (CIEP), antigen and antibody are placed into side-by-side wells. Application of an electrical current increases the rate of diffusion and induces linear movement of antigen and antibody so that a precipitin line forms more rapidly than with Ouchterlony procedures. CIEP is often used to demonstrate presence of microbial antigens in the body fluids of a patient.

5. Immune electrophoresis (IEP) is a two-stage procedure in which proteins are first separated by electrophoresis then allowed to diffuse toward a preparation of antibody. Precipitating immune complexes form arcs or bands wherever antigen encounters antibody of matching specificity. IEP is often used for qualitative or semiquantitative demonstration of proteins in serum, urine, or cerebrospinal fluids.

6. Immunofixation electrophoresis (IFE) is similar to IEP in that proteins are first separated by electrophoresis. Proteins are then exposed directly to antibody rather than forming precipitin lines by diffusion. After exposure to a specific antibody, a single band of precipitated immune complexes can be demonstrated on an electrophoretic gel strip. IFE procedures are largely replacing IEP because staining patterns produced by IFE are easier to read and interpret than the precipitin arcs formed with IEP.

7. Western blotting is a further modification of IFE. A complex mixture of proteins is electrophoresed. The separated proteins are then transferred or "blotted" onto nitrocellulose. Antiserum is added and immune complexes will form wherever antibody binds to antigen of matching specificity. Western blotting is the confirmatory test for HIV positivity. Patients with antibodies to HIV form multiple characteristic bands with the viral components that have undergone electrophoresis.

8. Single-diffusion procedures may use spontaneous or electrically modified movement of molecules through a supporting medium. In most single-diffusion procedures, antibody of known specificity and concentration is present in the medium. Antigen of unknown concentration is added to a well. After incubation, the presence and location of a precipitin line at the zone of equivalence are indicative of the amount of antigen present. With radial immunodiffusion (RID), the greater the amount of antigen, the larger the radius of the precipitin ring will be. With rocket electrophoresis, an electrical current stimulates movement of antigen through an antibody-containing gel. Precipitation occurs at the leading edge of antigen as it moves through the gel. The height of the rocket reflects the relative concentration of antigen. Absolute quantities must be extrapolated from comparisons with controls of known concentration. Rocket electrophoresis is used for detection and quantitation of protein such as alphafetoprotein in amniotic fluid or immunoglobulins (Igs) in cerebrospinal fluid.

9. Immune-complex formation in a solution alters the behavior of light transmitted through the fluid. Turbidity measures changes in light transmission; nephelometry measures light scatter at one or more defined angles. Under carefully controlled conditions, these techniques allow accurate quantitation of such proteins as complement components, serum Ig isotypes, and C-reactive protein.

REVIEW QUESTIONS

1. Serum IgG levels may be quantitated by _____.
   a. Ouchterlony procedures
   b. counterimmunoelectrophoresis (CIEP)
   c. radial immunodiffusion (RID)
   d. nephelometry
   e. c and d

2. Layering antigen and antibody solutions of matching specificities one on top of each other will generate _____.
   a. agglutination
   b. immune complexes
   c. a precipitin line
   d. a and b
   e. b and c

3. Mixing antigen and antibody solutions of matching specificity will result in _____ and can be measured by _____.
   a. changes in light transmission . . . turbidity
   b. changes in light scatter . . . nephelometry
   c. changes in light transmission . . . nephelometry
   d. changes in light scatter . . . turbidity
   e. a and b

4. Application of an electrical charge to enhance diffusion rates is used in _____ technique(s).
   a. CIEP
   b. Laurell's rocket procedure
   c. immunofixation
   d. a and b
   e. b and c

5. Precipitin lines formed between two separate wells surrounding a centrally placed well containing antibody join at the ends. This finding indicates _____.
   a. a reaction of identity
   b. antigen in both wells are identical
   c. antigen in both wells are different
   d. antigen in both wells are partially the same
   e. a and b

6. A patient's urine sample is subjected to immunoelectrophoresis (IEP) with anti–kappa antisera placed in the trough. A single heavy precipitin line forms in the gel. Which of the following is correct?
   a. The patient has free light chains in the urine.
   b. The patient likely has multiple myeloma.
   c. The patient has heavy chains in the urine.
   d. a and b
   e. b and c

7. If the above patient's urine was tested by IFE, which of the following is *not* necessary?
   a. Electrophoresis of patient's urine
   b. Transfer of proteins that have undergone electrophoresis to nitrocellulose
   c. Anti-kappa antiserum applied to gel strip
   d. Nonprecipitated proteins washed away
   e. Immune-complex formation stained for visualization

8. The precipitation test used most often to confirm HIV positivity is _____.
   a. Southern blot
   b. Northern blot
   c. Eastern blot
   d. Western blot
   e. immunofixation

9. Which of the following is *not* necessary for current HIV confirmatory testing.
   a. Electrophoresis of patient serum
   b. Electrophoresis of HIV antigen
   c. Transfer of proteins to nitrocellulose
   d. Removal of nonprecipitated immune complexes
   e. Staining of immune complexes for visualization

10. For quantitation of IgE in patient serum using RID, _____ is uniformly distributed in the supporting gel, and _____ diffuses outward from a single well.
    a. anti-IgE . . . IgE
    b. IgE . . . anti-IgE
    c. Coombs serum . . . IgE
    d. anti-IgG . . . IgE
    e. rabbit anti-human antiserum . . . IgE

ESSAY QUESTION

11. Given what you now know about the principle of Western blotting, why do you think this test is used as a confirmatory test of HIV positivity?

SUGGESTIONS FOR FURTHER READING

Cuiliere ML, Montagne P, Besson TH, et al: Microparticle-enhanced nephelometric immunoassay (Nephelia) for immunoglobulin G, A, and M. Clin Chem 1991;37(1):20–25
Garfin DE: Immunoblotting. In: Rose NR, DeMacario E, Fahey JL, et al, eds: Manual of Clinical Laboratory Immunology, 4th ed. Washington, DC: American Society for Microbiology, 1992:47–51

REVIEW ANSWERS

1. e	6. d
2. c	7. b
3. e	8. d
4. d	9. a
5. e	10. a

17 Methods Based on Agglutination

In agglutination, the antigen-antibody lattice incorporates particles, whereas the visible end result of precipitation is formation of macromolecular complexes. Agglutination can usually be observed with the naked eye, although discrimination is enhanced with a magnifying lens or low-power microscope. The relative concentration of antigen and antibody is less critical for agglutination than for precipitation, and agglutination techniques can detect reactants at lower concentrations. Therefore, agglutination procedures are generally more sensitive than those dependent on precipitation. Initially used to detect antibodies against bacterial or blood-cell antigens, agglutination procedures are now available for demonstration and sometimes quantification of a wide range of antigens and antibodies.

PRINCIPLES OF THE REACTION

Agglutination occurs in two stages. In the first stage, immunoglobulin (Ig) molecules attach to the antigen-bearing surface. Subsequently, if surrounding conditions are favorable, crosslinking into a visible lattice is observed. Specificity and reactivity of the antibody determine whether or not the first stage occurs; the second stage depends primarily on physical conditions.

Antibody Attachment

Attachment of antibody to antigen on a particle surface is called **sensitization** of the particle. Sensitization occurs only when specific antigen and antibody are present simultaneously. If the serum lacks antibody or if the antigens present are not recognized by the antibodies present, attachment will not occur (Fig. 17–1). However, even with the necessary elements present, characteristics of the antibody and the reaction conditions influence the rate and magnitude of sensitization (Fig. 17–2). With antigen-antibody systems of the same specificity, antibody molecules of higher affinity bind more rapidly than those with a lower binding constant. Temperatures other than the thermal optimum of the antibody may reduce or prevent association of antigen with antibody.

The nature of the antigen-bearing surface also affects sensitization. Antigenic sites may be inaccessible if overlaid or obscured by other surface molecules or if the epitopes are very sparse or very dense on the particle surface. Erythrocytes, bacteria, and other carrier particles express a net negative surface charge called the **zeta potential,** which may be sufficient to prevent effective steric interaction with antibody molecules. Surface charge can be modified by changing the ionic composition of the medium or by modifying the charge present on the particles (Fig. 17–3). Some agglutination procedures routinely include treating the particles with enzymes or other agents to modify surface properties.

Formation of the Lattice

Sensitization of particles does not guarantee agglutination. Before a lattice can form, antigen-combining (Fab) sites of antibody molecules must combine with anti-

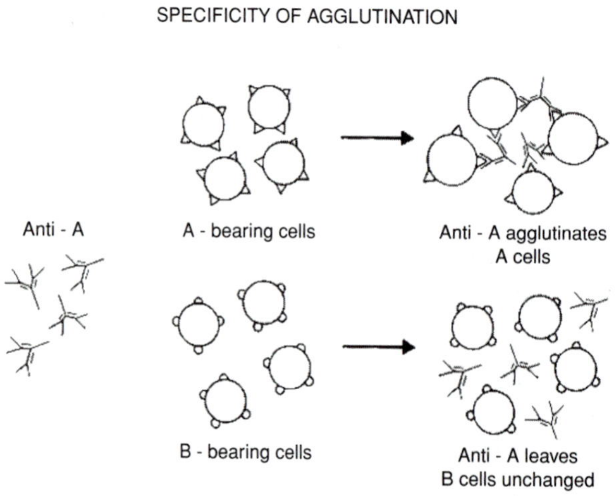

SPECIFICITY OF AGGLUTINATION

Anti - A

A - bearing cells

Anti - A agglutinates
A cells

B - bearing cells

Anti - A leaves
B cells unchanged

FIGURE 17–1. Agglutination occurs only when antibody encounters particulate antigen of the correct specificity. With a known antibody, agglutination reveals antigen specificity, as shown. If the antigen is known, the procedure can identify antibodies in an unknown serum.

FACTORS AFFECTING SENSITIZATION

A. Specificity

B. Antigen accessibility

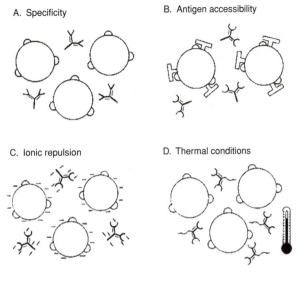

FIGURE 17–2. Antibody may not unite with particulate antigen under several circumstances. Specificity, shown in A, is the primary determinant. Reaction conditions also affect the combination of antibody with surface antigens. Steric interference by other molecules, shown in B, may impair immunoglobulin attachment. In a highly charged medium, shown in C, mutual repulsion may prevent antibody from uniting with surface proteins. If temperature is above (shown in D) or below thermal optimum for the antibody, reaction may not occur.

C. Ionic repulsion

D. Thermal conditions

gen expressed on different particles. If antigen sites are sparsely distributed on the particle surface, antibody molecules attached to one particle may fail to encounter, by chance association, epitopes on another particle. Conversely, if epitopes are densely present, the Fab sites of each antibody molecule may unite with several epitopes on a single particle, thus failing to form a lattice. Centrifugation is a physical process used to increase proximity of antibody and antigen-bearing surfaces. However, even after centrifugation, residual surface charge causes particles to maintain a certain space around themselves. Like charges repel, and individual units suspended in a medium remain measurably separate. Antibody with the same charge as the particle may succeed in combining with surface epitopes but, after attachment, may be unable to bridge the distance maintained between the particles. The IgG monomer, after binding to a surface antigen, often fails to agglutinate parti-

ALTERING CHARGE ALTERS REACTION

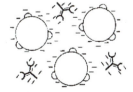

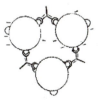

FIGURE 17–3. If ionic forces prevent engagement of antigen and antibody, lowering the ionic strength of the medium or altering the surface properties of the particles may permit sensitization and agglutination to occur.

Surface charge keeps particles and antibodies separated

Agglutination occurs with reduced surface charge

cles because the binding sites span a distance of only 25 nm. The IgM pentamer, with a diameter of about 100 nm and potentially 10 active combining sites, is far more effective in inducing agglutination than IgG molecules of the same specificity (Fig. 17–4).

Failure of Agglutination

Early serologists who observed this failure of agglutination theorized that such antibodies possessed only one combining site, and they described antibodies that caused sensitization but not agglutination as "incomplete." This interpretation was incorrect. Nonagglutinating antibodies are complete in all respects but may be unable to bridge the distance between antigen-bearing particles. Therefore, they cannot induce effective lattice formation. Agglutination can sometimes be promoted, after there has been sensitization without agglutination, by altering the ionic strength or viscosity of the suspending medium, the temperature of the reaction, or the nonantigenic surface properties of the particles.

If excessive numbers of antibody molecules attach to each particle, agglutination may not occur. Antibody excess can cause a prozone (see p. 346) in agglutination procedures as well as in precipitation. If individual antibody molecules attach to every available antigen site, no single molecule can combine with another particle to draw it into a lattice. The heavily sensitized particles remain suspended separately in the fluid medium. Diluting the serum to reduce the antibody concentration corrects the problem and allows agglutination to occur.

Use of Antiglobulin Reagents

Sensitization can be converted to visible agglutination by superimposing an additional antigen-antibody reaction onto the initial reaction. Ig molecules coating sensitized particles engage their Fab sites, but the constant portion (Fc) of the molecules remains exposed and accessible. Antibodies against the Fc portion of heavy chains or against constant domains of the light chain can unite with these surface-bound molecules. These antiglobulin antibodies can combine with target sites on separate Ig molecules linking them together. Because the target Igs are attached to particles, crosslinking the surface-bound target proteins brings the underlying parti-

IgM IS A BETTER AGGLUTININ THAN IgG

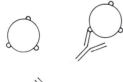

IgG is unable to link
widely separated particles

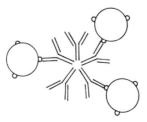

Larger IgM easily spans
distance between particles

FIGURE 17–4. Antigen-specific IgG antibodies often attach to surface antigen but fail to bridge the distance between suspended particles (*left*). IgM antibodies, with more combining sites and a greater diameter, readily agglutinate target material (*right*).

cles together in visible agglutinates (see Fig. 15–7). The antiglobulin reagent must be standardized to react only with globulin molecules and to have no effect on the particles or their antigens.

Unbound Globulins

Antiglobulin antibodies react with Ig wherever they encounter their target molecules. Ig molecules that are not bound into immune complexes combine more readily with antiglobulin antibodies than do Igs attached to a cell surface. If unbound Ig molecules are in the medium that contains antibody-coated particles, an antiglobulin reagent may unite so promptly with unbound Ig that little or no reactivity remains to crosslink the sensitized particles (Fig. 17–5). In procedures that use antiglobulin reagents, it is crucially important to remove all unbound proteins before adding antiglobulin serum.

Quantification

Agglutination is inherently qualitative. It is a reaction that occurs only if antigen and antibody bind to form a visible complex, and it cannot be quantified accurately. When temperature, suspending medium, and centrifugation are held constant, the rapidity with which agglutination occurs and the size of the clumps are roughly proportional to the intensity of the antigen-antibody reaction. Intensity can be recorded by assigning numeric values or according to a scale of +/−, 1+, 2+, 3+, and 4+. To compare the strength of several different preparations, the antigen or antibody used as an indicator material must be held stringently constant. With an antibody of known properties, reaction strength reflects antigenic characteristics of the cells or particles tested. Conversely, progressively stronger agglutination of standardized antigen-bearing particles occurs as antibody concentration increases, unless and until a prozone occurs.

NEUTRALIZATION OF ANTIGLOBULIN SERUM

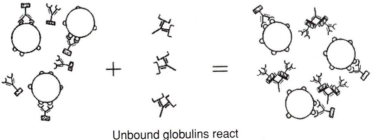

Unbound globulins react
preferentially with antiglobulin

FIGURE 17–5. Antiglobulin antibodies combine more rapidly with unbound than with bound immunoglobulin molecules. If all combining sites of the reagent antiglobulin are occupied by free immunoglobulin molecules as shown, indicator particles will not be agglutinated, whether or not there is antibody bound to their surface.

Performing and Interpreting Titration

Titration is a semiquantitative technique in which differential dilution provides approximate estimation of concentration. Titration can be useful in comparing activity levels of specimens collected at different times or from different sources. Each dilution is reacted against an indicator of reproducible properties. If antibody in serum is diluted many times and therefore becomes less and less concentrated, agglutination diminishes and eventually disappears. The result is reported as the **titer,** defined as the reciprocal of the highest dilution that causes agglutination. If agglutination occurs at 1:64 and not at 1:128, the titer is 64 (Fig. 17–6). It is not correct to report titer as dilution; in this example, the titer is 64, not 1:64.

The major problem with titration besides its necessarily inferential approach to quantity is difficulty of performing accurate dilutions and achieving precisely comparable results. Dilution intervals must be selected so that the expected results fall in an informative portion of the range. If, for example, doubling dilutions go from 1:128 to 1:256, and the critical distinction in concentration lies between 1:100 and

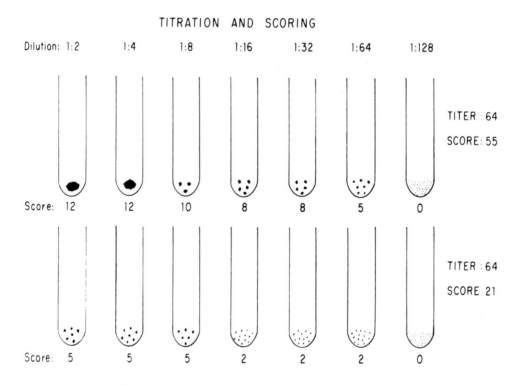

FIGURE 17–6. Both panels show dilutions of antibody ranging from 1:2 to 1:128. The upper specimen causes intense agglutination (score of 12) at the first two dilutions, and reactivity decreases sharply with increasing dilution. The lower specimen causes only modest agglutination (score of 5) at 1:2, but this reactivity changes relatively little at much higher dilutions. In both specimens, the highest dilution to show agglutination is 1:64, so both have a titer of 64.

1:150, the test loses much of its sensitivity. A more common problem is accuracy of dilution and reproducibility of results. As successive dilutions are made, incremental loss of very small volumes can produce enormous inaccuracy in concentration. Because of this imprecision, results in titrating two different specimens are considered significantly different only if end points differ by more than two dilution levels. With doubling dilutions of 1:8, 1:16, 1:32, and 1:64 and precision no better than plus or minus one dilution, an antibody truly detectable at 1:16 might, in three replicate tubes, give results at 1:8, 1:16, and 1:32. To be significant, there would have to be a difference of more than two tubes; for example, between 1:8 and 1:64. Prozones can present an artificial problem in titration. With highly concentrated antibody, serum that is undiluted or at the 1:2 dilution may cause little or no agglutination, whereas strong agglutination can occur at 1:4, 1:8, and so on. With the use of micropipettors, multiple-tip pipettors, calibrated dispensing pipettors, and automated instrumentation, greater accuracy and efficiency can be realized with procedures requiring titration.

Differences in Antibody Behavior

Combining titration with numeric scoring can give additional information. Antibodies that recognize the same antigens may express clinically significant differences in serologic behavior. The biologic properties of an antibody that gives 4+ agglutination when undiluted and declines progressively with increasing dilution are often different from those of a serum that gives consistently low levels of agglutination at every dilution over a wide range. Both might have the same titer, but the differences in intensity of agglutination suggest differences not only in serologic but also biologic behavior. Figure 17–6 illustrates this distinction.

AGGLUTINATION PROCEDURES

Agglutination was first used to demonstrate activity of antibody in unmodified serum, directed against unmodified red blood cells (RBCs) or bacterial cells. This type of agglutination continues to be useful in immunohematology and microbiology. However, procedures that use processed antigen or antibody or both have greatly expanded the applications of agglutination testing. In **passive agglutination** procedures, antigenic material is attached onto carrier particles. This allows antibody to encounter in particulate form an otherwise soluble antigen (Fig. 17–7). In **reverse passive agglutination,** the material linked to the carrier is antibody; the test is done to demonstrate presence of soluble antigen, which induces agglutination of the particle-linked antibody (Fig. 17–8).

Agglutination as an end point can be determined by visual inspection or with suitably calibrated instruments. With carrier particles of precisely reproducible characteristics and instrument-assisted test conditions, agglutination tests can give quantitative results. The particle-enhanced reaction can be quantified by measuring how agglutination affects the transmission or scatter of light, by counting the number of freely suspended particles before and after the immune reaction or by observing that the size of suspended material changes as individual particles agglutinate into cohesive clumps.

PASSIVE AGGLUTINATION

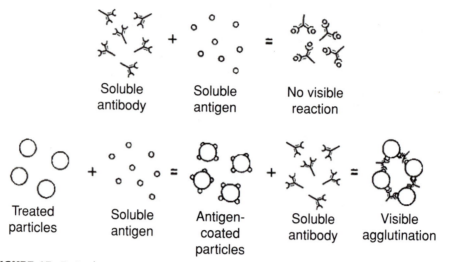

Soluble antibody	Soluble antigen	No visible reaction		
Treated particles	Soluble antigen	Antigen-coated particles	Soluble antibody	Visible agglutination

FIGURE 17–7. In the upper panel, reaction between soluble antigen and soluble antibody produces immune complexes too small to be detected. The lower panel shows how attaching soluble antigen to indicator particles converts immune complexes into particulate lattices readily detected as agglutination.

Direct Agglutination

Direct agglutination is most useful in the immunohematology and microbiology laboratories. Agglutination gives prompt, accurate, and reproducible information about surface antigens on blood cells and about blood group antibodies in serum. Agglutination of RBCs is referred to as **hemagglutination.** For ABO antigens and antibodies, immediate hemagglutination is characteristic. To demonstrate antigen-antibody reactions in the Rh system and most of the other systems such as Kell and Duffy, antiglobulin serum is often necessary. Agglutination tests are also used to demonstrate abnormal antibodies, like those in cold-agglutinin disease or infectious mononucleosis (IM). Cold agglutinins are antibodies that react better at cold temperatures (lower than body temperature). These types of antibodies may be present because of autoimmune disease or recent infection with *Mycoplasma pneumoniae*. Diagnosis of IM is dependent on detection of heterophile antibodies. Heterophile antibodies are antibodies produced in response to one antigen, yet can react with a sec-

REVERSE PASSIVE AGGLUTINATION

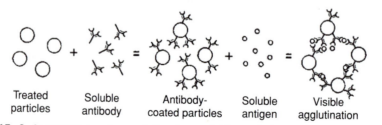

Treated particles	Soluble antibody	Antibody-coated particles	Soluble antigen	Visible agglutination

FIGURE 17–8. In reverse passive agglutination, soluble antibody is rendered particulate by adsorption to inert indicator particles. Contact with specific antigen brings the particles together into lattices visible as agglutination.

ond unrelated antigen. Direct agglutination immunoassays for IM contain horse or sheep RBCs or latex particles with adsorbed heterophile antigens on their surfaces.

The Coombs' Test

Modern antiglobulin testing began with Coombs and coworkers, who injected whole human serum into rabbits and used the resulting antihuman reagent to demonstrate anti-RBC antibodies that sensitized target cells but did not agglutinate them. Immunohematologists continue to find antiglobulin reactions invaluable, and several blood banking procedures bear the informal name **Coombs' test.** The reagents now used differ enormously from the anti–whole serum first used by Coombs and his colleagues, and the more correct term is **antiglobulin test.** The antiglobulin test reagent is often referred to as anti–human globulin.

Antibody Attached to Cells

In blood bank serology, antiglobulin serum has two different applications. The **direct antiglobulin test (DAT)** demonstrates whether antibody or complement components have attached to blood cells in the circulating blood of the living host (Fig. 17–9). Healthy individuals should not have large numbers of circulating globulin-coated RBCs. Attachment of antibody or complement to host blood cells usually indicates an autoimmune process, and the direct antiglobulin test is used to diagnose such hematologic or immunologic abnormalities. The test is called "direct" because RBCs are tested directly as they come from the body, processed only by washing to remove unbound globulins that might neutralize the antiglobulin reagent.

Antibody Present in Serum

A different application of antiglobulin testing is not as a single test but as a general procedure to detect antibodies in serum. The **indirect antiglobulin technique** is a

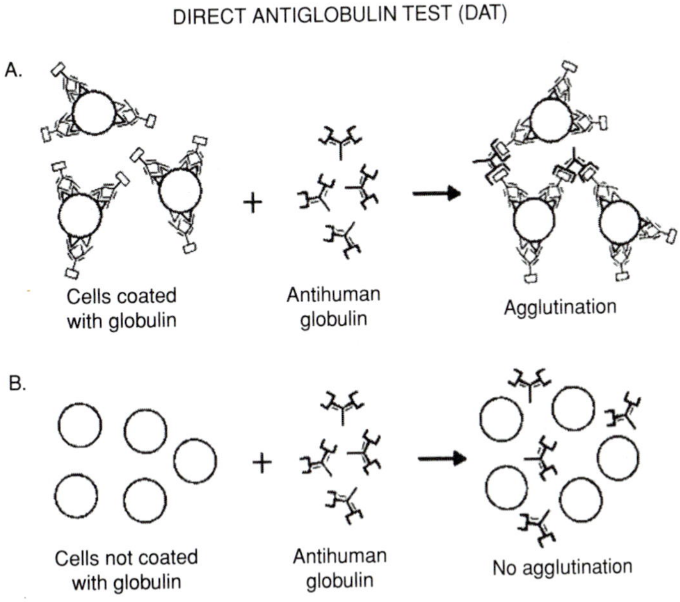

DIRECT ANTIGLOBULIN TEST (DAT)

FIGURE 17–9. The direct antiglobulin test demonstrates whether or not cells are coated with globulin. In *panel* A, antiglobulin reagent that combines with globulin molecules complexed to the cell surface causes agglutination of the underlying cells. In *panel* B, uncoated cells do not bind with the antiglobulin antibody and remain unagglutinated.

A.

Cells coated with globulin + Antihuman globulin → Agglutination

B.

Cells not coated with globulin + Antihuman globulin → No agglutination

two-stage procedure. First, serum is incubated with antigen-bearing cells so that antibody, if present in the serum, can combine with surface antigen and sensitize the cells. The incubated cells are then separated from the original serum, washed, and mixed with antiglobulin serum. If the original serum contained antibody that attached to antigens on the cell surface, the antiglobulin reagent will combine with the sensitizing Ig and agglutinate the coated cells. If the serum did not contain antibody against antigens on the test cells, addition of antiglobulin serum has no effect on the indicator cells (Fig. 17–10). The test detects the presence of antibody capable of causing agglutination of indicator cells. The indirect antiglobulin technique is used to demonstrate and to identify blood group antibodies and to crossmatch donor RBCs with recipient serum for safe transfusion.

RBCs are surrounded by a negative ion cloud that causes the cells to repel one another. The repulsive force is called the **zeta potential.** The zeta potential can be lowered with the addition of a dilute albumin solution or low-ionic-strength saline (LISS), and thus visible agglutination of antibody-coated RBCs is enhanced. Because of their size and configuration, IgM type antibodies are more effective than IgG in agglutinating RBCs. Some RBC antibodies such as the antibodies to the Rh antigen are exclusively of the IgG class. To enhance visible agglutination of the Rh antibody binding with Rh-positive RBCs, addition of albumin, LISS, centrifugation, or anti–human globulin may sometimes be necessary.

Microbiology Tests

Microbiology uses direct agglutination in two different diagnostic approaches. Reagent antibodies of known specificity can be used to identify **antigens on bacteria.** Agglutination is also the end point in **serodiagnosis** of infection, which depends on identifying antibodies in serum samples. An immunocompetent individual exposed to an organism characteristically develops antibodies against the infecting agent. The most accurate method of diagnosing infection is to culture the organism, but sometimes this is difficult or impossible. For example, it is possible that suitable material cannot be obtained, the patient is studied only after the organisms have left the body, the organism is difficult to grow, or handling the organism constitutes a threat to laboratory personnel. With the presence of any of these

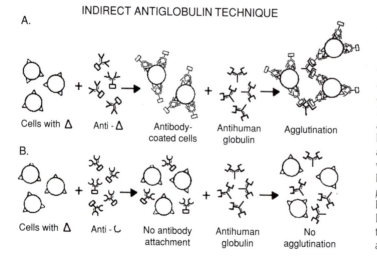

INDIRECT ANTIGLOBULIN TECHNIQUE

A.

Cells with Δ   Anti - Δ   Antibody-coated cells   Antihuman globulin   Agglutination

B.

Cells with Δ   Anti - ∪   No antibody attachment   Antihuman globulin   No agglutination

FIGURE 17–10. Indirect antiglobulin procedures require two steps: combination of antibody with specific antigen, followed by combination of antiglobulin reagent with cell-bound antibody. In *panel* A, antibody specific for the surface antigen sensitizes the cells, which are then agglutinated by antiglobulin serum. In *panel* B, antigen-antibody binding does not occur, leaving the cells unsensitized and unaffected by the antiglobulin serum.

difficult conditions, demonstrating antibodies against the suspected agent in the patient's serum provides important diagnostic information. Agglutination tests are often used to diagnose typhoid, brucellosis, tularemia, and leptospirosis. With the **Widal test,** *Salmonella* or *Brucella* antigen is mixed with patient's serum on a glass slide and macroscopically observed for agglutination.

Cross-reactive agglutination can be used in serodiagnosis of certain rickettsial diseases—Rocky Mountain spotted fever, typhus, and others. Infections with these rickettsiae provoke antibodies that coincidentally agglutinate suspensions of *Proteus vulgaris* bacteria, a completely unrelated organism. It is difficult to prepare rickettsial antigens and easier to make suspensions of various strains of *Proteus*. This examination for cross-reactivity, called the **Weil-Felix test,** can be used to detect rickettsial infections in which it is otherwise very difficult to identify the causative organism. Both the Widal and Weil-Felix tests, referred to as **febrile agglutinins,** should be interpreted with caution and used for screening purposes only.

Passive Agglutination

Passive agglutination is the same as direct agglutination except that the antigen has been adsorbed or attached onto a particle. Suitably purified solutions of many hormones, drugs, bacterial metabolites, and serum proteins can be adsorbed to indicator particles with little difficulty. RBCs are useful carrier particles because many proteins adhere spontaneously to the cell membrane. Treating the cells with tannic acid, various enzymes, or certain organic agents enhance the binding event.

Alternatively, carrier particles of uniform size and physical characteristics can be prepared from latex, charcoal, clay, and other substances. These inert particles circumvent one problem that carrier RBCs may create: the possibility that unsuspected antibodies may react against RBCs elements. Human sera sometimes contain heterospecific antibodies that can agglutinate nonhuman RBCs used in some test systems.

Clinical Applications

Rheumatoid factor is an autoantibody directed against the Fc portion of IgG. Serum that contains rheumatoid factor agglutinates indicator particles to which IgG has been attached. The original test for rheumatoid factor, the **Rose-Waaler test** used sheep erythrocytes to which rabbit antisheep antibodies had attached. Present tests for rheumatoid factor use latex particles coated with human IgG, a test system that is more sensitive and less liable to artifacts than the sheep-cell system. Other tests that use RBCs passively coated with antigen include those for antibodies to **thyroglobulin,** the hormone-containing storage protein of the thyroid. Penicillin, cephalosporins, or other pharmaceuticals can be adsorbed to allogeneic RBCs to demonstrate **drug antibodies** that cause immune-mediated RBC destruction.

The popular confirmatory test for syphilis, the microhemagglutination assay—*Treponema pallidum* (MHA-TP)—uses small quantities of tanned antigen-coated, RBCs reacted with serum in a special plastic microtiter tray. A positive serum reaction results in lattice formation at the bottom of the well. Nonagglutinated cells in a negative reaction settle to form a compact button. The screening tests for syphilis are also agglutination reactions dependent on cross-reactivity of syphilis antibodies to lipid (cardiolipin) found in high concentration in neural and cardiac tissue. For the VDRL (Venereal Disease Research Laboratory test for syphilis) test, purified cardiolipin particles are mixed with a dilution of the test specimen (serum or cerebrospinal fluid) and examined microscopically for visible aggregates. The rapid plasma reagin (RPR) is an improved modification of the VDRL, which allows visualization of macroscopic aggregates of charcoal particles coated with a stabilized mixture of cholesterol and cardiolipin. Serum dilutions are used to determine the titer of positive specimens detected with the VDRL and RPR tests.

Latex particles are used in test kits for diagnosis of many **autoimmune conditions.** Besides the latex test for rheumatoid factor mentioned above, there are preparations to detect autoantibodies against deoxyribonucleic acid (DNA), nucleoproteins, and a variety of cytoplasmic proteins. In many autoimmune conditions, antibodies develop against circulating hormones, and many assays are available that use hormone-coated particles. Other applications include testing for the group of liver-derived proteins characterized as **acute-phase reactants** and for antibodies against streptococcal enzymes and against a variety of fungal and protozoal antigens.

Reverse Passive Agglutination

An effective means of demonstrating presence of soluble antigen is to coat carrier particles with antibody and to allow the antigen to induce lattice formation. This kind of agglutination procedure is useful as a screening test for various materials that do not need to be precisely measured. It has found wide acceptance as a rapid procedure to demonstrate infection, replacing the time-consuming but definitive technique of culturing the invading organism. When multiplying organisms are present, soluble antigenic material often enters body fluids, where it can be detected through agglutination of particles coated with appropriate antibodies. This provides highly suggestive diagnostic information available within a few minutes and is useful for beginning treatment while more definitive diagnostic procedures are being undertaken.

Reverse passive agglutination is also suitable for semiquantitative assay of substances in body fluids. For example, under normal conditions, cleavage products of fibrinogen are not present at measurable levels in the serum. Presence of these abnormal products can be demonstrated through agglutination of particles coated with antibodies against fibrinogen-related peptides. The same approach can be used to detect threshold levels of drugs in body fluids. The coated carrier particles must be standardized so that agglutination occurs only at or above the desired concentration. Possibilities of cross-reactivity and nonspecific agglutination must be rigorously excluded.

INHIBITION OF AGGLUTINATION

Soluble antigen and soluble antibody often form complexes without visible evidence of binding. One way to demonstrate this combination is to show that antigen or antibody originally known to be present has been consumed or eliminated. **Agglutination inhibition** procedures require several steps. The first step is establishment of an indicator system. Reagent antibody and reagent antigen are standardized to produce agglutination of demonstrated intensity. Usually, the reagent antibody is soluble and the indicator antigen is in particulate form, but the reverse conditions can be used. After establishment of baseline agglutination, the next step is to incubate the test material and the soluble reagent to allow formation of immune complexes. The last phase is addition of the indicator particles. If incubating the test material with the known reagent abolishes agglutination, the inference is that soluble molecules are present in the specimen that have combined with test reagent to inhibit agglutination (Fig. 17–11). Appropriate controls are essential for agglutination inhibition tests to rule out the possibility of nonspecific interference.

Soluble Antigens

A familiar application of agglutination inhibition is **pregnancy tests,** which measure raised levels of human chorionic gonadotropin (hCG) in urine or blood. The test consists of latex particles coated with hCG and a solution of anti-hCG antibodies. First, urine or blood is incubated with the antibody; then the incubated mixture is added to the indicator particles. Persistence of agglutination at the previously established level indicates that the test material contained insufficient hCG to inactivate the reagent antibody. Abolition or pronounced reduction of agglutination indicates a level of soluble hCG sufficient to neutralize agglutinating activity of the reagent antibody and constitutes a positive result.

Agglutination inhibition can be used to estimate drug levels in body fluids. After establishment of baseline agglutinating action of reagent antibody on drug-coated particles, inhibitory effect of diluted serum samples can be determined. Titration of this sort gives semiquantitative results, but comparison against levels observed with known drug concentrations often provides clinically useful information.

Applications in Immunohematology

Many blood-cell antigens exist in soluble form as well as on cell membranes. For example, the ABO antigens are an integral part of cell membranes but are also present in plasma and other body fluids. Other antigens such as Lewis (Le^a, Le^b), Sid (Sd^n), and the major histocompatibility complex (MHC) class III proteins exist primarily in body fluids and attach only passively to cell surfaces. It is sometimes

AGGLUTINATION INHIBITION

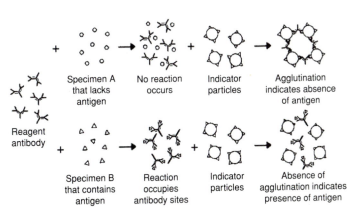

FIGURE 17–11. Antibody (*far left*) that is specific for antigens on the indicator particles will cause agglutination under standard conditions. Incubating the antibody with antigen in soluble form (*lower panel*) engages available Fab sites and prevents the antibody from causing agglutination. The upper panel shows agglutination occurring after incubation with material that lacks the specific antigen.

Reagent antibody + Specimen A that lacks antigen → No reaction occurs + Indicator particles → Agglutination indicates absence of antigen

Specimen B that contains antigen → Reaction occupies antibody sites + Indicator particles → Absence of agglutination indicates presence of antigen

desirable to demonstrate the presence or the concentration of these materials in body fluids, and agglutination inhibition is useful for this purpose. Because there are so many variables in concentration, in antibody behavior, and in cell-membrane properties, each test system must be carefully standardized before conclusions are drawn.

Soluble Antibodies

Certain antiviral antibodies can be demonstrated by their capacity to inhibit agglutination; the agglutination test depends on the biologic behavior of the virus involved. Viruses may agglutinate suspensions of RBCs that have specific receptors for their proteins. Different viruses can cause hemagglutination of cells from different animal species, so the tests have to be carefully selected and standardized. The principle of the test is simple: Antibodies stimulated by contact with a virus combine with viral antigens and interfere with viral attachment to RBC receptors. The two-stage test involves first incubating test serum with the virus preparation and, second, adding RBCs that the virus is known to agglutinate. Reduction or abolition of agglutination indicates presence of antibodies against the virus (Fig. 17–12). This technique is used to detect antibodies to a wide range of viruses: rubella, measles, mumps, influenza, adenoviruses, and several others. Controls are necessary to detect artifacts that affect the results, especially loss of agglutinating potency in the

HEMAGGLUTINATION INHIBITION

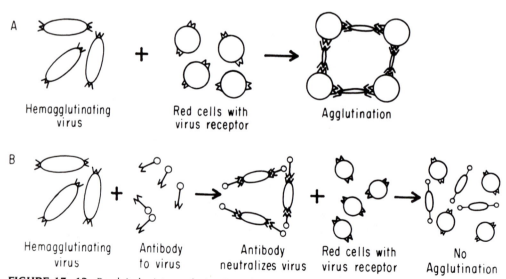

FIGURE 17–12. *Panel A* depicts agglutination of indicator red blood cells by a preparation of active virus. The presence of antibody specific for the virus can be demonstrated, as shown in *panel B*, by incubating serum with virus and then observing failure of the incubated virus to agglutinate the indicator cells.

reagent virus, and the presence in the test serum of antibodies capable of agglutinating the indicator cells.

Streptococcal infection often induces antibodies against the bacterial hemolysin called streptolysin O. Streptolysin O and S can cause lysis of both RBCs and white blood cells. Presence of the antibody, **antistreptolysin O (ASO),** in the serum is useful as an indicator of recent streptococcal infection. The classic test for ASO demonstrates that antibody-containing serum can neutralize effects of the hemolysin. A soluble preparation of streptolysin O is incubated with dilutions of patient serum. After incubation, reagent RBCs are added. If the serum contains antibodies against streptolysin O, an immune complex is formed and no streptolysin O is available to cause hemolysis. Because normal serum characteristically contains low to moderate levels of ASO, the test must be standardized so that inhibition occurs only at a concentration that is clinically significant. Agglutination procedures are far simpler. Instead of using RBCs and inhibition of hemolysis as an indication of infection, presence of antistreptolysin antibodies and other antistreptococcal antibodies can be demonstrated by direct agglutination. Serum can be mixed with latex particles coated with streptokinase, hyaluronidase, deoxyribonuclease (DNase), and nicotinamide adenine dinuclease (NADase). Antibody responses in patients vary according to different streptococcal antigens, and titration of sera and other confirmatory tests are usually necessary to positively establish streptococcal infection.

QUALITY ASSURANCE

Agglutination tests are rapid and can appear misleadingly simple. Both false-positive and false-negative results may occur if there are insufficient controls to detect common pitfalls.

The System Itself

Basic to agglutination testing is the behavior of the suspended particles. They must remain in a stable suspension, without spontaneous aggregation or excessive mutual repulsion. Particularly with RBCs, membrane characteristics that change with physiologic or artificial events may alter serologic behavior of the indicator particles. This is important both in immunohematology procedures that use unmodified RBCs and in passive systems that use RBCs as carriers. Changes in the ionic composition or the viscosity of the medium affect agglutination, as do changes in temperature, incubation period, or the quantity or concentration of the substances tested. It may be difficult to distinguish spontaneous association of particles caused by altered physical conditions from a low level of true agglutination. Using known positive and negative controls eliminates many artifacts, but the observer must always be alert to problems in interpretation.

When several specimens are to be compared, stringently uniform test conditions must be maintained. Variation in preparing reagents or timing the reactions can introduce errors of interpretation that are easily overlooked. Especially with titration, comparisons are most valid when all specimens are tested simultaneously by a single interpreter observing a single indicator system. Automated pipetting and diluting significantly improve reproducibility over manual manipulation.

Problems in Interpretation

Difficulty in observation and interpretation is more conspicuous and more significant in blood bank serology than in most other agglutination procedures. Known or unsuspected disease states often alter the behavior of serum or cells, and it may be difficult to distinguish subtle but significant disturbances from artifacts of the suspending medium, the incubation process, or the effect of centrifugation.

It is important to remember that several independent immune responses can occur simultaneously. An apparent positive result in an immunologic test may actually reflect an event completely different from the one under investigation. Several pitfalls apply, especially to agglutination procedures. In serum from patients with inflammatory or immunologic diseases, abnormalities of protein composition and concentration occur frequently; these changes often affect the behavior of suspended particles. Serum with increased globulins, decreased albumin, or various abnormal proteins may cause suspended particles to come together in stacked or clustered aggregates called **rouleaux.** Rouleaux form independent of antibody in serum or antigen on cell surface; they are simply the effect that the protein-containing fluid has on the charged particles.

Distinct from rouleaux formation is the problem of antibodies that agglutinate cells intended as inert indicator particles. Some patients have antibodies that agglutinate virtually all human cells—their own and those from nearly any other adult human. Other patients have antibodies that react with RBCs from other species. Tests that use carrier RBCs should include uncoated RBCs as a control to detect whether the test serum causes nonspecific agglutination.

Cross-reactivity is a problem in serodiagnosis of infections. Exposure to one organism may promote antibodies capable of agglutinating material from other organisms that share common surface configurations. Sometimes antigen reagents prepared from cell cultures express characteristics of the cells in which the organisms were grown. The test serum may have antibodies against this cellular material and thus give an apparent positive reaction against the microbial preparation.

Rheumatoid factor, an antibody directed against human IgG, can cause agglutination in any test that uses a human IgG reagent, either adsorbed to a carrier particle or as part of an agglutination inhibition system.

The preceding discussion, although far from exhaustive, should highlight the need for continuous care in performing agglutination tests and judgment in interpreting them. A vast array of test kits are available; the most important safeguard for accurate results is careful attention to the manufacturer's instructions.

SUMMARY

1. Incorporation of particles into an antigen-antibody lattice results in agglutination. Agglutination is generally easier to detect and more sensitive than the macromolecular complexes produced by precipitation. Agglutination occurs in two stages. (a) Antibody must attach to an antigen-bearing surface (sensitization). Many factors may affect antibody binding such as affinity, temperature, accessibility of antigenic sites, and surface charge. (b) The next stage is formation of the lattice. Adequate numbers of epitopes on antigen-coated particles are necessary to assure Fab sites of antibody combine with different

particles. Centrifugation may increase proximity of Fab and antigen. IgM is a more effective agglutinator than IgG because it is better able to bridge the distance between epitopes. Antibody excess can cause a prozone effect in both agglutination and precipitation.

2. Agglutination is inherently qualitative. However, if test conditions are constant, rapidity and size of clumps are proportional to the intensity of the antigen-antibody reaction. Antibody may be diluted and reacted with antigen. The reciprocal number of the highest dilution at which agglutination still occurs is considered the titer. The higher the titer number, the greater is the concentration and strength of antibody. Accuracy of dilution technique is critical to the accuracy of the titer.

3. Agglutination of red blood cells (RBCs) by antibody (hemagglutination) is useful for determination of blood type and identification of other RBC antigens. Cold agglutinin and heterophile antibody of infectious mononucleosis can also be detected by hemagglutination.

4. The direct antiglobulin test (DAT) demonstrates whether antibody or complement components have attached to blood cells in the circulation of the patient. RBCs of the patient are washed and incubated with anti–human globulin (Coomb's serum). Hemagglutination usually indicates presence of autoimmune antibody.

5. The indirect antiglobulin test detects antibody in the serum not attached to host cells. Patient serum is incubated with antigen-bearing RBCs to allow attachment, washed to remove unbound antibody, and reacted with antiglobulin serum. If antibodies are present in patient serum, hemagglutination occurs. To enhance visible agglutination of RBCs, the zeta potential can be reduced by addition of reagents such as albumin or low-ionic-strength saline (LISS).

6. Agglutination tests in microbiology can detect presence of antibody to a suspected microorganism. Patient serum is reacted directly with the microorganism or antigen from the microbe or with antigen from the microbe attached to a particle (passive agglutination).

7. Instead of microbial antigens, rheumatoid factor, drugs, hormones, and other clinically relevant antigens can be attached to particles for detection of antibodies.

8. With reverse passive agglutination techniques, carrier particles are coated with antibody for detection of soluble antigen. Infectious microorganisms may shed antigenic material that is detectable by agglutination of particles coated with appropriate antibodies. Semiquantitative detection of other substances in body fluids such as drugs, hormones, or fibrinogen cleavage products is also possible with this technique.

9. Agglutination inhibition procedures use standardized reagent antibody and antigen to produce agglutination of demonstrated intensity. Test material containing either antigen or antibody is incubated with the appropriate reagent. Indicator particles are added. If agglutination is inhibited, then test material contains the suspected antigen or antibody. Application of agglutination inhibition procedures have been adapted for detection of antigens such as human chorionic growth hormone (an indicator of pregnancy), streptococcal antigens, and soluble antibodies to various viruses.

Continued on the following page

10. Although agglutination tests are rapid and seem simple to perform, many factors must be considered in interpretation and assurance of test accuracy. Particles must remain in stable suspension without spontaneous aggregation or excessive repulsion. Test conditions such as ionic composition, temperature, viscosity of the suspending media, and length of incubation must be optimal and consistent. Positive and negative controls must be included. Possible presence of interfering proteins and cross-reactive antibodies must be considered in interpretations of positive results.

REVIEW QUESTIONS

1. Factors affecting the sensitization stage of agglutination include _____.
   a. temperature
   b. antigen accessibility
   c. specificity
   d. ionic repulsion
   e. all of the above

2. _____ can more easily cause agglutination because _____.
   a. IgM . . . it has more combining sites
   b. IgG . . . binds to epitopes better
   c. IgM . . . it spans distances between particles better
   d. IgM . . . it has less surface charge
   e. a and c

3. A pregnancy test based on the agglutination inhibition principle is performed. Mixing of reagents with a patient's urine sample results in agglutination of latex principles. Is the patient pregnant?
   a. Yes
   b. No
   c. Possibly

4. The microhemagglutination assay–*Treponema pallidum* (MHA-TP) confirmatory test for syphilis uses _____ for observing agglutination.
   a. purified cardiolipin
   b. stabilized charcoal particles
   c. tannic acid treated red blood cells (RBCs) coated with antigen
   d. tannic acid treated RBCs coated with antibody
   e. latex particles coated with anti-TP antibodies.

5. *Cryptococcus neoformans* (CN), a fungal microbe that causes cryptococcosis sheds capsular material into the bloodstream. Serum from a patient with suspected cryptococcosis was mixed with latex particles coated with CN antibody. Positive agglutination would indicate that _____.
   a. the patient does *not* have CN
   b. the patient has CN
   c. the patient has a nonspecific agglutinating protein
   d. b and c

6. The type of agglutination test mentioned in question 5 is called _____.
   a. direct agglutination
   b. passive agglutination
   c. reverse passive agglutination
   d. agglutination inhibition
   e. indirect antiglobulin

7. Titration is performed on the serum sample of the patient in question 5. The highest dilution at which agglutination is still visible is 1:64. The titer is
   a. 1:16
   b. 1:32
   c. 1:64
   d. 32
   e. 64

8. In the presence of _____ number of antibody molecules, agglutination may nor occur. This is called _____.
   a. increased/prozone
   b. decreased/prozone
   c. increased/prezone
   d. decreased/prezone

9. Use of antiglobulin to demonstrate agglutination requires _____.
   a. bound antibody with accessible Fc
   b. removal of all unbound protein
   c. free immunoglobulin with specificity for antiglobulin
   d. a and b
   e. a, b, and c

10. RBCs from a patient were tested with specific antisera to detect surface antigens and establish blood type. Agglutination results were as follows.

Anti-A	Anti-B	Anti-AB
+	−	+

    The patient's blood type is _____.
    a. A
    b. B
    c. AB
    d. O

11. A direct antiglobulin test was also performed on this patient's blood. Positive agglutination was seen. This result indicates _____.
    a. antibody is bound to patient's RBCs
    b. antigen is present in patient's serum
    c. patient may have an autoimmune disease
    d. a and c
    e. b and c

12. To lower the zeta potential and enhance agglutination, _____ may be used.
    a. low-ionic-strength saline (LISS)
    b. albumin
    c. an electric current
    d. pepsin
    e. a and b

ESSAY QUESTION

13. What are the differences between the direct and indirect antiglobulin tests and how are these two tests performed?

SUGGESTIONS FOR FURTHER READING

Macario AJL: Infectious disease immunology: Bacterial, mycotic and parasitic diseases. In: Rose, NR, Macario, EC, Fahey JL, et al, eds: Manual of Clinical Laboratory Immunology, 4th ed. Washington, DC: American Society for Microbiology, 1992;426–529

Walker RH, ed: Technical Manual, 11th ed. Bethesda: American Association of Blood Banks, 1993

Widmann FK, ed: Standards for Blood Banks and Transfusion Services, 15th ed. Bethesda: American Association of Blood Banks, 1993

REVIEW ANSWERS

1. e	5. d	9. d
2. e	6. a	10. a
3. b	7. e	11. d
4. c	8. a	12. e

18 Receptor-Ligand Assays

Receptor-ligand assays use interaction with a specific binding molecule to detect and measure target material. Immune reactions, with their exquisite sensitivity and the close steric association of antigen and antibody, are ideal for this form of assay, but other binding proteins and receptor molecules can be used for selected measurements.

INTERACTION OF RECEPTOR AND LIGAND

The definitions of receptor (or binder) and ligand are somewhat circular. A **receptor** is material with one or more sites that bind a specific target molecule; a **ligand** is a molecule capable of complexing with its specific binder. In this usage, the term receptor goes far beyond the concept of receptor molecules on cell membranes and encompasses many diverse chemical and biologic materials.

Necessary Conditions

The receptor-ligand reaction must have high affinity and specificity. **Specificity** of receptor means reaction with a single ligand and absence of reaction with similar but nonidentical molecules. **Cross-reactivity** connotes the tendency to bind molecules other than the primary ligand. **Affinity** is the strength of the forces that maintain association between the ligand and the receptor. In cross-reactions, when receptor interacts with material other than its primary ligand, the affinity is much lower than that of the primary interaction. In general, the higher the affinity between receptor and ligand, the greater the specificity and sensitivity of the assay system.

Analytic Use of Antibodies

Antibodies have many desirable properties as receptors: they can be produced against selected targets; they exhibit high specificity and affinity; they can be prepared to a high degree of purity and stability; and they can be manipulated, labeled, and otherwise modified without loss of reactivity. Some analytic techniques, instead of using antibodies, use binding proteins naturally present in serum. For example, there are naturally occurring receptors for corticosteroids, thyroglobulin, estrogens, vitamin D, and intrinsic factor. However, only a few binding proteins occur naturally, and their affinity is often too low for optimum sensitivity at low concentrations. Analysis by receptor-ligand interaction was independently developed in the late 1950s and early 1960s by Yalow and Berson, who used anti-insulin antibodies in an immunoassay for insulin, and by Ekins, who used naturally occurring thyroid-binding globulin to measure thyroid hormone.

Combination of antigen with antibody in the first stage of an immune reaction characteristically generates no immediately detectable effect. For adaptation as an assay, reacting elements must be labeled to make the end point visible. Either receptor or ligand can be labeled; however, specificity and reactivity must be preserved. For quantitative results, the magnitude of the receptor-ligand reaction must correlate with concentration of the target material to be measured. Quantitative results are obtained by constructing an activity curve with standards of known concentration. Standards are unlabeled compounds, usually the target material to be measured or substances that behave in the immunoassay very similarly to the target material. Known concentrations of the standard are added to the immunoassay, results are obtained, and the test results from the unknown analyte can then be compared with the standard.

Reactivity Without Biologic Function

One problem with immunoassays is that immunologic behavior is not always the same as biologic behavior. A molecule may express the epitope recognized by reagent antibody but may lack the configuration necessary for biologic activity. Examples of this phenomenon are frequently encountered. Immunoassays for fibrinogen can measure dysfunctional fibrinogen molecules or degradation fragments that lack coagulation activity. Partially cleaved complement components may combine with reagent antibodies but lack elements necessary to perpetuate the cascade. Tissue fluids may contain antigenic material from previously infective microorganisms despite current absence of viable organisms.

Direct Assays

Direct union of receptor and ligand is the simplest test system. If labeled receptor binds with ligand, the quantity of ligand can be directly calculated from the quantity of labeled material that is bound. The principle is simple, but it can be very difficult to control volume, concentration, and conditions of the reaction. Limits must be imposed so that units of measurement can be derived. Frequently, one reactant is immobilized on a solid phase, such as inert particles or the walls of a tube, well, or column. Most often the receptor is immobilized, and the material containing ligand is added as the unknown. It may be difficult to demonstrate union of ligand with the immobilized receptor, so a second binding agent can be added in a "sandwich" technique. After ligand completes its interaction with immobilized receptor, the system is washed to remove everything except those ligand molecules that have bound to the receptor. The "sandwich" indicator must react only with the ligand, not with the receptor or any of the solid-phase elements, and its reaction with bound ligand must not disturb the original receptor-ligand bond. When these conditions are met, the amount of labeled indicator that attaches will be directly proportional to the quantity of previously bound ligand (Fig. 18–1).

If the ligand is fixed in quantity and location, receptor can be labeled and added directly. This is done to demonstrate antigens on cell surfaces or in sections of tissue (Fig. 18–2). The label can be a fluorochrome, an enzyme, a radionuclide, or some material visible by electron microscopy. Either the specific antibody to a cell surface antigen can be labeled for **direct** demonstration. Or, a labeled antiglobulin serum can be used in an **indirect technique** to identify the site at which unlabeled reagent antibody has attached. This is discussed more fully on pages 408–411.

Competitive Binding

A **competitive binding** assay is a technique that uses, as a baseline, a known measured interaction between reagent receptor and reagent ligand. The end point or test result is the change imposed on this interaction by addition of the unknown sample.

SANDWICH TECHNIQUE
DEMONSTRATES BINDING

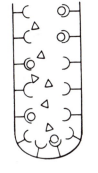

Remove
Unbound
Ligand
→
Add
Indicator

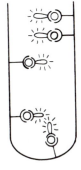

FIGURE 18–1. When mixed antigens are incubated with a single receptor, only the corresponding ligand binds to the solid-phase material (*left*). Presence of the ligand can be demonstrated by "sandwiching" with a labeled indicator material that recognizes a separately accessible binding site (*right*).

Fixed receptor binds
specific ligand

Labeled indicator
forms "sandwich" with
bound ligand

LABELED RECEPTOR BINDS TO FIXED LIGAND

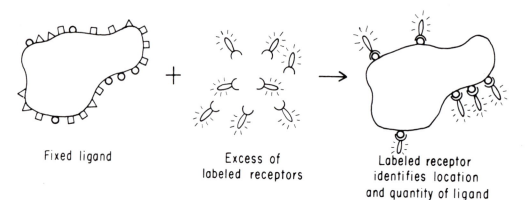

Fixed ligand

Excess of
labeled receptors

Labeled receptor
identifies location
and quantity of ligand

FIGURE 18–2. If the ligand is present in a fixed tissue preparation, direct application of a labeled receptor demonstrates the location and the quantity of the target ligand.

The degree to which the unknown alters or "competes" with the indicator reaction is proportional to the quantity of unknown. Competitive binding depends on random interaction of individual receptor and ligand molecules according to the laws of mass action. In a system containing ligand molecules that are identical in every respect except that some are labeled and some are not, the number of labeled and unlabeled molecules that bind to the receptor depends entirely on the number of labeled and unlabeled molecules in the starting material (Fig. 18–3). It is essential that the label

COMPETITIVE BINDING

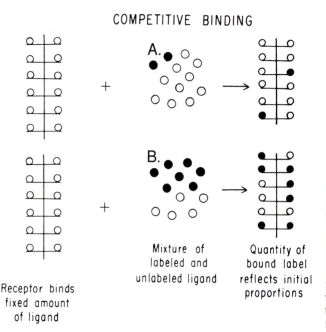

Receptor binds
fixed amount
of ligand

Mixture of
labeled and
unlabeled ligand

Quantity of
bound label
reflects initial
proportions

FIGURE 18–3. Competitive binding procedures require that the limited amount of receptor (*left*) bind labeled and unlabeled materials equally. Provided there is no preferential binding, the number of labeled and unlabeled molecules that fix to the receptor will be exactly proportional to the number present in the starting material (*center* and *right*).

not interfere or bias the binding interaction either positively or negatively. If 75 percent of ligand molecules are unlabeled and 25 percent are labeled, the receptor will bind 75 percent unlabeled molecules and 25 percent labeled. If the starting proportion changes to 50 percent labeled and 50 percent unlabeled, the bound material will be 50 percent labeled and 50 percent unlabeled, regardless of absolute concentration.

Measuring the Analyte

A limited amount of receptor can bind only a limited amount of ligand. Competitive binding procedures are standardized by determining how much label is bound after the receptor interacts with ligand that is 100 percent labeled. Ligand molecules in the unknown specimen will necessarily be unlabeled. In the test, the unknown specimen is added to a system containing a limited quantity of binder and an excess of labeled reagent ligand. The receptor binds labeled and unlabeled ligand molecules in proportion to their concentration in the starting mixture (Fig. 18–4). Unlabeled ligand molecules in the specimen will compete for receptor sites and therefore reduce the number of labeled molecules that attach to the receptor. If the unknown contains no ligand at all, the receptor will bind as much label as it did under control conditions. If the unknown contains small numbers of ligand molecules, the quantity of label binding to the receptor will be modestly reduced. If the unknown contains large amounts of the ligand, unlabeled molecules will occupy so many of the available binding sites that fixation of labeled material is markedly reduced. Competitive binding tests have been developed that use a wide range of labels, materi-

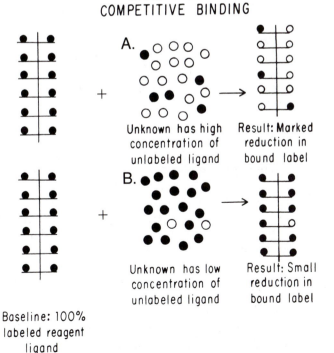

INTERPRETING COMPETITIVE BINDING

A. Unknown has high concentration of unlabeled ligand → Result: Marked reduction in bound label

B. Unknown has low concentration of unlabeled ligand → Result: Small reduction in bound label

Baseline: 100% labeled reagent ligand

FIGURE 18–4. The baseline is the quantity of label bound when the receptor is saturated with labeled reagent ligand (*left*). Labeled reagent is mixed with the unknown, in which ligand is unlabeled. Unknown sample A contains a large amount of unlabeled ligand, which severely dilutes the labeled material. A low concentration of unlabeled ligand in sample B dilutes the reagent material very little and causes little reduction in the amount of bound label available for measurement.

als that receive label, receptors, fixation procedures, and ways of measuring the end point.

Properties of Labels

A wide choice of labels can be used for either receptor or ligand. Three major categories are in use, each with advantages and disadvantages. Essential features are that the label remain attached throughout the entire test, that it not alter reactivity of the native material and that it retain its activity throughout the shelf life of the reagents.

Radioisotopes as Label

Radioactivity was the label used in the first immunoassays with the end point determined by counting radioactive emissions. The nature and number of emissions vary with the isotope used, but measurement affords a high degree of precision and sensitivity. Variables significant in selecting radioactive labels include the half-life of the radioactive element; the specific activity, which is the number of emissions per unit mass of the material; and the nature of the emission, either gamma or beta. It is usually easier to measure gamma emissions. One of the most frequently used isotopes is iodine-125 (^{125}I), a gamma emitter with a half-life of 60 days and a relatively high specific activity. ^{125}I can be linked to a variety of proteins in a stable association that damages the protein relatively little. Another gamma emitter with narrower applicability is cobalt-57 (^{57}Co), which has a half-life of 270 days. The beta emitters hydrogen-3 (^{3}H) and carbon-14 (^{14}C) have much lower specific activity than ^{125}I, and half-lives of 12.3 years and 5730 years, respectively.

Disadvantages of radioactivity as a label are that reagents lose potency as radioactivity decays; radioactivity may alter the test materials; and disposal of spent or unused materials creates problems in waste management. Fixed material must be separated from unbound material before tests are counted, because the counter cannot distinguish whether emissions come from complexed or residual label. Equipment to quantify radioactivity is expensive, and the procedures require that personnel be knowledgeable in the principles of physics and capable of stringent adherence to safety requirements.

Fluorochromes as Label

Fluorescent labels are stable and inexpensive and pose no health threat. In addition, not only fluorescence, but phosphorescence, chemiluminescence, and delayed fluorescence techniques have been developed. Both heterogeneous and homogeneous fluoroimmunoassay (FIA) procedures are available. Fluorescence is a phenomenon in which light energy is absorbed at one wavelength and then energy is dissipated with the release of light at another longer wavelength. In phosphorescence, there is a delayed release of energy. With chemiluminescence, energy in the form of light is the product of a chemical reaction. The most commonly used chemiluminescent molecules are the luminals, acridinium esters and dioxetanes. These compounds emit light when they are oxidized.

Delayed fluorescence or time-resolved fluorescence uses fluorophores with extended decay times. A fast light pulse excites the fluorophore. Fluorescence is then measured after a certain time interval has elapsed. Background and nonspecific fluorescence decays during this time interval allowing more accurate "separated" or "resolved" measurement of fluorescence associated with the immune complex.

Fluorescent techniques have several limiting factors in that they are sensitive to temperature and viscosity and biologic specimens may contain substances with natural fluorescence. Bilirubin is a good example of a serum protein with considerable natural fluorescence. Time-resolved fluorescent techniques help to minimize problems with background fluorescence, but do not completely eliminate them.

Enzymes as Label

With **enzyme labeling,** enzymatically active protein is conjugated to antigen or antibody. After immune binding occurs, the quantity of enzyme-labeled material is determined by adding substrate and measuring the intensity of the enzyme reaction—usually a color reaction. The enzyme must have specific activity that persists after conjugation and must not act on the material to which it is conjugated. The enzyme-substrate reaction must be one that is easy to observe and quantify. Enzymes are stable, inexpensive labels that can be attached to many antigens and antibodies, and they provide an end point suitable for measurement by readily available photometric equipment. One potential problem is the difficulty of conjugating one protein to another without alteration of either. Enzymes are large molecules; in some cases, their mass imposes a physical obstacle between antigen and antibody. Enzymes are highly sensitive to conditions of temperature, pH, substrate concentration, and the presence of other materials—variables that may affect accuracy and reproducibility of the quantitative assay.

Separation Systems

The principle of most immunoassays is the discrimination between bound and unbound reactants. Often these must be physically separated before the end point can be measured, but in some cases, immune-complex formation sufficiently alters the characteristics of the label so that bound and unbound constituents can be discriminated without separation. Procedures that determine the end point without separating the reactants are called **homogeneous assays.** Those requiring separation are described as **heterogeneous assays.** An example is shown in Figure 18–5. Homogeneous assays are generally more useful for small analytes such as drugs and thyroid and steroid hormones. Heterogeneous immunoassays are more versatile. The required separation step eliminates interfering substances. A larger sample size can be used, and therefore greater sensitivity can be obtained.

Physical Manipulation

Bound and unreacted materials may have different physical properties that facilitate separation. Bound material characteristically forms larger complexes and can often be isolated by centrifugation. Some assays measure unbound label remaining in the supernatant, whereas others measure the quantity of label incorporated in the bound material sedimented by centrifugation. More elaborate separation techniques exploit differences in molecular size, as in gel filtration, or differences in charge and configuration, as in electrophoresis. Either the complexed or the unre-

HETEROGENEOUS ASSAY

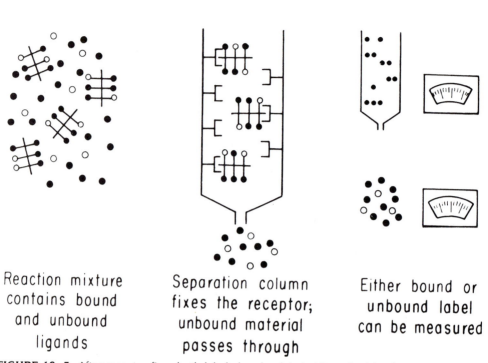

| Reaction mixture contains bound and unbound ligands | Separation column fixes the receptor; unbound material passes through | Either bound or unbound label can be measured |

FIGURE 18–5. After receptor fixes both labeled and unlabeled ligands (*left*), it is often necessary to separate ligand that remains unbound from the molecules attached to the receptor. A separation column (*center*) is one way to effect physical separation. Labeled material is present in both the bound and unbound fractions (*right*). The magnitude of the receptor-ligand interaction can be determined by measuring either fraction.

acted materials may preferentially adhere to solid-phase material like charcoal, resins, or silicates, which facilitate removal by centrifugation or filtration. Various types of membranes can be used to trap reactants. Physical differences can sometimes be induced if they do not occur spontaneously, as, for example, by precipitating proteins with nonspecific agents such as ammonium sulfate or various alcohols.

Immune Manipulation

A common technique is to introduce a second antibody that engages either a bound or unbound phase of the reaction mixture. Sometimes soluble antibody is introduced to induce precipitation or agglutination, but more often the separating antibody is in a solid phase, bound to particles or to the walls of a column, tube, well, or disk. Staphylococcal protein A, which has receptors specific for the Fc portion of IgG, can be used as a separatory binder if IgG is one of the reactants (Fig. 18–6).

STAPHYLOCOCCAL PROTEIN A BINDS IgG

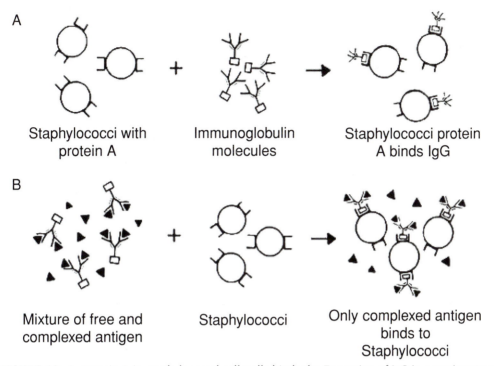

A

Staphylococci with
protein A

Immunoglobulin
molecules

Staphylococci protein
A binds IgG

B

Mixture of free and
complexed antigen

Staphylococci

Only complexed antigen
binds to
Staphylococci

FIGURE 18–6. Protein A in staphylococcal cell walls binds the Fc portion of IgG in a nonimmune fashion (*panel* A). This phenomenon can be used as a separation technique. Immunoglobulin adheres to the organisms, bringing with it antigen bound to the Fab sites (*panel* B). Removing the particulate organisms removes the antigen-antibody complexes and leaves behind antigen that has not combined with antibody. Antigen bound to protein A via IgG can be isolated and quantitated.

SOME SELECTED PROCEDURES

Immunologists and immunochemists have displayed remarkable ingenuity in adapting receptor-ligand interactions to analytic purposes. This section considers a few widely used techniques, but the list is far from exhaustive.

Radioimmunoassay

Radioimmunoassay (RIA) is a general term comprising several different applications. Radioimmunoassay is used for competitive-binding techniques and for direct demonstration of antigen-antibody attachment.

Labeled Ligand

The most common RIA is a **competitive binding procedure** in which the unknown is measured as ligand. The test system consists of a limited amount of antibody and a radiolabeled reagent ligand (Fig. 18–7). The ligand or antigen is commonly labeled with a gamma emitter such as ^{125}I. The first step in RIA testing is to determine the amount of radioactivity bound when the limited number of antibody sites combine fully with labeled ligand. Because antibody binds labeled and unlabeled molecules in whatever proportions exist in the reaction mixture, adding unlabeled unknown to the reaction mixture reduces fixation of radioactivity. After the reaction reaches equilibrium, bound and unbound material is separated.

Measurement can determine either the level of radioactivity complexed to antibody or the activity that remains unbound. If bound material is measured, the radioactivity count will vary inversely with the amount of ligand in the unknown. Small amounts of unlabeled ligand allow large amounts of activity to remain as captured reagent label, whereas high levels in the unknown compete successfully for most of the binding sites. If the end point is radioactivity left unbound, the number of counts is directly proportional to the quantity of the unknown; increasing levels of unlabeled material occupy increasing numbers of binding sites, causing progressively more radioactive material to remain unbound and to be counted. A standard curve is plotted of the percentage of bound labeled antigen versus known concentration of unlabeled antigen. From the standard curve, unknown concentrations of unlabeled antigen can be determined.

Competitive binding RIA can be used to screen for the presence of hepatitis B in donor blood for transfusion purposes. Microtiter wells are coated with a constant amount of antibody specific for a surface antigen on the hepatitis B virus (HBsAg). A

COMPETITIVE RADIOIMMUNOASSAY

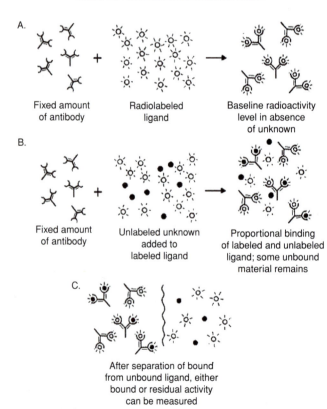

A.

Fixed amount
of antibody

Radiolabeled
ligand

Baseline radioactivity
level in absence
of unknown

B.

Fixed amount
of antibody

Unlabeled unknown
added to
labeled ligand

Proportional binding
of labeled and unlabeled
ligand; some unbound
material remains

C.

After separation of bound
from unbound ligand, either
bound or residual activity
can be measured

FIGURE 18–7. (*Panel* A) The first step in competitive radioimmunoassay is determining baseline radioactivity when receptor antibody is saturated with labeled ligand. *Panel* B shows how incubation with a mixture of labeled and unlabeled ligand alters the level of bound radioactivity. *Panel* C shows that the result can be expressed as the change in level of bound label or as the quantity of label left unbound.

serum sample and ^{125}I-labeled HBsAg are added to a microtiter well. After incubation, the supernatant is removed, and the amount of radioactivity bound to the antibody in the well is determined. An infected serum sample with HBsAg will displace labeled HBsAg and the amount of radioactivity measured will be less than in control wells with uninfected serum.

Labeled Antibody

If label is attached to antibody rather than to ligand, the term **immunoradiomimetric assay (IRMA)** is sometimes used. The competitive binding principle is the same, but the baseline is the amount of labeled antibody that fixes to a limited amount of solid-phase antigen. The test begins by incubating soluble labeled antibody with soluble unknown ligand. If there is antigen in the unknown, it will bind to Fab sites of the labeled antibody. The incubated mixture is then added to the immobilized reagent antigen; only those labeled antibody molecules that have not already bound antigen present in the unknown can combine with the fixed antigen. Labeled antibody is allowed to bind with the solid-phase antigen, and unbound material is washed away. The radioactivity bound to the solid-phase antigen is inversely proportional to the amount of ligand present in the unknown (Fig. 18-8).

The **sandwich** form of RIA characteristically starts with unlabeled antibody immobilized to a solid phase. The unknown specimen is added, and any ligand present binds to the solid-phase antibody. After attachment of ligand molecules and removal of unbound material, a radiolabeled second antibody is added. The ligand must have at least two epitopes, one that binds to the solid-phase antibody and the other available to react with the labeled indicator antibody. Indicator antibody adheres wherever a ligand molecule has attached to the original antibody; the amount of radioactivity bound is directly proportional to the quantity of unknown ligand. Two separation steps are necessary: one after incubation of ligand with solid-phase antibody and the other to remove indicator antibody that has not attached to the immobilized ligand.

Sandwich RIA can be used to measure unknown antibody by reversing the positions of the reagents. Unknown serum is incubated with unlabeled antigen prepared as the solid phase. Antibody molecules in the serum unite with fixed antigen. Immunoglobulin (Ig) that binds to the solid-phase antigen can be detected with radiolabeled antiglobulin serum. If the test is performed twice—once with labeled anti-IgM and once with anti-IgG—the levels of each antibody class can be compared.

Enzyme-Labeled Procedures

The two principal applications of enzyme labeling are **enzyme-linked immunosorbent assay (ELISA)** or **(EIA)** and **enzyme-multiplied immunoassay test (EMIT)**. In the ELISA, enzyme performs exactly the same labeling function as the radioactivity in RIA. Enzyme is coupled to one of the immune reactants; addition of substrate after the primary reaction indicates how much labeled material has entered the complex (Fig. 18-9). ELISA procedures are heterogeneous; unbound labeled material must be removed before measuring the end point. The procedure called EMIT is homogeneous. The enzyme used is one that changes reactivity depending on the bound or unbound state of the underlying molecule. Alteration in enzyme function thus reflects the degree of immune binding, and the materials need not be physically separated.

IMMUNORADIOMIMETRIC ASSAY

(IRMA)

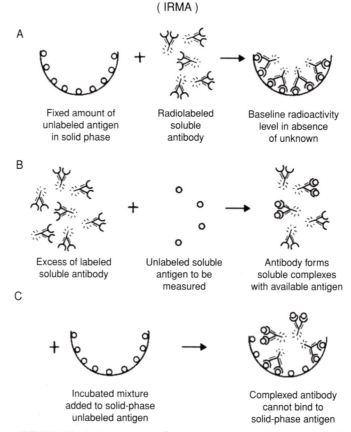

FIGURE 18–8. In immunoradiomimetric assays, the receptor is labeled and both the reagent ligand and the ligand present in the unknown are unlabeled. *Panel* A shows the baseline level of radioactivity when labeled antibody combines with a limited quantity of fixed, unlabeled ligand. In *panel* B, the antibody reacts with unlabeled material in the unknown solution. All the antigen present unite with Fab sites of the labeled antibody. *Panel* C shows that antibody molecules complexed with ligand from the unknown are unable to react with the solid-phase antigen. The reduction of bound radioactivity reflects the amount of soluble ligand in the unknown.

ELISAs are replacing RIAs in the laboratory because of simplicity and versatility. Their use in physicians' offices and even home test kits has expanded. ELISAs are similar in sensitivity to RIAs and do not have the problems of short half-life of isotopes and disposal and handling of radioactive wastes. Increasing use of ELISA techniques is also due to availability of monoclonal antibodies and antigens produced by recombinant DNA techniques, and abilities to automate steps in ELISA procedures.

Competitive ELISA Techniques

Like RIA, ELISA can be used for competitive binding or direct reactions. In competitive binding assays, the reactant in limited quantity is usually solid-phase bound antibody. Enzyme-labeled reagent ligand and unlabeled ligand in the unknown are

ENZYME - LABELED IMMUNOSORBENT ASSAY (ELISA)

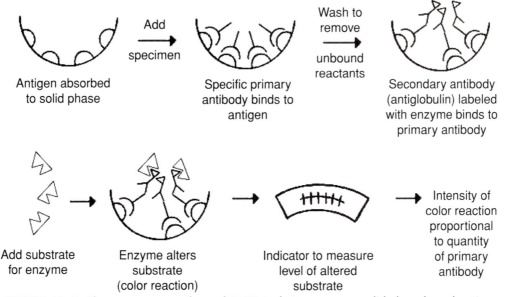

FIGURE 18–9. The most common form of ELISA techniques uses a solid-phase bound antigen and enzyme-labeled secondary antibody. Labeled secondary antibody (antiglobulin) will bind only to primary antibody. With addition of substrate and chromogen, a colored reaction product is formed, which can be measured. A color reaction occurs only if primary antibody is present in the specimen. The amount of primary antibody is directly proportional to the intensity of the color reaction.

incubated with a limited quantity of antibody. After immune binding occurs, unbound material is removed. Enzyme is thus immobilized on the solid phase at sites where reagent ligand has combined with antibody; substrate is then added to determine the amount of enzyme-labeled ligand present (Fig. 18–10). The end point of the enzyme-substrate reaction must be readily quantifiable, usually a color change but sometimes a change in state of fluorescence.

Sometimes the solid-phase material is antigen, the unknown to be measured is antigen, and antibody carries the enzyme label. The baseline is the binding of la-

FIGURE 18-10. In competitive binding ELISA, the end point is the degree to which admixture with unlabeled ligand reduces the previously established level of enzyme activity. Only two steps are necessary: (1) incubating the fixed receptor with a mixture of reagent and unknown ligand and (2) adding the substrate to determine the level of enzyme present.

COMPETITVE BINDING ELISA

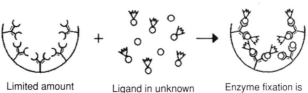

Limited amount of fixed binder

Ligand in unknown mixed with labeled ligand

Enzyme fixation is proportional to labeled-to-unlabeled ratio

beled antibody to the limited quantity of immobilized antigen. The labeled antibody is incubated with a solution of the unknown material, providing an opportunity for antigen molecules to complex with Fab sites of the labeled antibody. After incubation, only unoccupied Fab sites are left to bind with the reagent antigen; the amount of enzyme bound to solid-phase antigen is inversely proportional to antigen concentration in the unknown.

Noncompetitive Indirect ELISA Techniques

Noncompetitive indirect ELISAs are the most widely used of ELISA techniques. They can be used to detect and quantify antibody or antigen. When used for detection of antibody, serum or another source of antibody is added to an antigen-coated microtiter well. Antibody is allowed to bind with solid-phase bound antigen. Unbound antibody and other proteins are washed away, and the presence of antibody bound to antigen is detected with an enzyme-labeled antiglobulin secondary antibody. Any free secondary antibody is washed away and a substrate for the enzyme is added. Enzymatic activity on the substrate produces a colored reaction product that can be measured in a spectrophotometer. Intensity of the color reaction is directly proportional to the number of antibody molecules combined with solid-phase antigen.

Noncompetitive indirect ELISA is the method most commonly used for detection of serum antibodies to HIV. Recombinant forms of viral envelope and core proteins are adsorbed onto beads in microtiter wells. Individuals infected with HIV produce antibodies that will bind to epitopes on the viral proteins. HIV antibodies are then detected with enzyme-labeled anti–human Ig.

If antibody is attached to a solid phase and antigen is then bound and quantitated, these assays are referred to as **capture** or **sandwich assays.** A sample containing antigen is added to a well and allowed to react with solid-phase–bound antibody. The well is washed to remove unbound reactants, and a second enzyme-labeled antibody specific for a different epitope on the antigen is added and allowed to bind. Any free second antibody is then removed by washing. Substrate is added and the colored reaction product measured. Capture ELISAs can be used for detection of innumerable types of antigen as long as the antigen has at least two epitopes and as long as antibodies for binding to these epitopes are available. Examples of assays using this technique are ELISAs for detection of cytokines. Capture ELISAs for interleukin-1 (IL-1), IL-2, IL-6, and tumor necrosis factor (TNF) are commercially available.

Immunohistochemical Staining

Enzyme-labeled or fluorescent-labeled antibodies can be used to identify and localize antigens in tissue sections. Polyclonal or monoclonal antibodies labeled with a fluorescent dye have been in use for many years. Immunofluorescent staining is generally not as sensitive as enzyme-labeled staining techniques and is difficult to perform on fixed tissue. A fluorescence microscope is also required for visualization of fluorescent antibody bound to tissue antigens. Enzyme-labeled antibodies useful for histologic staining include those conjugated with peroxidase, alkaline phosphatase, or glucose oxidase. With immunohistochemical staining, direct or indirect techniques may be used. Enzyme-labeled antibody may be bound directly to antigens in tissue sections, or unlabeled antibody is bound to tissue antigen. The immune complex is then detected by binding of a second labeled antibody (antiglobulin). Subsequent addition of substrate and color reagent results in deposition of colored reaction product at the site of antibody binding. Use of biotin as a label allows amplification of the initial antibody binding site because biotin will bind a glycoprotein called **avidin.** Avidin has four binding sites for biotin; therefore, aggregates of avidin-biotin complexes with attached enzymes will bind to biotinylated antibody (Fig. 18–11). Most staining techniques using avidin-biotin are indirect with the secondary antibody or antiglobulin biotinylated. Indirect labeling techniques are particularly useful if primary antibody is in limited supply. Binding of a small amount of diluted primary antibody is then detectable by usually a much cheaper and readily available enzyme-labeled antiglobulin.

Detection of tissue antigens is more sensitive with frozen sections. However, techniques have been developed with enzyme-labeled antibodies that allow localization of antigen in formalin-fixed paraffin sections. Tissue sections stained with enzyme-labeled antibody can be permanently mounted, cover-slipped, and observed with a regular light microscope. Antibodies associated with autoimmune diseases and detection of cell-surface markers and tumor antigens are common applications of enzyme-labeled immunohistochemical techniques.

Immunoelectronmicroscopy

Labeled antibody techniques have also been applied to electron microscopy. To visualize binding of antibody, an electron-dense label such as ferritin or colloidal gold must be conjugated either to the primary antibody or to an antiglobulin reagent antibody. The electron-dense ferritin or colloidal gold absorb electrons and appear as small black dots wherever antibody binding has occurred. Immunoelectronmicroscopy has been very useful for localizing intracellular proteins, elucidating trans-

IMMUNOHISTOCHEMICAL STAINING
USING AVIDIN AND BIOTIN

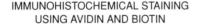

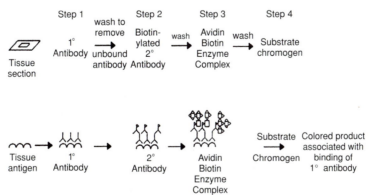

FIGURE 18–11. Immunohistochemical staining is a multistep procedure. Use of a biotinylated secondary antibody allows for amplification and therefore easier detection of the binding site for primary antibody. Immunohistochemical detection and localization of antigens and antibodies in tissue are primarily qualitative evaluations; however, with computer-assisted image analysis, quantitative evaluation is also possible.

port mechanisms within a cell, and understanding major histocompatibility complex (MHC) class I and II antigen-processing pathways.

Enzyme-Multiplied Immunoassay Techniques

The term **enzyme-multiplied immunoassay technique (EMIT)** is misleading; the antigen-antibody reaction is not multiplied. The enzyme-multiplied immunoassay test is a competitive binding assay in which the enzyme label is applied to reagent antigen. Its widest use is the measurement of drug levels. Enzyme is attached to the reagent drug in a configuration that allows the enzyme to remain active when drug molecules are free in solution but causes it to lose activity if the underlying drug molecule complexes with its antibody. The material present in limited quantity is unlabeled antibody specific for the drug. Competition for antibody sites occurs between the labeled reagent drug and unlabeled drug molecules in the unknown. As with all competitive assays, binding of labeled reagent diminishes as the concentration of ligand in the unknown increases.

With EMIT assays, which are homogeneous, binding of labeled drug can be measured without a separation step because enzyme on the bound molecules loses its ability to convert substrate (Fig. 18–12). Enzyme activity declines with increasing fixation of labeled reagent. Increasing levels of drug in the unknown reduces fixation of labeled reagent, so the measurable level of enzyme activity is directly propor-

BINDING STATE AFFECTS LABEL ACTIVITY

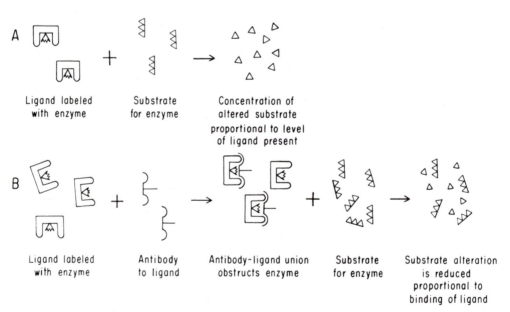

FIGURE 18–12. With molecules of suitable configuration, activity of the enzyme changes if the underlying molecule enters an immune complex. *Panel* A depicts an enzyme-labeled molecule that retains full activity. *Panel* B shows how antibody to the ligand molecule can hinder activity of the attached enzyme. In *Panel* B, two-thirds of the labeled ligand molecules have united with antibody, and a corresponding proportion of substrate remains unaffected.

tional to the drug level in the unknown. If the unknown has low concentration, most of the labeled reagent unites with antibody, loses its reactivity, and exhibits low substrate conversion. A high level of unknown prevents reagent drug from entering a complex, so the numerous unbound molecules retain ability to convert large amounts of substrate.

Fluorescent-Labeled Procedures

Fluorescence is emission of light at one wavelength after electrons of the susceptible substance have been excited by exposure to light at a different wavelength. In fluorescent compounds, called **fluorophores** or **fluorochromes,** the electrons oscillate to produce energy detectable as emission of longer wavelengths than the light absorbed. The exciting wavelengths are usually in the ultraviolet spectrum, and emitted light is in the visible spectrum. Fluorophores useful in the laboratory include **fluorescein isothiocyanate (FITC),** which emits a green light, and **rhodamine,** which emits red light. Equipment for detection and measurement uses filters to remove all but the desired excitation wavelength and to provide optimum detection of the emitted light.

Types of Tests

Fluorochromes can be conjugated to antibody so that fluorescence will be directly proportional to the number of antibody molecules present. Antibody-mediated fluorescence can be evaluated in qualitative, semiquantitative, or quantitative fashion, depending on the fluorometric devices used. Quantitative fluorescence procedures use sandwich or competitive principles, which are the same as those for radioactive or enzyme-labeled assays. Fluorescence often varies with physical conditions and with the configuration of the underlying protein. These variables can be exploited to develop homogeneous assays, in which bound and unbound materials need not be separated before measuring the end point.

Fluorescent-labeled antibodies are useful in qualitative procedures to identify and to locate antigens in tissue or on microorganisms. For example, immune complexes deposited in tissue can be demonstrated and characterized with fluorescence-labeled antibodies to Ig or to complement. Labeled antibody attaches wherever the proteins have deposited and can be observed with a fluorescence microscope. Goodpasture's syndrome is an autoimmune disease characterized by binding of autoantibodies specific to basement-membrane antigens in the kidney glomeruli and alveoli of the lung. Autoantibody in biopsy tissue from kidney or lung of a patient with Goodpasture's syndrome can be detected by immunohistochemical staining with a fluorescence-labeled anti-IgG.

Direct versus Indirect

It is customary to classify fluorescence microscopy into **direct** and **indirect** techniques. In direct procedures, the fluorescent label is attached to the specific antibody directed against target antigen. These are one-step tests: fluorescent antibody is layered on the slide preparation where it combines with its target antigen. Be-

DIRECT IMMUNOFLUORESCENCE

IS ANTIGEN ON CELL OR TISSUE?

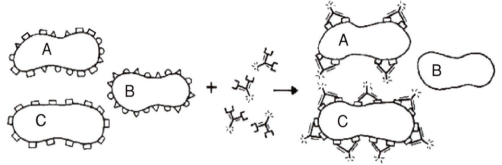

FIGURE 18–13. When fluorescent-labeled antibody is incubated with fixed cells or tissue, it attaches where its antigen is expressed in the specimen. In the drawing, fluorescence completely outlines structure B but adheres at only a few locations to structure A. Structure C has many surface antigens, but none has the specificity recognized by the labeled antibody.

cause the antibody recognizes no other target, no other tissue elements will be labeled and fluorescence outlines exactly where antigen is present (Fig. 18–13). This requires a separate labeled antibody specific for each target antigen. Indirect fluorescence procedures require two steps. First, unlabeled antibody is applied to the slide where it can recognize and combine with specific antigen. The slide is then washed to remove unbound antibody and all other extraneous proteins. The second step is addition of fluorescence-labeled antiglobulin serum, which combines with the Fc portion of bound antibody molecules. Only one reagent needs to be labeled, the fluorescent antiglobulin, which will react with any antibody that has bound to antigens on the slide (Fig. 18–14). An example is the identification of tubulin in a mitotic cell. Monoclonal antitubulin antibodies are made from mouse hybridoma cells. Antitubulin antibodies bind to mitotic spindle formations in cells, but can not be detected until fluorescence-labeled antiglobulin to mouse IgG is added.

Characterizing Antigens

Direct fluorescence is used in diagnosing conditions characterized by antibody attachment or deposition of immune complexes or abnormal proteins. Testing requires knowledge of which proteins are likely to be present, so as to select labeled antibodies of those specificities. Most commonly used are antibodies against Ig isotypes; against complement components; and against fibrinogen, amyloid, and other materials associated with inflammation. Direct fluorescence microscopy is also used to diagnose and to identify microorganisms. Because the fluorescent label is easy to locate, the technique is helpful in demonstrating small numbers of organisms in tissue preparations or in mixed microbial populations. Direct fluorescence microscopy also identifies individual strains of organisms by their reactions with a battery of selected specific antisera (Fig. 18–15). An example is a direct technique

INDIRECT IMMUNOFLUORESCENCE

IS ANTIGEN PRESENT IN TISSUE?

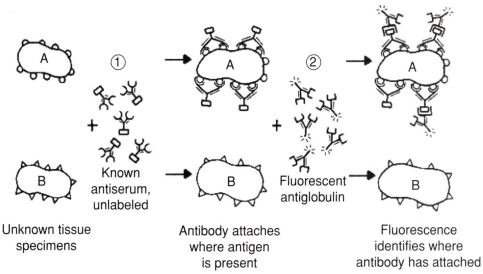

FIGURE 18–14. Indirect immunofluorescence requires two steps. Adding fluorescent-labeled antiglobulin serum is the second; the first is incubating unknown material with unlabeled antibody of known specificity. In the example here, the antibody combines, in a reaction that cannot be observed, with antigen present on structure A but not on structure B. The reaction is made visible when fluorescent antiglobulin serum unites with antibody bound to A, but fails to react with structure B.

DIRECT IMMUNOFLUORESCENCE

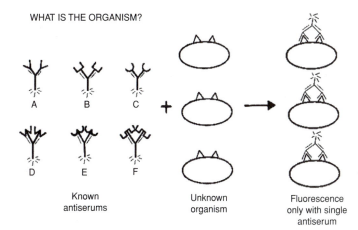

FIGURE 18–15. Immunofluorescent identification of unknown microorganisms uses a battery of known antiserums, each labeled with fluorochrome. Separate preparations of the unknown are incubated with each antiserum. In this example, the organism is strain A. The other antibodies do not encounter antigens with which they can react.

is the use of a labeled antibody for identification of the fungus *Coccidioides immitis* in a clinical specimen. Highly specific antibodies are available commercially that eliminate cross-reactions with related fungal antigens.

Identifying Antibodies

Indirect fluorescence is used to examine serum for the presence of antibodies, especially those associated with autoimmune conditions. Specificities often studied include antibodies against tissue-specific antigens such as pancreas, colon, or thyroid, or against internal cellular elements such as deoxyribonucleic acid (DNA), ribonucleic acid (RNA), mitochondrial constituents, or smooth muscle antigens. Indirect fluorescence for antibody testing requires a preparation of tissue or fixed cells on which antigen is expressed. Serum is incubated with the slide to allow antibodies, if present, to combine with their antigen; unbound proteins must be washed away before antiglobulin serum is added. If the serum contained antibodies against antigens on the slide, the fluorescent antiglobulin reagent finds bound Igs with which to unite. If no antibodies are present, the antiglobulin serum finds no suitable target and no fluorescence will adhere (Fig. 18–16). Detection of antinuclear

INDIRECT IMMUNOFLUORESCENCE

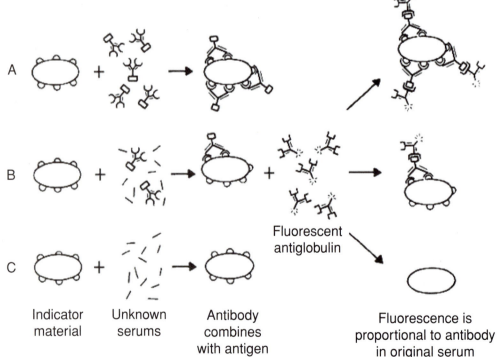

FIGURE 18–16. Indirect immunofluorescence can demonstrate and quantify antibody in an unknown serum. After serum is incubated with an indicator preparation of known antigen, fluorescent antiglobulin serum unites with whatever antibody has attached to the reagent material. In this example, serum A contains a large amount of antibody, serum B contains a small amount of antibody, and serum C contains no immunoglobulin that reacts with the reagent material.

antibodies (ANA) in systemic lupus erythematosus commonly uses an indirect fluorescence procedure. Patient serum is incubated with animal or human cells fixed to a slide. Unbound antibodies are carefully washed from the slide preparation, and presence of ANA is visualized with addition of a fluorescence-labeled antihuman Ig. If the patient is negative for ANA, no fluorescence is observed. Positive nuclear fluo-

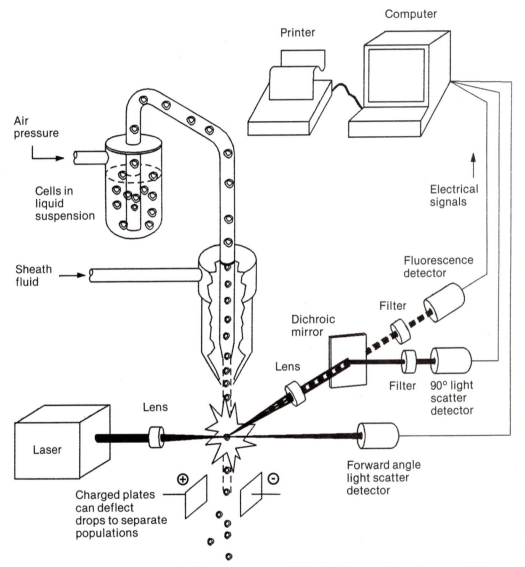

FIGURE 18–17. Components of a flow cytometer include a fluid system for cell transportation, a laser for cell illumination, photodetectors for signal detection, and a computer to collect and analyze data. Cells introduced into the instrument are suspended in a sheath fluid and then flow in single file past the laser beam. As each cell interrupts the laser beam, it is counted, associated fluorescence detected, or the cell characterized as to size and type based on its forward and sidelight scattering properties. As cells exit the detector, they can be enclosed in a droplet that is electrically charged in proportion to their fluorescence. The charged droplets are then separated (sorted) as they flow past deflector plates. (From Stevens: Clinical Immunology and Serology: A Laboratory Perspective. Philadelphia: FA Davis Company, 1996:37, with permission.)

rescence can appear in a variety of patterns, which requires additional training for interpretation.

The **fluorescent treponemal antibody (FTA)** test, a serologic test for syphilis, uses indirect immunofluorescence. The reagent slide containing a fixed suspension of organisms is incubated with the patient's serum. Fluorescent antiglobulin serum adheres to any antibody molecules that have bound to the organisms. Problems with this procedure, as with all indirect fluorescence tests, are nonspecific adherence of unwanted proteins and the possible presence of antibodies that cross-react with the intended antigen or organism.

Fluorescence in Flow Cytometry

Direct and indirect immunofluorescence techniques have proved very useful in **flow cytometry.** A flow cytometer is an instrument that identifies cells by their distinctive light-scattering profiles as they flow in single file past a laser beam. Cells are transported in a sheath fluid through a small opening (aperture). As a cell passes through a laser beam, light is scattered in many directions. Optical detectors are positioned at different angles to detect this scattered light. The amount of forward scattered light can be correlated with cell size, whereas side scatter is associated with granularity. In addition, cell-associated fluorescence can be detected. Fluorescence-labeled antibodies can bind to antigens expressed on cell membranes. Flow cytometers are also known as fluorescence-activated cell sorters (FACS). Flow cytometers can quantify the fluorescence emitted as individual cells flow through the aperture. With appropriate wavelengths and filters it is possible to measure two different emission spectrums at the same time, allowing simultaneous use of two different fluorescence reagents (Fig. 18–17).

Direct fluorescence is extremely useful for characterizing cell-surface and cytoplasmic properties. Cell suspensions can be prepared from body fluids or from solid tissues carefully dissociated into individual cells and can be labeled with a fluorescent antibody. The most common application of fluorescence flow cytometry is enumeration of CD4 and CD8 lymphocytes, but almost any antigen can be studied if a specific antibody exists and the target cells can be suspended in a carrier fluid.

SUMMARY

1. A receptor has one or more sites that will specifically bind a ligand. This interaction between receptor and ligand can be used for the assay of many diverse chemical and biologic materials. Conditions necessary for receptor-ligand assays are specificity without cross-reactivity, high affinity and capability to label one or the other reactants without affecting reactivity.

2. For direct assay, the receptor is usually immobilized on a solid phase. Ligand is added as the unknown. The quantity of ligand is then calculated from the quantity of labeled material that is bound. Binding of ligand to receptor can be detected by a second binding agent to form a "sandwich." All unbound ligand must be removed so that the amount of bound second agent is proportional to the quantity of previously bound ligand.

3. With competitive binding assays, a baseline must be established for known amounts of reagent receptor and ligand. Addition of unknown sample will "compete" with binding of reagent receptor and ligand. The degree to which the reaction is altered is proportional to the quantity of unknown reactant.

4. Labels to detect the interaction of receptors and ligands must remain attached throughout the test, must not alter the reactivity of the native material, and must retain activity throughout the shelf life of the reagent. Types of labels include radioisotopes, fluorochromes, and enzymes, which produce a detectable, quantifiable reaction product on reaction with a suitable substrate.

5. With some assays, it is necessary to physically separate bound and unbound reactants to measure the end point (heterogeneous assay). With other assay systems, separation may not be necessary because immune-complex formation sufficiently alters the characteristics of the label (homogeneous assay). Methods of separation include centrifugation, gel filtration, electrophoresis, adherence to a solid phase, and use of a second antibody (antiglobulin) or staphylococcal protein A to a solid phase.

6. Radioimmunoassays use a radioactive label to detect immune-complex formation or displacement by unlabeled reactant as in competitive binding assays. If a limited amount of antibody is combined with a known amount of radioactively labeled ligand, addition of unlabeled ligand will reduce the amount of bound labeled ligand. Increasing amounts of unbound radioactivity is directly proportional to the quantity of unknown unlabeled ligand. Hepatitis B antigen in patient serum can be measured using this procedure.

7. Immunoradiomimetric assay (IRMA) is a modification of competitive binding radioimmunoassays (RIAs) whereby soluble labeled antibody is incubated with an unknown quantity of ligand. The mixture is added to immobilized reagent antigen. Any labeled antibody that has not bound antigen from the unknown sample will bind to reagent antigen. Amount of radioactivity associated with immobilized reagent is inversely proportional to the amount of ligand.

8. Sandwich RIAs consist of unlabeled antibody immobilized to a solid phase. An unknown quantity of ligand is added. With addition of a second radiolabeled antibody, which binds to another epitope of the ligand, the amount of bound radioactivity is directly proportional to the amount of unknown ligand. Sandwich RIAs can also consist of solid-phase antigen to which serum antibody binds. Bound antibody is then detected with radiolabeled antiglobulin serum.

9. Enzyme-linked immunosorbent assays (ELISAs) are similar to RIAs except that an enzyme is used in place of a radioactive label. ELISAs avoid the problems of disposal and handling of radioactive wastes. Competitive binding, sandwich, and EMIT techniques all can be used with enzyme-labeled reactants. Noncompetitive indirect ELISA is the technique most commonly used for detection of serum antibodies to HIV. Viral proteins are immobilized to a solid phase. Individuals infected with HIV produce HIV antibodies that bind to viral epitopes. HIV antibodies are then detected with enzyme-labeled anti–human immunoglobulin (Ig).

Continued on the following page

10. Antigens may also be localized in tissue sections using enzyme-labeled antibody. Immunohistochemical staining with labeled polyclonal or monoclonal antibody binds antibody directly to antigenic sites in the tissue, or antigenic sites can be visualized with an indirect technique using a second labeled antibody (antiglobulin). Immunohistochemical staining is applicable to light and electron microscopy. Cell-surface markers, tumor antigens, and hormones are only a few of the possible molecules that can be identified and localized.

11. Fluorochromes such as fluoroscein isothiocyanate (FITC) and rhodamine can be conjugated to antibody and used in direct and indirect assay procedures. Fluorometric devices for quantitating the amount of bound antibody are available. Fluorescence-conjugated antibody can also be used to localize antigen on cells and in tissue sections. Individual cells in suspension labeled with a fluorescent antibody can be characterized and quantitated in a flow cytometer.

REVIEW QUESTIONS

1. In general, the higher the _____ between receptor and ligand, the greater the sensitivity of the assay system.
   a. specificity
   b. cross-reactivity
   c. affinity
   d. reactivity
   e. connectivity

2. To identify the presence of immune complexes in the kidney of a patient with Goodpasture's syndrome, _____ reagent(s) is/are needed.
   a. monoclonal antibodies to human CRI conjugated to fluoroscein isothiocyanate (FITC)
   b. ^{125}I-labeled antiglobulin
   c. antihuman IgG conjugated to FITC
   d. peroxidase coupled to antitubulin antibodies
   e. latex particles coated with protein A

3. Reagent(s) necessary for performing the HIV screening test by ELISA include(s) _____.
   a. enzyme-labeled antihuman globulin
   b. anti-HIV antibody bound to microtiter wells
   c. electrophoretic gel
   d. protein A bound to a separation column
   e. a and b

4. What is the first step in competitive radioimmunoassays (RIAs) or enzyme-linked immunosorbent assays (ELISAs)?
   a. After separation of bound from unbound ligand residual, bound antibody is measured.
   b. Determine baseline radioactivity when antibody is saturated with labeled ligand.
   c. Add unlabeled unknown to labeled ligand.
   d. Proportional binding of labeled and unlabeled ligand occurs.
   e. Add second antibody.

5. A blood sample is positive for hepatitis B surface antigen (HBsAg) as measured by competitive binding RIA. The amount of radioactivity bound to antibody in the well is _____ compared with that of baseline controls.
   a. increased
   b. decreased

6. A blood sample is positive for HIV using a noncompetitive indirect ELISA technique. Positivity is determined by _____.
   a. presence of colored reaction product in the well
   b. presence of precipitated immune complex in the well
   c. absence of color in the well
   d. increased light scatter
   e. emission of fluorescent light

7. Avidin-biotin labeling is used for _____ and produces _____.
   a. immunohistochemical staining for light microscopy . . . colored compound
   b. immunoelectronmicroscopy staining . . . an electron-dense precipitate
   c. enzyme-multiplied immunoassay (EMIT) procedures . . . precipitate
   d. flow cytometry . . . fluorescent green light
   e. a and b

8. Disadvantages of radioactive labels include _____.
   a. loss of potentency with radioactive decay
   b. expensive detection equipment
   c. necessity for heterogeneous test procedure
   d. a and b
   e. a, b, and c

9. With _____, energy in the form of light generated by a chemical reaction is measured.
   a. fluorescence
   b. phosphorescence
   c. chemiluminescence
   d. EMIT procedures
   e. immunoradiomimetric assay (IRMA) procedures

10. Examples of fluorescent label(s) include:
    a. FITC
    b. rhodamine
    c. luminals
    d. a and b
    e. a, b, and c

11. Limiting factor(s) for fluorescence labeling techniques include _____.
    a. sensitivity to temperature
    b. expensive equipment for fluorescence detection
    c. presence of natural fluorescent materials
    d. a and b
    e. a, b, and c

ESSAY QUESTIONS

12. Explain what the following statement means: Immunologic behavior in an immunoassay may not always reflect biologic behavior.

13. What is the difference between a homogeneous and a heterogeneous assay? Provide an example of each and describe how each assay is performed.

14. What is the difference between a competitive and noncompetitive binding assay. Provide an example of each and describe how each assay is performed.

SUGGESTIONS FOR FURTHER READING

Betts Carpenter A: Enzyme-linked immunoassays. In: Rose NR, Demacario EC, Fahey JL, et al, eds: Manual of Clinical Laboratory Immunology, 4th ed. Washington, DC: American Society for Microbiology, 1992:2–9

Chan DW: Immunoassay Automation: A Practical Guide. San Diego: Academic Press, 1992:3–11

Gosling JP: Introduction to immunoassay. In: Gosling JP, Basso LV, eds: Immunoassay: Laboratory Analysis and Clinical Applications. Boston: Butterworth-Heineman, 1994:1–25

Stevens CD: Clinical Immunology and Serology: A Laboratory Perspective. Philadelphia: F. A. Davis Company, 1996:37–38

Yalow RS: Radioimmunoassay: A probe for fine structure of biologic systems. Science. 200:1231–1245, 1978.

REVIEW ANSWERS

1. c   7. a
2. c   8. e
3. a   9. c
4. b   10. d
5. b   11. e
6. a

19 Complement in Laboratory Testing

Laboratory tests involve complement in three different contexts. The oldest technique is to induce complement-mediated biologic events as a method of detecting antibodies. Development of a complement-mediated end point is essential, but the purpose of these tests is to **demonstrate that antibody is present.** The usual end points are red blood cell (RBC) hemolysis in complement fixation tests and complement-mediated killing of lymphocytes in lymphocytotoxicity testing. A second manner in which complement is involved in laboratory testing is **identification of complement components at the site of immune reactions.** This usually involves C3 cleavage fragments on cell membranes or complement-containing immune complexes in biologic fluids. The **quantity** or the **characteristics of complement** components themselves, either in the entire cascade or as individual components and detection of complement receptors (CRs), may also be measured in the laboratory.

COMPLEMENT IN THE DEMONSTRATION OF ANTIBODIES

Activation of the entire complement cascade generates the "membrane attack unit," which lethally damages cell membranes. If RBCs are the target, liberated hemoglobin provides an end point that is easy to observe and to measure. Demonstrating

421

lethal damage to lymphocytes requires a different, inherently semiquantitative end point.

Complement Fixation Technique

When they combine with antigen, all IgM antibodies and many IgG antibodies activate the first component of complement. Union with antigen is an independent event, but if C1 is present and functional, it will attach to the Fc portion of the bound immunoglobulin (Ig) molecule. If a membrane was the site of antigen-antibody reaction, C4 and later components attach to the surface. If the antigen-antibody combination generates a fluid-phase aggregate, complement components accumulate in or on the macromolecular complex. Neither the specificity of the antibody nor the nature of the antigen affect the cascading activation of complement proteins.

In complement fixation (CF) testing, the end point is hemolysis; the indicator system requires (1) RBCs already coated with a complement-activating antibody, (2) a preparation containing reagent complement, and (3) reaction conditions that allow the antibody under investigation to combine with its antigen. Antibody action alters the baseline level of hemolysis generated when reagent complement is added to the coated reagent cells. Most CF procedures test for the presence of a specific antibody, and the reagent system includes a standardized preparation of known antigen. Figure 19–1 illustrates the principle of CF testing.

Two-Stage Procedure

After the indicator system has been standardized for baseline level of hemolysis, the test requires two steps. First, the unknown serum and the known antigen are allowed to interact in the presence of complement. If complement-activating antibody is present, it combines with the antigen and causes C1 to enter the immune complex. This is described as "fixing" complement components. Antibody present in the unknown material reacts with antigen and causes the level of free complement in the system to drop significantly. If the serum contains no antibody, no immune reaction occurs, no complement is fixed, and the level of available complement remains unchanged.

The second step is addition of indicator RBCs already coated with a complement-fixing antibody to the incubated mixture. The reagent antibody that coats the indicator cells must not agglutinate the cells but must strongly and invariably interact with complement. If the sensitized reagent cells are exposed to free complement, C1 interacts with the bound Ig and the hemolytic cascade proceeds; the sensitized cells will not hemolyze in the absence of complement.

Interpretation

If antibody is present in the test serum, it combines with reagent antigen in the first step. The resulting immune complexes bind complement, which is then unavailable for subsequent reactivity. If the unknown specimen contains no antibody, the complement in the incubation mixture persists at its previously calibrated level. In a positive test, the complement-depleted incubation mixture lacks the factors needed to hemolyze the sensitized indicator cells; therefore, a positive end point is absence of hemolysis, as shown in Figure 19–1. In a negative test, the serum lacks antibody,

COMPLEMENT FIXATION TEST

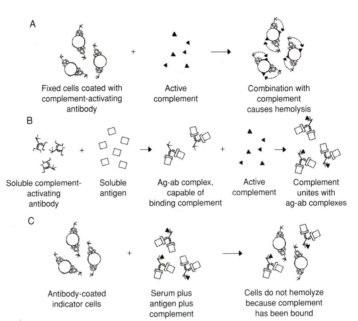

FIGURE 19-1. *Panel* A shows the indicator system for complement fixation tests: hemolysis when reagent complement is added to red blood cells sensitized with a complement-activating antibody. *Panel* B shows the first step of the test, in which serum containing soluble antibody is allowed to complex with soluble antigen. When reagent complement is added, Cl binds to the complexed antibody. *Panel* C shows that the complement, now "fixed" in the soluble complexes, is no longer available to unite with the sensitizing antibody on the indicator cells. Absence of hemolysis thus indicates that an antigen-antibody reaction has occurred in the soluble phase depicted in panel B.

no complexes form, and no complement is removed from the medium. Sensitized cells are then hemolyzed at the same intensity as in the baseline control. The degree to which complement is fixed and hemolysis diminished is directly proportional to the concentration of antibody in the test serum.

Potential Problems

Most CF procedures use guinea pig complement and antibody-coated sheep RBCs as the indicator. The range of potential problems is enormous; accurate CF testing requires numerous painstaking steps to standardize all reagents and to avoid artifacts and misinterpretation. The complement preparation must be tested before each use because several components are labile on storage. Reactivity of the indicator RBCs may change over time and may also be affected by environmental conditions. The sensitizing antibody must behave consistently. The concentrations of all materials, including the ionic and macromolecular composition of the suspending medium, must be stringently reproducible.

Variables exist not only in the indicator system but also in the test materials. The reagent antigen must have uniform specificity and reactivity. The serum must be examined for effects on complement that occur without regard to antibody presence. Serums that impair complement reactivity are described as "anticomplementary." Immune complexes or aggregated Igs in serum are anticomplementary because they bind complement through the alternative pathway. Chelating agents bind the cations necessary for complement interactions, and heparin, if present in even small amounts, will inhibit the complement cascade. CF procedures must include a control of serum and complement without added antigen and of complement and antigen without added serum.

Applications

Although CF tests demand a large amount of time and technical proficiency, they are highly sensitive and are useful in detecting antibodies difficult to demonstrate with other systems. The earliest serologic test for syphilis was a CF procedure, the **Wasserman test.** Syphilis testing has long used other techniques, and routine tests for many other antibodies have switched from CF testing to simpler procedures. However, CF testing is still used as a reference against which newer and less demanding techniques are compared. It also remains useful in identifying and quantifying antibodies against certain viral, fungal, and protozoal antigens.

Lymphocytotoxicity

Lymphocytotoxicity tests are used to demonstrate antibodies against HLA antigens. These antibodies mediate various serologic effects, but lymphocytotoxicity gives consistent and accurate reactions for serums with a wide range of specificities. In the presence of complement, the union of cytotoxic antibody with HLA antigen irreversibly damages the cell membrane, which cannot then perform its barrier functions. This lethal damage is detected by showing that materials normally excluded from the cell interior can cross the damaged membrane and penetrate the cell.

Three-Stage Procedure

Cytotoxicity testing is a three-stage procedure. Serum and cells must first be incubated together. After optimal opportunity for antibody to attach to surface antigens, a standardized preparation of complement is added. If antibodies have bound to the cell membrane, the added complement unites with the bound Ig, the cascade is activated to completion, and the cell is irreversibly damaged. The last step is to introduce a dye that penetrates the membrane of nonviable cells but cannot enter intact cells. Viable cells remain unstained, but cells to which the complement-binding antibody attached will be suffused with the intracellular dye. This principle is illustrated in Figure 13–1.

The proportion of viable to damaged cells indicates the magnitude of antigen-antibody reaction. Reactivity is affected by the concentration and avidity of the antibody and the intensity with which antigen is expressed on the membrane, as well as by the specificity of antibody for membrane antigen.

Biologic Variables

The test is easier to explain than to interpret. Variations in serum-cell reactivity are much greater for HLA antibodies and their antigens than for RBC antigens and antibodies. Individuals who form HLA antibodies seldom exhibit a single, monospecific reactivity; a serum specimen often reacts to a variable degree with many different cells. Conversely, cells of a single phenotype may show variable reactivity with a number of different sera. Even reagent antisera licensed for typing purposes may produce results that are not always clear-cut. Lymphocytotoxicity tests are usually performed in trays that contain numerous microtiter wells, allowing reactivity patterns of different cell suspensions and different serum samples to be observed and to be compared.

DEMONSTRATION THAT ANTIGEN-ANTIBODY REACTION HAS OCCURRED

Many events initiate the complement cascade but do not provoke membrane attack and do not cause immediate cell damage. Activation of classical or alternative pathways often causes cleavage products of C3 to accumulate, either on cell membranes or in the fluid-phase complex of antigen and antibody. In these settings, the presence of C3b or other C3 fragments indicates that an immune reaction of some sort has occurred. In immunohematology, cell-bound C3 indicates that there has been reaction between antibody and cellular antigens. When soluble antigen and antibody form complement-containing immune complexes, the complexes may behave in various ways. They may remain free in body fluids, they may adhere to circulating blood cells, or they may settle on membranes of blood vessels, renal glomeruli, pulmonary air spaces, or other locations.

Antibodies Against Blood-Cell Antigens

Antibodies that react with blood-cell antigens often activate the complement cascade through cleavage of C3, but inhibition then outstrips activation and the process stops. Only for activation of C1 is the physical presence of Ig molecule essential. Even after antibody dissociates from the complex, subsequent complement interactions can continue on the cell membrane. The presence of C3 or its conversion products can be demonstrated with an antiglobulin specific for these cleavage products. Whether or not antibody has dissociated, the presence of residual C3 fragments signals that antibody had previously combined with antigen. The action of antibodies active against RBCs, granulocytes, or platelets can be demonstrated in this way. The technique is easiest for RBC antibodies, but can be adapted for platelets and neutrophils through measurements adapted for low levels of complement fragments.

Anticomplement Testing

When suitably specific, anticomplement serum does not react with any membrane antigen or any part of the Ig molecule; its sole target is the complement protein. Anticomplement serum agglutinates RBCs that have complement attached to their membranes, but has no effect on unmodified cells or on cells sensitized only with Ig. Tests for platelet antibodies cannot use agglutination as an end point because platelets tend to agglutinate spontaneously. A radioactive label or an immunofluorescence system is often used to demonstrate complement bound to platelets by previous antibody activity.

Anticomplement globulin is used to demonstrate either *in vivo* or *in vitro* events. A direct antiglobulin test (see p. 383) positive with anticomplement demonstrates that a complement-activating autoimmune reaction has occurred within the patient's circulation. Autoantibodies with a low thermal optimum characteristically activate complement but do not persist in their attachment to the cell surface; examining the cell membrane for bound antibody is unrewarding after these reactions.

Even transient antibody attachment causes irreversible attachment of complement. Finding complement on circulating cells thus indicates that antibody activity has been directed against antigens of the individual's own cells.

Tests for Antibody in Serum

Anticomplement antiglobulin also can be used in an indirect antiglobulin procedure to demonstrate *in vitro* antibody activity. Most blood group antibodies that react with cellular antigens either cause agglutination or remain as sensitizing adherent molecules; a few interact so briefly or in such small numbers that they cannot be detected with anti-immunoglobulin reagent. If the brief antigen-antibody encounter has caused complement attachment, it is possible to demonstrate that serum contains antibody by demonstrating complement components on the cell membrane after serum has been incubated with cells (Fig. 19–2).

Detecting Immune Complexes

Immune complexes play a significant role in autoimmune diseases such as rheumatic or collagen-vascular diseases, many hematologic disorders, some forms of glomerulonephritis, and some infectious diseases. Tissue changes result from the inflammation-promoting effects of complement incorporated into deposited im-

USE OF ANTICOMPLEMENT ANTIGLOBULIN

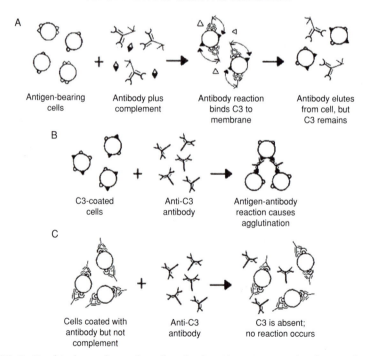

FIGURE 19–2. *Panel* A shows that union of antibody with antigen can bind C3 to the cell membrane, even if the immunoglobulin dissociates after interacting with C1qrs. *Panels* B and C show how antiglobulin serum with specificity for C3 can demonstrate that C3 is present. The surface-bound C3 demonstrated by agglutination with anti-C3 is evidence that a complement-binding reaction has occurred, whether or not the immunoglobulin remains attached to the cells.

mune complexes. Tests for immune complexes characteristically use an indicator system that detects the presence of complement, using antiserum specific for C3 fragments or for earlier components in the classical pathway.

Tissue versus Serum

It is easy to apply fluorescence-labeled anticomplement serum to sections of tissue. If complement has been deposited in the tissue, attachment of the labeled indicator identifies the location. The presence of complement in tissue undergoing acute inflammation is considered diagnostic of immune-mediated inflammatory disease. Demonstrating complement-containing complexes in body fluids is less definitively diagnostic. Immune complexes initiate type 3 hypersensitivity conditions, but serum or other fluids may contain complexes when there are no manifestations of disease and active type 3 disease can exist when the fluids available for testing contain no demonstrable complexes. Very sensitive enzyme-linked immunosorbent assay (ELISA) procedures using monoclonal antibodies as capture antibodies for immune complexes have been developed. How useful they are for clinical evaluation remains to be determined.

Other tests for immune complexes depend on the interaction of free C1q with the Fc of bound Ig molecules and the interaction of C3 fragments with complement receptors on the membranes of indicator cells. The first application uses the same principle as the complement fixation procedure described earlier in this chapter. Test serum is incubated with reagent serum known to contain hemolyzing quantities of complement. If the test serum contains antigen-antibody complexes, they incorporate available C1q, which is then unavailable for participation in the standardized cascade provoked by sensitized reagent cells. A positive result is reduction in previously established hemolytic activity, through consumption of C1q by immune complexes in the test material.

Exploiting C3 Receptors

Many cells, including RBCs, B lymphocytes, macrophages, and many tumor cells, have membrane receptors for C3b or its degradation products (see pp. 156–157). Tests use suspensions of these cells to bind immune complexes that may be present in the test material. One procedure uses peripheral blood B lymphocytes, with inhibition of membrane-receptor events as the indicator of immune complex and C3b binding. Another procedure uses a line of tumor cells called **Raji cells,** which have large numbers of receptor sites for C3d, iC3b, and C1q. Serum to be tested for presence of immune complexes with associated complement fragments is incubated with the Raji cells. ^{125}I-labeled rabbit antihuman IgG antibodies are then added to the Raji cells to detect the amount of immune complex attached to the Raji cell membranes.

MEASUREMENT OF COMPLEMENT

Serum complement activity can be low because of rare congenital deficiencies of individual component proteins or because of acquired pathophysiologic events. Congenital deficiencies are usually encountered during investigation of aberrant immune function or defective antibacterial defenses. Acquired conditions are usually evaluated during investigation of immune-mediated diseases. Events that may depress functioning complement include consumption of components during immune-complex formation, increased levels of protein destruction with or without decreased protein production, and development of inhibitors. Overall complement function is screened by measuring either the hemolytic properties of native serum or other complex physiologic events, such as opsonization and chemotaxis. Assay of individual proteins can be undertaken if screening indicates significant abnormality.

CH_{50} Assay

Hemolysis is the end point of the entire complement cascade. Demonstrating reduced hemolytic capacity cannot indicate the nature of the defect, but demonstrating that normal hemolytic activity exists suggests functional integrity of the entire system. However, wide latitude exists minor deficiencies in C4, C5, C8, or C9 do not affect overall hemolytic activity, and major deficiencies (up to 50%) in factors C1, C2, C3, C6, or C7 may not depress overall hemolysis. The curve that relates complement activity to observed hemolysis is S-shaped. Tests for overall hemolytic activity use 50 percent hemolysis (CH_{50}) as the indicator because changing levels of complement exert maximal visible effect at the midpoint of the curve.

Technical Considerations

The CH_{50} assay uses RBCs presensitized with an antibody that strongly initiates hemolysis when complement is present (Fig. 19–3). Different dilutions of test serum are added to the sensitized cells, and the amount of hemoglobin that the test serum releases is compared with hemolysis induced by pooled normal serum at the same dilutions. Collection and storage of test serum and control pools must be stringently standardized because *in vitro* events can rapidly damage the balanced system. Other artifacts that may affect reproducibility include the condition of the sensitized RBCs; the activity of the indicator antibody; and the time, temperature, and ionic conditions of the reaction.

When CH_{50} is reduced, the assay can be modified to pinpoint the factor at fault,

CH_{50} DETERMINATION

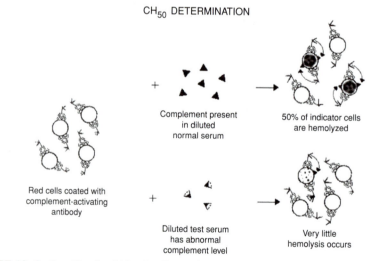

Complement present
in diluted
normal serum

50% of indicator cells
are hemolyzed

Red cells coated with
complement-activating
antibody

Diluted test serum
has abnormal
complement level

Very little
hemolysis occurs

FIGURE 19–3. Sensitized red blood cells used as an indicator in the CH_{50} test will hemolyze if complement is added. The upper drawings show that complement in diluted normal serum induces hemolysis at the 50 percent level. The lower drawings show that a similar dilution of abnormal serum contains reduced amounts of complement and induces very little hemolysis.

provided that preparations of individual components are available. However, this cumbersome approach is seldom used, and individual components are better evaluated by specific assays.

Individual Complement Components

When there is congenital or, more often, acquired deficiency of overall function, it may be useful to measure levels of specific complement components. Components normally present in large quantities are most easily measured. C3 is the component measured most often. C3 is the most abundant component and is associated with activation of both the classical and alternative pathways, therefore playing a pivotal role in most complement-mediated activities. Other components that can be quantified are C2, C1q, and factor B of the alternative pathway. Nephelometry (see p. 371) is often used for these milligram-level measurements. Radial immunodiffusion (see pp. 367–369) is useful for these proteins as well as for others present at or above 25 μg/mL. A low-concentration product that can provide useful information about systemic events is C5a, the anaphylatoxin cleaved from C5 by either classical- or alternative-pathway generation of C3b. ELISA procedures to detect individual components or fragments, as well as activated complement complexes (C3bBbP or C3BP), have also been developed.

Protein Polymorphisms

In addition to quantitative measurement, qualitative evaluation of complement components is becoming increasingly important. The genes that regulate manufacture of complement components exhibit allelic variation, and significant polymorphism has been noted for the proteins. Structural variants of some components may depress overall complement activity, but a more significant finding is that immune dysfunction of various sorts, especially predisposition to autoimmune diseases, often accompanies these abnormal products.

Both immunologic and functional techniques are used to identify these protein polymorphisms. Ouchterlony double diffusion (see Chapter 16) is used to compare the patient's proteins with the precipitin arcs given by normal components. Immunoelectrophoresis and immunoblot techniques allow similar direct comparison against patterns characteristic of normal proteins. In multistage assays, proteins are first separated by electrophoresis and then overlaid with antibody-containing gels that allow both qualitative and quantitative characterization. An interesting variant is to overlay the separated proteins with a gel containing sensitized cells that undergo hemolysis at the migration sites of functional components.

When polymorphism is suspected or demonstrated, molecular techniques can be used for precise characterization. Endonucleases (see Chapter 5, Molecular Genetic Techniques) are used to cleave the nucleoproteins, and a library of probes are used to characterize the variant forms present. The proteins that manifest the highest degree of polymorphism are associated with genes of the major histocompatibility complex (MHC) locus, namely the class III products C2, C4, and factor B of the alternative pathway.

MEASUREMENT OF COMPLEMENT RECEPTORS

Complement fragments interact with specific surface receptors on phagocytic cells, lymphocytes, and many other cell types. Through this interaction, various aspects of inflammation and the immune response are generated. Complement receptors (CRs) on these cell types may be detected by rosette formation. Complement-coated erythrocytes or some other types of particles adhere to cells bearing CR, forming a cluster or rosette around the CR-positive cell. The number of rosettes present in a preparation can be viewed and counted under a microscope. With the availability of polyclonal and monoclonal antibodies to CRs, new techniques for analyzing the activity and structural relationships of CRs on various cell types have been developed. Monoclonal antibodies, because of their exquisite specificity, have been used to detect minute structural differences in receptors. These antibodies can be labeled with radioisotopes, fluorochromes, or enzymes for quantitative immunoassay or localization and visualization of CRs on cells and in tissues.

SUMMARY

1. Laboratory tests involving complement include those that are actually for detection of antibody, tests to detect complement at immune reaction sites, and actual measurement of complement components and complement receptors.

2. The complement fixation (CF) test demonstrates that suspected antibody is present in a serum sample. A baseline level of hemolysis must be established by incubating red blood cells (RBCs) (coated with complement-activating antibody) with known antigen and reagent complement. To perform the CF test, unknown serum and known antigen are incubated in the presence of complement. If antibody is present, complement is fixed and is no longer available to interact with the indicator system of antibody coated RBCs. Therefore, in a positive CF test, baseline hemolysis is reduced or absent. In a negative test, no antibody is present in the unknown serum, no complement is fixed and with addition of known antigen and antibody-coated RBCs, original baseline levels of hemolysis occur. CF tests are difficult and time-consuming, and numerous steps must be taken to ensure that all reagents are behaving optimally. However, this test is highly sensitive and useful for detecting antibodies difficult to demonstrate with other systems.

3. Lymphocytotoxicity tests are used to demonstrate antibody against HLA antigen. In the presence of HLA antibody, lymphocytes with matching HLA antigen are susceptible to activated complement membrane damage. These cells can be visualized by the addition of a viability stain that only penetrates damaged cells. Because of variations in serum and cell reactivity, lymphocytotoxicity tests can be difficult to interpret.

4. The complement cascade may be initiated by antigen-antibody binding, but may not necessarily go to completion with formation of the membrane attack complex. However, C3 cleavage products accumulate with activation of either the classical or alternative pathways, and these products can be detected with anticomplement antibodies. Anticomplement antibodies cause agglutination of RBCs that have complement attached to their membranes. Other cell types with membrane-bound complement can be visualized with immunofluorescence labeling or an indirect, second-labeled antibody technique.

5. Immune complexes in tissues with associated complement components

can be detected with fluorescence-labeled anticomplement antibodies. Presence of complement indicates immune-mediated inflammatory disease. Breakdown products of C3 can also be detected by a line of tumor cells called Raji cells which have a large number of receptors for C3d, iC3b, and C1q.

6. Decreased levels of complement due to various congenital deficiencies or elevations of complement due to immune-mediated disease may be detected by measuring the hemolytic activities (CH_{50} assay) or the physiologic activities of complement in opsonization or chemotaxis. Individual components or presence of activated complexes can be measured with nephelometry, radial immunodiffusion, or ELISA using specific complement antibodies.

7. Structural variation of complement components may result in reduced activity and associated immune dysfunction and predisposition to autoimmune disease. Both immunologic and molecular techniques have been developed to identify these protein polymorphisms.

8. Presence of complement receptors on various cell types can be detected by rosette formation or immunolabeling techniques with monoclonal antibodies.

REVIEW QUESTIONS

1. Reagents necessary to perform the complement fixation test include _____.
   a. red blood cells (RBCs) coated with antibody
   b. complement
   c. antigen
   d. a and b
   e. a, b, and c

2. An early serologic test for syphilis called the Wasserman test used a complement fixation procedure. A serum sample tested by this procedure showed reduced hemolysis when compared with the baseline control. The sample is _____ for syphilis.
   a. positive
   b. negative

3. Variable(s) that can affect the outcome of the complement fixation test include

   _____.
   a. lability of the complement preparation
   b. variation of indicator RBCs
   c. lability of reagent antibody
   d. lability of reagent antigen
   e. all of the above

4. Lymphocytes from a potential donor are being tested for HLA-A antigen. Lymphocytes incubated with anti-A1, anti-A2, and anti-A3 show staining reaction with anti-A3. HLA-A antigen(s) present on this donor's lymphocytes is/are

   _____.
   a. HLA-A1
   b. HLA-A2
   c. HLA-A3
   d. a and b
   e. a, b, and c

5. Reagents necessary to perform lymphocytotoxicity include _____.
   a. complement
   b. anti−HLA antibodies
   c. anti−human antibody conjugated with fluorescein isothiocyanate
   d. a and b
   e. a, b, and c

6. RBCs from a patient incubated with anticomplement globulin are observed to form agglutinates. This observation suggests that _____.
   a. complement or complement components are bound to the RBC membrane
   b. an autoimmune reaction has occurred in the patient's circulation
   c. if complement is bound, likewise antibody is also bound.
   d. a and b
   e. a, b, and c

7. To determine whether immune-mediated inflammatory disease is occurring in the kidney of a patient with systemic lupus erythematosus (SLE), tissue sections from a kidney biopsy can be incubated with _____.
   a. antihuman IgG conjugated with FITC
   b. anticomplement serum conjugated with FITC
   c. monoclonal antibody to human complement receptor or C3b conjugated with FITC
   d. Raji cells
   e. a and b

8. Serum levels of C2 in a patient with a suspected deficiency can be determined by _____.
   a. ELISA
   b. nephelometry
   c. CH_{50} assay
   d. a and b
   e. a, b, and c

SUGGESTIONS FOR FURTHER READING

Fredrickson GN, Truedsson L, Sjoholm AG: New procedure for the detection of complement deficiency by ELISA. J Immunol Methods 1993;166:223−268

Gaither TA, Frank MM: Complement receptors. In: Rose NR, DeMacario EC, Fahey JL, et al, eds: Manual of Clinical Laboratory Immunology, 4th ed. Washington, DC: American Society for Microbiology, 1992:142−152

Marcus-Bagley D, Alper CA: Methods for allotyping complement proteins. In: Rose NR, DeMacario EC, Fahey JL, et al, eds: Manual of Clinical Laboratory Immunology, 4th ed. Washington, DC: American Society for Microbiology, 1992:124−141

REVIEW ANSWERS

1. e	5. d
2. a	6. d
3. e	7. e
4. c	8. d

Glossary

Absorption: Removal of antibody from fluid by causing it to bind antigen-bearing material and then separating the solid-phase complex from the fluid phase.

Accessory cells: Cells that enhance immune interactions but do not express antigenic specificity; usually monocyte, macrophages, or antigen-presenting cells.

Activation: 1. For lymphocytes, stimulation by antigen or mitogen, leading to immunoblast transformation and often to clonal expansion and synthesis of antibodies or lymphokines. 2. For complement components, cleavage or configurational change leading to altered functional state. 3. For macrophages, heightening of functional state after stimulation by cytokines.

Acute-phase reactants: Serum proteins that exhibit altered concentration in systemic inflammatory states. Examples: fibrinogen and C-reactive protein.

Addressins: Proteins on endothelial surfaces that bind to homing receptors on leukocyte cell membranes and thereby regulate lymphocyte and other leukocyte migration from the blood.

Adjuvant: Material that does not elicit an independent immune response but, when given with a specific antigen, enhances immune reactivity.

Adsorption: Adherence of material to a solid surface, especially the association between antigen-bearing particles or surfaces and specific antibody.

Affinity: The strength of interaction between a single antigenic determinant and a single immunoglobulin combining site; expressed as K, the association (or binding) constant.

Agglutination: Clumping of antigen-bearing particles by formation of a lattice in which combining sites of the corresponding antibody incorporate previously suspended particles.

Agglutination inhibition: Abolition of agglutination by soluble antigen molecules that complex with combining sites before the immunoglobulin can bind to solid-phase antigen.

Allele: Any of the two or more alternative forms of a gene that can occupy a single chromosomal locus.

Allelic exclusion: The phenomenon whereby active expression of an allele on one member of a chromosome pair prevents the corresponding allele on the other chromosome from generating a product.

Allergen: An antigen that provokes hypersensitivity reactions in a susceptible individual, especially those agents that provoke immediate-type hypersensitivity.

Allergy: A harmful immunologic reaction to extrinsic material; often applied to immediate-type hypersensitivity reactions.

Allogeneic: Material originating from individuals of the same species but different genetic constitution.

Allograft: Grafted or transplanted tissue from a donor of the same species but different genetic constitution from that of the recipient.

Allotype: The form of a protein synthesized under direction of any single allele determining that polypeptide; connotes antigenic difference among products made by different individuals of the same species.

Alternative pathway: Activation of the complement cascade by interaction of C3, factors B and D, and properdin; initiated by contact with appropriate surfaces and occurring independently of antigen-antibody reactions. Also called **properdin pathway.**

Ames test: *In vitro* test for carcinogenicity of a substance using an enzyme-deficient bacterial strain of *Salmonella typhimurium.*

Amyloid: Extracellular fibrous proteins that usually derive from precursors present in the blood and that accumulate as amorphous deposits in individuals suffering from chronic inflammation or myeloma.

Analyte: Material that is measured or analyzed.

Anamnestic: Pertaining to immunologic memory, whereby second or subsequent contact with an antigen provokes an immune response different in nature or intensity from that elicited by the first contact.

Anaphylatoxins: Cleavage fragments of complement that promote release of cellular products that induce increased vascular permeability, enhanced inflammatory reactivity, and increased smooth-muscle and epithelial cell activity.

Anaphylaxis: Systemic manifestation of immediate-type hypersensitivity, mediated by widespread release of cellular mediators following interaction between antigen and cell-bound antibody.

Anergy: Loss of previously present immune reactivity; usually disappearance of delayed-type hypersensitivity against antigens that previously induced a positive skin test.

Antibody: An immunoglobulin capable of specific combination with an identifiable antigen.

Antibody-dependent cell-mediated cytotoxicity (ADCC): Damage inflicted on antibody-coated cells by lymphocytes and macrophages that do not recognize specific antigen but have Fc receptors that combine with the Fc portion of antibody already bound to the target cell.

Anticomplement activity: Capacity to inhibit activation of the complement cascade in a complement fixation test.

Antigen: A material capable of provoking an immune response when introduced into an immunocompetent host to whom it is foreign.

Antigen-binding site: The portion of the immunoglobulin molecule, comprising the variable domains of heavy and light chains, that expresses a configuration complementary to that of antigen.

Antigenic determinant: The configuration of antigen material that elicits a specific immune response; the site that interacts with the idiotypic portion of the antigen receptor.

Antigen-presenting cell: Any cell capable of retaining, on its membrane, processed antigen in a form accessible to the receptors of T or B lymphocytes; primarily cells of epithelial or of monocyte/macrophage origin.

Antigen receptor: Molecules, present on membranes of T and B lymphocytes, which express a configuration complementary to that of a specific antigen and through which the appropriately presented antigen initiates immune activation.

Antiglobulin serum: A preparation of antibody for which the specific target is globulin, either a wide range of globulins (e.g., polyspecific antihuman globulin serum) or a single molecule (e.g., anti-C3b or antitransferrin). An informally used synonym in **Coombs' serum.**

Apoptosis: Programmed cell death characterized by nuclear fragmentation, blebbing, and phagocytosis of cell residue. In contrast, necrosis may result in damage to surrounding tissue.

Arthus reaction: Localized complement-mediated acute inflammation induced when injected antigen unites with circulating antibody to form complexes that precipitate at the injection site.

Atopic: Pertaining to immediate-type hypersensitivity reactions induced by contact with widely distributed environmental antigens such as pollens, yeast, and animal proteins.

Atopy: A constitutional state of predisposition to immediate-type hypersensitivity reactions.

Autograft: Grafted or implanted tissue that originates from the individual in whom it is placed.

Autoimmunity: Immune manifestations directed against self (autologous) antigens.

Autologous: Deriving from self.

Autosomes: All the chromosomes except the two sex chromosomes.

Avidity: The cumulative strength of interaction between all the antigen combining sites in a preparation of antibody and all the epitopic determinants of a complex antigen.

B-cell receptor (BCR): Antigen-binding molecule expressed on surface of B cells; an immunoglobulin. On activation, the B cell produces antibody of the same specificity as the expressed BCR.

B lymphocytes: The lymphocyte population that possesses the membrane characteristics of major histocompatibility complex (MHC) class II products and immunoglobulin molecules that serve as antigen receptor.

Bence Jones protein: Monoclonal immunoglobulin light chains, either kappa or lambda, characteristic of several neoplasms of B-cell origin, especially multiple myeloma; usually found in urine, but also present in serum.

Blocking antibody: Antibody in body fluids that interferes with other manifestations of immunity; especially IgG antibodies that prevent association of antigen with cell-bound IgE and antibodies that inhibit the cytolytic reaction of NK cells with tumor cells.

B_2-Microglobulin: A small (11.6-kD) glycoprotein that constitutes one chain of the major histocompatibility complex (MHC) class I heterodimers and is synthesized under the control of a gene on chromosome 15.

Bradykinin: A small polypeptide (nine amino acids) that evolves from a plasma precursor during activation of the kinin system and induces increased vascular permeability, contraction of smooth muscle, and perception of pain.

Bursa equivalent: The tissue or organ in mammals that performs the function served by the bursa of Fabricius in birds; probably the fetal bone marrow and possibly also the fetal liver.

Bursa of Fabricius: An outpouching of lymphoid tissue, in the cloaca of immature birds, that is the site at which avian B lymphocytes differentiate and mature.

CALLA: Common acute lymphoblastic leukemia antigen.

Carcinogen: Any substance or agent that can cause cancer.

Carcinoma: Cancer originating from tissue of epithelial origin.

Cardiolipin: A phospholipid in neural tissue, heart muscle, and mitochondrial and bacterial enzymes against which autoreactive antibodies develop in syphilis and in many of the dysfunctional conditions known as "collagen-vascular diseases"; the antigen used in nontreponemal serologic tests for syphilis.

Carrier: A macromolecule that combines with a smaller molecule, called a **hapten,** to render the hapten immunogenic.

Carrier particles: Otherwise inert particles to which either antigen or antibody can be adsorbed, functioning to induce agglutination as an end point for union of otherwise soluble immune reactants.

Cell-mediated immunity (CMI): Immune reactivity for which the participation of viable T lymphocytes is essential, manifested either by secretion of lymphokines or exercise of direct cell-to-cell toxicity.

CH$_{50}$: Complement-mediated hemolysis of 50 percent of a preparation of indicator red blood cells; used to evaluate hemolytic complement level in whole serum.

Chemokines: Cytokines involved in the selective migration of immune and inflammatory cells; important role in inflammatory responses.

Chemotaxis: Migration of cells in response to a stimulus, often to the presence of cytokines, anaphylatoxins, or cell-derived mediator substances.

Class: 1. For immunoglobulins, the category determined by identity of the heavy chain. 2. For products of the major histocompatibility complex (MHC), the structural characteristics of the complex proteins synthesized under direction of individual alleles.

Class I: Products of the major histocompatibility complex (MHC) that constitute the HLA-A, HLA-B, and HLA-C series; all class I products are dimers containing the β_2-microglobulin chain in addition to a large, polymorphic alpha chain.

Class II: Products of the major histocompatibility complex (MHC) that constitute the HLA-DP, HLA-DQ, and HLA-DR series; class II products are heterodimers in which both polypeptides are determined by alleles in the MHC.

Classical pathway: Activation of the complement cascade by enzymatic and steric interactions initiated after reaction with antigen by an antibody that expresses a site to which C1q can bind.

Clonal selection: A key theory of adaptive immunity that states that individuals have many lymphocyte clones that can each react with only one epitope. These clones are generated at random, but cells responsive to self epitopes are destroyed during fetal life.

Clone: A population of genetically identical cells derived from successive divisions of a single parent cell.

Cluster determinants: The term CD (see **clusters of differentiation**) is sometimes interpreted to denote **cluster determinant.**

Clusters of differentiation (CD): Antigenic features characteristic of leukocytes of various types and maturational phases, identified by groups (clusters) of monoclonal antibodies that express common or overlapping reactivity.

Codon: The set of three adjacent bases in a segment of deoxyribonucleic acid (DNA) that codes for individual amino acids and for initiation and termination signals.

Collagen: The dense white protein that constitutes the bulk of connective tissue and scar tissue.

Competitive binding: An assay principle in which two different forms of the same material, usually labeled and unlabeled, compete for binding sites on a limited quantity of receptor.

Complement (C′): A system of serum proteins that interact in a prescribed sequence to initiate many effector functions of immune reactions and other events that involve the inflammatory and coagulation systems.

Complement fixation: An assay principle in which occurrence of an antigen-antibody reaction is revealed through binding of complement components to the immune complex.

Constant region: The carboxy-terminal portion of immunoglobulin heavy or light chains, comprising the unvarying polypeptide sequence characteristic of all chains of a given class or subclass.

Contact sensitivity: A form of cell-mediated hypersensitivity manifested by redness, itching, and other symptoms at the site where allergens have been in contact with skin.

Coombs' serum: An informal designation for antiglobulin preparations, especially those used in agglutination procedures.

Coombs' test: An informal designation for agglutination procedures that use antiglobulin serums to demonstrate prior attachment of antibody or complement to antigen-bearing cells.

Cortex: The outer portion of an organ or structure.

Counterimmunoelectrophoresis (CIE): A precipitation assay in which the diffusion of antigen and antibody through the supporting medium is given speed and direction by an applied electrical field.

CR proteins: The diverse group of plasma and membrane proteins that serve as receptors for individual components or cleavage fragments of the complement system.

Crossing-over: Interchange of genetic material between the two members of a single chromosome pair.

Crosslink: In immunology, the simultaneous engagement of several adjacent receptors by multiple examples of a single ligand.

Crossmatch: A procedure to detect previously established immune reactivity between serum or cells of a recipient and the antigens present in tissue or blood of a prospective donor.

Cross-reactivity: Reactivity of an antibody with material other than the antigen that elicited its secretion.

Cytokine: A protein, secreted by a stimulated cell, which affects the function or activity of other cells.

Cytophilic: The property of antibodies, especially IgE but sometimes also IgG, to bind to receptors on the membrane of certain cells, especially basophilic granulocytes.

Cytotoxic T lymphocytes (Tc): CD8-positive T cells that exert lethal contact effects on target cells expressing the correct major histocompatibility complex class (MHC1-I) products and the appropriate antigenic specificity.

Degranulation: Release of preformed materials from cytoplasmic granules, as occurs, for example, after antigen recognition by IgE bound to a basophilic granulocyte.

Delayed-type hypersensitivity (DTH): A cell-mediated immune response that reflects the actions of lymphokines released when CD4-positive T cells encounter their specific antigen.

Dendritic cells: A diverse population of cells with branching cytoplasmic processes, lying close to aggregates of B lymphocytes and serving to present antigens.

Differentiation: Process whereby cells acquire new proteins, new surface markers, and new functions. Cells become more specialized and lose proliferative capacity.

Diffuse: To spread through a medium from an initial site of high concentration.

Diploid: Characterized by two complete sets of chromosomes, as found in normal somatic cells.

Direct antiglobulin test (DAT): A procedure that demonstrates *in vivo* attachment of antibody or complement to circulating blood cells; performed by adding antiglobulin reagent directly to a preparation of washed cells.

Disulfide bond (S-S bond): A strong covalent bond formed by oxidation of two contiguous sulfhydryl (SH) groups; can be cleaved by reduction, that is, restoring the electrons so that the S-S bond breaks down to two separate SH groups.

Domain: A folded segment within a complex protein, for example, a segment of the immunoglobulin light or heavy chain composed of approximately 110 amino acids and held in a globular configuration by disulfide bonds.

Double diffusion: A precipitation technique in which preparations of both antigen and antibody diffuse through an inert supporting medium.

DR antigens: Major histocompatibility complex (MHC) class II antigens, identified by serologic reactions and originally noted to be related to, but not identical with HLA-D antigens, which can be identified only by cell-culture techniques; now believed to be the most important histocompatibility antigens for most tissue allografts.

Dysplasia: Development of abnormal cells.

Effector: A cell, protein, or other agent that produces a specific effect.

Effector cells: The cells that mediate a specific activity, distinct from accessory cells that enhance a variety of effects.

Electrophoresis: A procedure to separate mixed molecules by differences in migration patterns during application of an electrical field.

ELISA: Enzyme-linked immunosorbent assay.

Endocytosis: Process whereby a cell ingests macromolecules by enclosing them in a small portion of the cell membrane, which invaginates to form an intracellular vesicle.

End point: The detectable event that demonstrates occurrence of a given interaction.

Enzyme-linked immunosorbent assay (ELISA or EIA): An assay procedure in which either antigen or antibody is adsorbed to a solid phase and the end point is determined by the activity level of an enzyme label bound to one of the reactants.

Enzyme-multiplied immunoassay (EMIT): A homogeneous immunoassay in which the bound or unbound state of the labeled reactant is measured by changes in the activity level of the enzyme used as label.

Epitope: A single, discrete configuration with antigenic activity.

Equivalence: The proportion between antigen and antibody concentration at which maximal precipitation occurs.

Fab: The fragment, generated by papain cleavage of an immunoglobulin monomer, which contains one antigen-binding site. Original term meant **f**ragment, **a**ntigen-**b**inding, but now often used as an adjective, as in the terms **Fab fragment** or **Fab segment.**

Fc: The fragment, generated by papain cleavage of an immunoglobulin monomer, which consists of the hinge region and the linked C-terminal ends of both heavy chains. Original term meant **f**ragment, **c**rystallizable, but often used as an adjective, as in the terms **Fc fragment** or **Fc region.**

Fc receptor (FcR): Any receptor molecule that binds with the Fc region of immunoglobulin molecules; often modified by designating the heavy-chain isotype for which the receptor is specific.

Flow cytometry: Any procedure that counts cells or particles by subjecting the fluid-borne material to an analytic procedure during flow through an aperture.

Fluid-phase: Refers to particulate or soluble material suspended in a fluid medium.

Fluorescein isothiocyanate (FITC): The form of fluoroscein, an orange-red material that fluoresces green in alkaline conditions, which can be complexed to antibodies and other proteins.

Fluorescence: Emission of light at a wavelength slightly longer than that of the absorbed light source; hence, emission of a color different from that of the original material or the light source applied.

Fluorescent treponemal antibody test (FTA): A test in which specific antitreponemal antibodies are demonstrated by indirect immunofluorescence, with fixed treponemal organisms used as targets.

Fluorometric: Assay technique in which a fluorescent end point is subjected to quantitative analysis.

Follicle: A saclike mass; used to describe aggregates of lymphocytes in lymph nodes, spleen, or tissue undergoing immune-mediated inflammation.

Foreign: In immunology, pertaining to material of genetic constitution different from that of the host; of "nonself" origin.

Freund's adjuvant: A preparation widely used to enhance immunogenicity of injected antigens; consists of a water-in-oil emulsion of mineral oil (called **Freund's incomplete adjuvant**) to which killed mycobacteria may be added (then called **Freund's complete adjuvant**).

Gamma globulin: Plasma proteins with the slowest (gamma) migration pattern on electrophoresis at pH 8.6. Because most immunoglobulins have gamma mobility, term is sometimes used to denote immunoglobulin concentration or antibody content.

Gammopathy: Any condition of abnormal immunoglobulin synthesis, including global and partial deficiencies, global and monoclonal excesses, and synthesis of abnormally constituted immunoglobulins.

Gene: The segment of deoxyribonucleic acid (DNA) that directs synthesis of an individual protein.

Gene rearrangement: Modification of DNA sequence within a gene locus to select certain segments for expression and to delete material unnecessary for synthesis of the specific polypeptide.

Genome: The entire complement of genes possessed by an individual; all the information encoded in a complete set of chromosomes.

Genotype: Often used to denote the allele on both chromosomes at an individual locus or segment; more general meaning synonymous with genome.

Germ line: The sequence of genes in their unmodified state before rearrangement for active synthesis of the relevant protein.

Germinal center: Sites in secondary lymphoid tissue where rapidly dividing B cells form a pale-staining spherical mass surrounded by a zone of dark-staining cells; the location of somatic mutation and memory-cell formation.

Gm markers: Allotypic differences in amino acid sequence in specific segments of the gamma heavy chain. Individual Gm sequences are associated with specific subclasses.

Graft-versus-host disease (GVHD): The pathophysiologic consequences of cell-mediated immunity occurring when engrafted immunocompetent T cells recognize as foreign and react against antigens of an immunodeficient host.

Haploid: Characterized by a single set of chromosomes, as found in normal ova and sperm.

Haploidentical: Having in common one haplotype.

Haplotype: A sequence of closely linked alleles in a defined segment of a single chromosome and characteristically transmitted as a genetic unit.

Hapten: A small epitope that cannot, by itself, elicit an immune response but that, when linked to a larger carrier molecule, is recognized by an antigen-specific receptor. Molecules of hapten can interact with antibody, once formed.

Heat shock proteins (hsp): Class of proteins synthesized by cells when subjected to physiologic stresses.

Heavy chain: The larger of the two paired polypeptide chains that constitute the immunoglobulin monomer. Heavy chains are composed of approximately 440 amino acids, arranged in one variable domain and three or four constant domains.

Helper cells: The subpopulation of T lymphocytes that possess the CD4 antigen and cooperate with B lymphocytes or other T lymphocytes to generate immune reactivity.

Hemagglutination: Agglutination or antigen-bearing red blood cells.

Hematopoiesis: Formation and development of blood.

Hemolysis: Damage to the membrane of red blood cells that results in escape of hemoglobin.

Heterodimer: A compound molecule consisting of two dissimilar units.

Heterogeneous assay: A receptor-ligand assay in which the bound material must be separated from the unbound material before the end point is measured.

Heterologous: Deriving from a species different from that of the host.

Heterophile antibody: An antibody that binds to epitopes on a variety of unrelated molecules.

Heterozygous: Possessing different alleles at a given locus on the two members of a chromosome pair.

High endothelial venules (HEV): The postcapillary portion of venules, characterized by membrane markers that allow lymphocytes to escape from the bloodstream into lymphoid tissue or tissue fluids.

Hinge region: The flexible portion of the immunoglobulin heavy chain lying between the first and second constant domains; shape change necessary for binding with antigen occurs in this area; is the site of the disulfide bonds that link the two heavy chains and may be the target of enzymic cleavage.

Histamine: A small molecule present in many sites, including the granules of mast cells and basophils, which upon release causes short-lived increased vascular permeability, vasodilation, smooth muscle contraction, and secretion by several types of epithelial cells.

Histocompatibility: The degree to which two individuals share antigens important for survival of tissue grafts.

HLA: The antigens, determined by numerous genes within the major histocompatibility complex, which most significantly affect survival of engrafted tissue. The initials stand for "human leukocyte antigens" because they were first detected on white blood cells.

Homing receptors: Lymphocyte cell membrane receptors that bind to addressins (ligands) on endothelial surfaces, thus promoting cell adhesion and migration.

Homogeneous assay: A receptor-ligand assay in which it is unnecessary to separate the bound and unbound materials before measuring the end point.

Homologous: In immunology, deriving from an individual of the same species as, but of different genetic composition from, the host.

Homozygous: Possessing the same alleles at a given locus on the two members of a chromosome pair.

Host: The individual exposed to immune stimulation.

Humoral: Referring to material in body fluids (the "humors" of the body); used especially to denote antibodies, the fluid-borne products of immune reactivity, in contrast to cell-mediated immune effects.

Hyperacute rejection: Rejection of a tissue graft occurring within minutes or hours of transplantation, owing to actions of preformed antibodies in the host against antigens on the donor tissue.

Hyperplasia: Increased proliferation of cells that may be a premalignant change in a tissue.

Hypersensitivity: A general term denoting harmful effects of immune actions. Often classified as "immediate," resulting from release of preformed substances after interaction of antigen with cell-bound antibody, and "delayed-type," resulting from effects of lymphokines released by T cells after contact with antigen.

Hypertrophy: Increase in size of cells, thereby contributing to an increase in the size of a tissue or organ; does not involve tumor formation or increase in the number of cells.

Hypervariable regions: Short segments within the variable domains of immunoglobulin light and heavy chains, in which different immunoglobulin molecules exhibit pronounced differences in amino acid sequence. These sequences (three in light chains and four in heavy chains) determine the idiotypic specificity of the molecule.

Hypogammaglobulinemia: Low levels of gamma globulins in the serum.

Iccosome: Small beaded structure containing immune complexes and membrane from follicular dendritic cells; may be shed and endocytosed by B cells and antigen presented to T cells in a secondary or subsequent immune response.

Idiotope: The antigenic determinant that resides in the idiotypic configuration of an antigen-receptor molecule.

Idiotype: The structural configuration unique to that portion of an antigen receptor molecule that recognizes a specific antigen. The unique amino acid sequence can, itself, serve as an antigen. By extension, the term denotes the specificity of the antigen-recognition part of the receptor.

Immediate hypersensitivity: The form of immune-mediated pathophysiologic event that reflects actions of mediator substances released from the localized cells after cell-bound antibody unites with antigen.

Immune: Pertaining to the presence and actions of cells and proteins of the lymphoreticular system in its responses to antigenic stimulation.

Immune complex: The macromolecular complex formed when antibody unites with antigen.

Immune memory: Ability of the immune system to "remember" a previous exposure to an antigen. This phenomenon is mediated by memory cells that promote a heightened state of immune reactivity on reencounter with antigen.

Immune surveillance: A theory that lymphocytes constantly circulate, surveying the body for cancerous or abnormal cells and then eliminating them.

Immunity: The consequences of immune reactivity, in which the occurrence and nature of the response depend on the specificity of the agent inducing the reaction.

Immunoblast: The enlarged form of a lymphocyte that is undergoing DNA synthesis preparatory to cell division.

Immunoblot: A procedure similar to the Western blot. A mixture of complex antigens is separated by electrophoresis, transferred to nitrocellulose paper, and reacted with antisera. Identification of antibodies to known antigens is possible, or demonstration of differences in antigen is also possible when reacted against known antibodies.

Immunodominant: The portion of an epitope that most significantly affects its specificity.

Immunoelectrophoresis (IEP): A semiquantitative technique in which proteins are first separated by electrophoresis and then participate in double diffusion with one or several antibodies against the individual proteins.

Immunofixation electrophoresis (IFE): A technique to identify proteins by inducing precipitin bands at the site where a specific antibody interacts with proteins that have first been separated by electrophoresis.

Immunogen: A material capable of eliciting an immune response.

Immunoglobulin (I_g): The category of glycoproteins composed of two identical light chains and two identical heavy chains, attached in a longitudinally symmetric fashion to create two identical sites capable of combining with antigen.

Immunoglobulin superfamily: Group of proteins that contain structurally related domains (immunoglobulin-fold domains); includes immunoglobulins, T-cell receptors, major histocompatibility complex (MHC), adhesion, and other surface membrane molecules. The degree of homology in amino acid sequences of these proteins suggests derivation from a common ancestral gene or genes.

Immunotherapy: Manipulation of immune actions or products to achieve therapeutic goals; includes active and passive immunization, transplantation of immunologically active tissue, immunosuppression, immune enhancement with adjuvants or pharmacologic agents, and hyposensitization.

Inflammation: A cellular, vascular, and chemical reaction to injury in which the occurrence and nature of the response are not affected by the specificity of the agent inducing the injury.

Innate immunity: Nonspecific, host defense mechanisms that include anatomic, barrier, physiologic, phagocytic, and inflammatory responses.

Interferon: A group of small polypeptide cytokines produced either by nonspecific cells after viral infection or other stimuli, or by antigen-stimulated T lymphocytes. Interferons can induce cells to resist viral infection.

Interiorization: Incorporation into the cell cytoplasm of material that was on the external membrane surface.

Interleukins: A group of cytokines produced by macrophages, T lymphocytes, and other cells that affect the activation, proliferation, and function of many different target cells, but especially of lymphocytes and hematopoietic cells.

Interstitial fluid: The fluid, normally low in proteins and cells, which is outside of blood and lymphatic vessels and surrounds the cells and structural elements of all tissues.

Isoantibody: Antibody that reacts with antigens derived from individuals of the same species but of different genetic constitution as the host.

Isograft: Grafted or transplanted tissue between two genetically identical individuals.

Isotype: Structural and potentially antigenic elements characteristic of all molecules of a given class or subclass.

Isotype switch: Attachment of the genetic material determining immunoglobulin idiotype from one segment that determines isotypic constant region to a segment determining a different isotype.

J chain: A 15-kD glycoprotein present in all polymeric immunoglobulins, hence present in IgM and secretory IgA but not in IgD, IgE, or IgG.

Kappa chain: One of two light-chain isotypes, synthesized under direction of a gene on chromosome 2 and present in approximately two-thirds of human immunoglobulin molecules.

Kinin system: A system of precursor and activator proteins that culminates in the formation of kinin–polypeptides that promote increased vascular permeability, contraction of smooth muscle, and activation of the coagulation and fibrinolytic systems.

Knock-out mouse: A slang term for a mouse strain in which a single gene is inactivated or disrupted.

Kuppfer's cells: Cells of the monocyte/macrophage system located in the sinusoids of the liver and active in phagocytizing and processing material present in blood brought to the liver by the portal venous system.

Lactoferrin: Iron-binding protein that appears to be necessary for hydroxyl radical formation and has a role in cell adhesion and granulopoiesis; an important component of secondary granules in neutrophils.

Lambda chain: One of two light-chain isotypes, synthesized under control of a gene on chromosome 22; present in approximately one-third of human immunoglobulin molecules.

Langerhans' cells: Dendritic cells present in skin, lymph nodes, spleen, and thymus; derived from the monocyte/macrophage lineage, they express major histocompatibility complex (MHC) class II products and serve as antigen-presenting cells.

Large granular lymphocytes: Lymphocytes that lack receptors for specific antigen; characterized by numerous granules in abundant cytoplasm and responsible for most killer (K) and natural killer (NK) cell activities.

Lectins: Proteins that can be extracted from plants and that bind to various sugars and glycoproteins on cell membranes, inducing agglutination, mitosis, or activation of cells that express the appropriate receptor.

Ligand: A molecule that binds to a receptor molecule of complementary configuration.

Light chain: The smaller of the two paired polypeptide chains that constitute the immunoglobulin monomer. Containing approximately 220 amino acids, light chains have a variable domain that contributes to the antigen-combining site and a single constant domain.

Linkage disequilibrium: Simultaneous presence of alleles on the same chromosome at a frequency greater than that dictated by the distribution of those alleles in the population.

LISS: Low-ionic-strength saline used to reduce the zeta potential and enhance agglutination of antibody-coated red blood cells.

Locus: The position on a chromosome occupied by the gene for a specific characteristic.

Lymph fluid: The fluid present in lymphatic vessels, derived from interstitial fluid and reentering the bloodstream when the thoracic duct empties into the venous system.

Lymph nodes: Aggregates of lymphocytes and macrophages present in groups along the course of lymphatic vessels; the site of much antigen processing and presentation, antibody production, and lymphocyte proliferation.

Lymphocyte: A small mononuclear cell with dense nuclear chromatin and sparse cytoplasm, present in blood, lymphatic fluid, and tissues of the lymphoreticular system; effector cells for immune reactivity and for certain types of chronic inflammation.

Lymphocyte-defined antigens: HLA antigens that cannot be identified with antibodies and can be detected only by appropriate reagent lymphocytes in cell-culture techniques.

Lymphocytotoxicity: An end point used in serologic examination for HLA antigens, in which complement-binding antibodies cause lethal damage to lymphocytes expressing the appropriate antigens.

Lymphoid: Pertaining to lymphocytes, lymphatic fluid, or the tissues of the lymphoreticular system.

Lymphokines: Soluble small polypeptides (cytokines) secreted by antigen-stimulated lymphocytes and capable of affecting functional events in other cells and tissues.

Lymphokine-activated killer cells (LAK cells): Large granular lymphocytes that have been exposed, *in vitro*, to the lymphokine interleukin-2 (IL-2) and are then reintroduced into the host, where their heightened state of activation exerts more effective natural killer (NK) cell actions.

Lysozyme: An enzyme in tears, saliva, breast milk, other secretions, and phagocytic cells; aids in degradation of mucopeptides in gram-positive bacterial cell walls.

M spike: The sharply defined peak on a densitometer tracing of protein electrophoresis that reflects the presence of monoclonal protein in the fluid examined.

Macrophage: A phagocytic cell derived from monocytes originating in bone marrow and exhibiting greater phagocytic, secretory, and chemotactic capacity than monocytes, which are less fully differentiated.

Major histocompatibility complex (MHC): Linked genes that determine cell-membrane antigens necessary for antigen presentation and significant in survival of allogeneic tissue grafts. In humans, MHC is on chromosome 6 and includes genes for at least six series of HLA antigens, for several proteins of the complement system, and for other activities associated with immunity.

Mannose-binding protein (MBP): Acute-phase protein that binds to mannose. MBPs are potent opsonins and can activate the complement system.

Mast cells: Basophilic granulocytes present in tissues; characterized by receptors for the Fc portion of IgE antibodies and by cytoplasmic granules that contain histamine and other mediators of inflammation.

Mediator: A substance that exerts a characteristic effect on a target cell, usually through combination with a specific receptor.

Medulla: The inner portion of an organ or structure.

Meiosis: The process of cell division in which one diploid precursor cell generates four haploid gametes.

Memory cells: Clonal progeny of an antigen-stimulated T or B lymphocyte, which exist in a state of potential activation and respond to antigen exposure with increased speed and intensity of immune response.

Metaplasia: Replacement of one type of tissue by another type that is not normal for that site.

MHC restriction: The phenomenon in which T lymphocytes recognize their specific antigen only when it is presented on a cell expressing the same major histocompatibility complex (MHC) class I or class II antigens as those of the host. CD4-positive T cells require class II antigens, and CD8-positive cells are restricted by class I antigens.

Micelle: A molecular aggregate that retains discrete existence suspended in plasma or other aqueous media.

Mitogen: Material that combines with specific non–antigen receptors on cell membranes to stimulate DNA synthesis and cell division.

Mitosis: The process of cell division in which a diploid cell reproduces into two diploid daughter cells with the same genetic characteristics.

Mixed lymphocyte culture (or **reaction**) **(MLC or MLR):** A laboratory procedure in which lymphocytes of different genetic composition are cultured together and allowed to exert antigenic stimulation that promotes DNA synthesis and immunoblast transformation.

Monoclonal: Pertaining to or arising from daughter cells of a single clone, all of which have the same genetic composition and the capacity to synthesize the same products.

Monoclonal antibody (Mab): Homogeneous antibody of a single specificity produced from a single clone of hybrid cells called a **hybridoma.** A hybridoma is a result of fusion of a myeloma cell with a plasma cell.

Monocyte: A large leukocyte with an ovoid or indented nucleus, derived from the same hematopoietic precursor as netrophils and capable of differentiation into macrophages characteristic of many different tissue locations.

Monokine: A cytokine secreted by monocytes or macrophage.

Monomer: A molecule consisting of a single, nonrepeated structural unit.

Motility: Ability to move spontaneously. Macrophages and neutrophils exhibit motility; in response to injury and inflammation.

Mucosa-associated lymphoid tissue (MALT): The stratified mass of lymphocytes beneath the epithelial surface of respiratory, alimentary, excretory, and reproductive tracts.

Myeloid: Pertaining to the bone marrow, particularly to cells of the granulocytic series.

Myeloma (often, **multiple myeloma**): A neoplasm of immunoglobulin-secreting plasma cells, usually characterized by aggregates of neoplastic cells in bones or other sites and by the presence in serum or urine of monoclonal protein produced by these cells.

Neoplasm: A synonym for cancer or tumor.

Nephelometry: Measurement of the turbidity of a fluid, used to quantify precipitated immune complexes in a fluid medium.

NK cells: Natural killer cells. Large granular lymphocytes that exert cytotoxic effects on target cells without expressing specific antigenic receptors or B-cell or T-cell markers.

Null cells: Lymphocytes and other cells (stem cells) that lack surface markers that allow assignment to T or B categories.

Oligo: A combining form that means "few." Oligosaccharides, for example, have no more than 10 sugar residues.

Oncofetal tumor antigen: Fetal antigen expressed on a tumor cell.

Oncogene: A gene capable of producing neoplastic transformation, if suitably activated. The normal mammalian genome contains many oncogenes in unactivated form; also present in many viruses.

Opsonins: Substances that, when present on the surface of a cell or particle, enhance phagocytosis. IgG antibodies and cleavage fragments of C3 are the major opsonins in humans.

Opsonization: Enhancement of phagocytosis by the presence, on the surface of a cell or particle, of molecules for which the phagocytic cell has receptors.

Ouchterlony double diffusion: A qualitative precipitation technique in which antigen and antibody diffuse from wells cut in a gel. The resulting precipitate pattern indicates whether antigens are present or identical.

Papain: The proteolytic enzyme used to cleave the immunoglobulin monomer into two Fab and one Fc segment.

Passive agglutination: A laboratory technique in which soluble antigen is adsorbed to the surface of inert particles. Combination with antibody thus induces agglutination rather than precipitation.

Passive immunity: Immune protection achieved by transfer of effector material, usually antibody, from an immunized individual into an individual not previously exposed to the antigen.

Patching: Movement of molecules on a cell membrane from a diffuse distribution into discrete clusters.

Pepsin: The proteolytic enzyme used to cleave the immunoglobulin monomer into a single F(ab')$_2$ fragment plus immunologically inert fragments of heavy chain.

Peptide bond: The covalent bond that links amino acids into protein chains. Formed between the COOH group of one amino acid and the NH$_2$ group of the other.

Phagocytosis: Ingestion of particulate material by macrophages, neutrophils, and other leukocytes.

Phenotype: The aggregate of genetically determined characteristics expressed by an individual.

Phytohemagglutinin (PHA): Extract derived from the kidney bean plant that provokes lymphoblast transformation in T lymphocytes, independent of contact with specific antigen.

Pluripotential: Having the capacity to express any of several different developmental characteristics.

Poly-: Combining form meaning "many." Sometimes used to denote anything above one, but usually denotes a number greater than "several."

Polymer: In immunology, immunoglobulin molecules consisting of more than one immunoglobulin monomer joined covalently.

Polymorphism: The presence, in a population, of different forms of a characteristic determined by alleles at a single locus.

Postzone: An informal term used to describe failure of agglutination or precipitation occurring when there is pronounced antigen excess.

Precipitation: Formation of an insoluble immune complex after combination of soluble antigen with soluble antibody.

Precipitin line: The deposit of precipitated immune complex seen in the supporting medium when soluble antigen and soluble antibody meet in suitable proportions.

Presentation: In immunology, display of processed antigen on the surface of a cell capable of engaging in productive contact with effector cells that express the appropriate antigen receptor.

Primary immune response: The immune events, humoral or cell-mediated or both, which occur when an immunocompetent host encounters an antigen for the first time.

Processing: The modifications exerted on native antigen to render it effectively immunogenic.

Progeny: Descendants or offspring; describes cells that evolve from a single precursor.

Properdin: Factor P of the alternative pathway of complement activation. Present at serum concentration of approximately 25 μg/mL, it stabilizes the C3 convertase activity of C3b associated with activated factor B.

Proteolytic: Having the property to cleave proteins by dividing polypeptide bonds.

Proto-oncogene: Normal cellular gene often involved in regulation of growth. If mutated or aberrantly expressed, it can contribute to malignant transformation of the cell and development of cancer.

Prozone: The failure to achieve visible agglutination or precipitation that occurs when antibody is present in excess.

Pseudogene: Gene that is incapable of being expressed.

Psychoneuroimmunology (PNI): Study of the interactions among the nervous, endocrine, and immune systems.

Radial immunodiffusion: A single diffusion technique in which antigen can be quantified by the size of the precipitin ring formed when antigen diffuses radially from a well cut into antibody-containing gel.

Radioimmunoassay (RIA): An analytic procedure in which a radioisotope is used to label antigen or antibody participating in an immune reaction.

Radioisotope: An unstable form of an element, which emits radiation in decaying to a stable state.

Reagin: A term used for two different antibodies: (1) the anticardiolipin antibody demonstrated in nontreponemal tests for syphilis; (2) any antibody that binds to basophilic granulocytes and elicits immediate-type hypersensitivity.

Receptor: A molecular configuration that interacts with a molecule, usually smaller, and exhibits a complementary configuration. The combination of receptor with its ligand mediates subsequent biologically significant events.

Restriction endonuclease: An enzyme of bacterial origin that cleaves DNA at specific sequences, generating fragments of reproducible properties that can be used to detect the presence of complementary sequences in unknown specimens being tested.

Retrovirus: A virus that uses the enzyme reverse transcriptase, to transcribe its ribonucleic acid (RNA) into viral DNA, which is then inserted into the host cell's DNA.

Rheumatoid factor: Autoantibody directed against the Fc portion or IgG and present in the serum of patient's with rheumatoid arthritis and other autoimmune conditions.

Rhodamine: A fluorescent dye that emits in the red spectrum after excitation by ultraviolet lightwaves.

Ribosomes: The spherical bodies in cytoplasm that are the site of ribonucleic acid (RNA)-directed protein synthesis.

Rocket electrophoresis: An analytic technique in which antigen moves in an electrical field through antibody-containing gel, leading to precipitation in tapered columns, the height of which is proportional to the concentration of antigen.

RPR Test: Rapid plasma reagin test; an agglutination test for antibodies associated with syphilis.

Sarcoma: Cancer cells originating from tissue of mesodermal or connective tissue origin.

Secondary immune response: Immune events, either humoral or cell-mediated which occur on second or subsequent exposure to an antigen and reflect the existence and activity of memory cells.

Secretory component: The glycoprotein chain that epithelial cells add to polymerized IgA as it traverses the cell to enter secreted fluid.

Self: In immunology, the cellular and soluble configurations characteristic of the host's genetic constitution.

Sensitization: 1. Induction of an immune response, especially one with deleterious consequences to the host. 2. Attachment of antibody to the surface of antigen-bearing particles without formation of the lattice that constitutes agglutination.

Series: A group of protein products of essentially similar nature but differing in characteristics determined by different alleles at the locus that directs their synthesis.

Seroconversion: Development of positive results on a test for specific antibody after previous demonstration that antibody was absent.

Serodiagnosis: Diagnosis of infectious or other diseases from the results of tests for appropriate antibodies.

Serologically defined antigen: In the HLA system, an antigen that can be detected and identified through reactions with antibodies, without the need for tests of cell-mediated immunity.

Serology: The study of serum, especially tests for the presence of antibodies.

Single diffusion: A precipitation technique in which one reactant is uniformly dispersed in the suspending medium and one reactant diffuses through the immunologically active material.

Sinusoid: A vascular channel, carrying either blood or lymph fluid, which has a lumen wider and more irregular than that of capillaries and often allows prolonged or intimate contact between the moving fluid and the cells lining the channel.

Solid phase: The portion of a heterogeneous system that consists of solid material, as opposed to fluid or gaseous constituents.

Somatic mutation: Gene mutation occurring in non–germ-line cells. In B cells, it is a process whereby point mutations occur in the variable region of the immunoglobulin genes during activation and proliferation. This process aids in the generation of antibody diversity and enhanced antigen binding.

Specificity: In immunology, characterized by a unique, reproducible configuration that restricts steric interaction to a molecule of complementary configuration. The identifying term applied to individually characterized immune reactants.

Stem cell: An undifferentiated cell whose progeny can evolve along different lines of differentiation under suitable internal or external conditions.

Staphylococcal protein A: A cell-wall protein of *Staphylococcus aureus*, which interacts with the Fc portion of IgG through a receptor-ligand association.

Subclass: In immunology, the categories of immunoglobulin determined by isotypic variants within heavy-chain classes.

Superantigen: A molecule capable of binding to major histocompatibility complex (MHC)-II and the V beta domains of certain T cells causing these cells to divide with subsequent clinical disorders.

Suppressor cells: A subset of T lymphocytes that express the CD8 antigen and act to inhibit the effector actions of B cells or other T cells.

T-cell receptor (TCR): Antigen-binding molecule expressed on the surface of T cells associated with CD3; composed of highly variable alpha and beta chains or gamma and delta chains.

Terminal deoxynucleotidyl transferase (TdT): An enzyme that catalyzes rearrangement of DNA in the nucleus of immature T and B cells, and in approximately 2 percent of cells in the normal bone marrow.

Th-1 cells: CD4-positive T cells that engage in inflammatory reactions.

Th-2 cells: CD4-positive T cells that help in humoral responses.

Thoracic duct: The collecting vessel that connects the central accumulation of lymphatic fluid with the bloodstream. It passes from the region of the lumbar vertebrae upward through the diaphragm to enter the venous system at the left internal jugular or subclavian vein.

Thymocytes: Cells of lymphoid origin present in the thymus, where they undergo progressive differentiation and maturation before exiting to become T lymphocytes.

Thymosins: A collective term for proteins intrinsic to the thymus that have the capacity to promote differentiation and maturation of lymphoid precursors into immunocompetent T lymphocytes.

Thymus-dependent antigen: Any antigen that elicits antibody only when there is concomitant stimulation of B lymphocytes by T lymphocytes or their secreted products.

Thymus-independent antigen: Any antigen capable of promoting antibody production in the absence of concomitant T-cell activity.

Titer: A figure that denotes the relative concentration of an antibody or other reactant; reciprocal of the highest dilution that produces a reaction.

Titration: In serology, the process of testing serially diluted material to determine relative concentration. Each dilution is tested against a standard indicator to demonstrate the highest dilution at which reaction occurs. The reciprocal of this dilution is the titer of the test material.

Tolerance: In immunology, the state in which an otherwise immunocompetent host fails to react against a specific antigen.

Transformation: In immunology, the change that T or B lymphocytes exhibit after stimulation by specific antigen or by a suitable mitogen. The stimulated cell transforms into an immunoblast, characterized by increased nuclear size and synthesis of DNA.

Transgenic mouse: A mouse strain carrying a foreign gene in its genome; genetic technique used to study the function of the inserted gene.

Tuberculin test: An *in vivo* test for established cell-mediated immunity to proteins of the tubercle bacillus. Intradermal injection of the prepared antigen elicits a delayed hypersensitivity reaction in individuals who have had previous immunizing exposure to the organisms.

Turbidimetry: A technique for analyzing the concentration of precipitated material suspended in a fluid medium, by measuring the reduction of light transmitted through the material.

Tumor necrosis factor (TNF): Cytokines produced by macrophages (TNF-α) and some T cells (TNF-β) that are cytotoxic to tumor cells, but not normal cells. TNFs have multiple functions in inflammation and immune responses.

Tumor suppressor gene: Normal genes involved in regulation of cell proliferation, which inhibit or suppress cancerous cell changes.

Vaccination: Used as a general term describing introduction of microbial antigens with the intent of inducing immunity; originally, introduction of cowpox (vaccinia) antigens to induce cross-reactivity that protected against smallpox.

Van der Waals forces: Weak but universally present attractive forces exerted between molecules, arising from oscillation of electrical forces.

Variable region: The amino-terminal half of the light chain and approximately quarter of the heavy chain in which pronounced variations in amino acid sequence confer idiotypic specificity.

Variolation: Introduction of material from a smallpox (variola) lesion, with the intent of inducing immunity to the disease and avoiding disabling or fatal native infection.

VDRL: Agglutination test for antibodies associated with syphilis; first designed by the **V**enereal **D**isease **R**esearch **L**aboratories.

Wasserman test: The first serologic test for syphilis; a complement fixation procedure that is now known to demonstrate presence of an anticardiolipin antibody strongly associated with syphilis, and not antibody to any specific antigen of *Treponema pallidum.*

Western blot: An immunoprecipitation procedure in which the test serum is reacted with a preparation of antigens separated by electrophoresis and then transferred (blotted) to a supporting medium.

Xenogeneic: Originating from a source other than the species to which the host belongs.

Xenograft: Grafted or transplanted tissue from another species.

Zeta potential: Electrostatic potential existing between cells when suspended in a solution containing electrolytes.

Zone of equivalence: Relative concentration of antigen and antibody in which the number of multivalent binding sites are approximately equal, resulting in maximal lattice formation and precipitation.

Appendix

SOME COMMON ABBREVIATIONS

ACTH	adrenocorticotropic hormone
ADA	adenosine deaminase
ADCC	antibody dependent cell mediated cytotoxicity
AIDS	acquired immunodeficiency syndrome
ALL	acute lymphocytic leukemia
ANA	anti-nuclear antigens
BALT	bronchial associated lymphoid tissue
BCR	B cell receptor
BFU-E	burst forming unit-erythroid
C1INH	C1 esterase inhibitor
CALLA	common ALL antigen
cAMP	cyclic adenosine monophosphate
CD	cluster designation
CFU-S	colony forming unit-spleen
CGD	chronic granulomatous disease
CIEP	counter immunoelectrophoresis
CLL	chronic lymphocytic leukemia
CMI	cell mediated immunity
CMV	cytomegalo virus
CR1	complement receptor 1
CRP	C reactive protein
CTL	cytotoxic T lymphocyte
DAT	direct antiglobulin test
DTH	delayed type hypersensitivity
EBV	Epstein Barr virus
ECF-A	eosinophil chemotactic factor of anaphylaxis
ELISA or EIA	enzyme linked immunosorbent assay
EMIT	enzyme multiplied immunoassay test
FAB	French American British system of acute leukemia classification
Fab	immunoglobulin fragment with antigen binding capacity
FACS	fluorescent activated cell sorter
Fc	immunoglobulin fragment with complement binding capacity or crystallizable

453

FISH	fluorescent in situ hybridization
FITC	fluorescein isothiocyanate
FTA	fluorescent treponemal antibody test
GALT	gut associated lymphoid tissue
GVHD	graft versus host disease
HDN	hemolytic disease of the newborn
HEV	high endothelial venules
HIV	human immunodeficiency virus
HLA	human leukocyte antigen
HTLV	human T cell lymphotrophic virus
HSP	heat shock protein
ICAM	intracellular adhesion molecule
IEP	immunoelectrophoresis
IFA	immunofluorescent assay
IFE	immunofixation electrophoresis
IFN	interferon
Ig	immunoglobulin
IL	interleukin
IRMA	immunoradiomimetric assay
ISG	immune serum globulin
LFA	leukocyte function antigen
LISS	low ionic strength saline
Mab	monoclonal antibody
MAH-TP	microhemagglutination assay for *Treponema pallidum*
MALT	mucosa associated lymphoid tissue
MGUS	monoclonal gammopathy of undetermined significance
MHC	major histocompatibility complex
MLC	mixed lymphocyte culture
MLR	mixed lymphocyte reaction
NK	natural killer cell
PA	pernicious anemia
PABA	paramino benzoic acid
PAF	platelet activating factor
PCR	polymerase chain reaction
PDGF	platelet derived growth factor
PMN	polymorphonuclear neutrophil
PNI	psychoneuroimmunology
RA	rheumatoid arthritis
RFLP	restriction fragment length polymorphism
RIA	radioimmunoassay
RID	radial immunodiffusion
RS	Reed Sternberg cell
SCID	severe combined immunodeficiency disease
sIg	surface immunoglobulin
SLE	systemic lupus erythematosus
TCR	T cell receptor
TdT	terminal deoxynucleotidyl transferase
TH1	T helper type 1 cell
TH2	T helper type 2 cell
TNF	tumor necrosis factor

GREEK LETTERS

α	alpha
β	beta
δ	delta
ϵ	epsilon
γ	gamma
μ	mu
ζ	zeta

Index

Bold page numbers denote illustrations; page numbers followed by a "t" denote tables.